Society, Medicine and Politics in Colonial India

The history of medicine and disease in colonial India remains a dynamic and innovative field of research, covering many facets of health, from government policy to local therapeutics. This volume presents a selection of essays examining varied aspects of health and medicine as they relate to the political upheavals of the colonial era. These range from the micro-politics of medicine in princely states and institutions such as asylums through to the wider canvas of sanitary diplomacy as well as the meaning of modernity and modernization in the context of British rule.

The volume reflects the diversity of the field and showcases exciting new scholarship from early-career researchers as well as more established scholars by bringing to light many locations and dimensions of medicine and modernity. The essays have several common themes and together offer important insights into South Asia's experience of modernity in the years before independence. Cutting across modernity and colonialism, some of the key themes explored here include issues of race, gender, sexuality, law, mental health, famine, disease, religion, missionary medicine, medical research, tensions between and within different medical traditions and practices and India's place in an international context. This book will be of great interest to scholars and researchers of modern South Asian history, sociology, politics and anthropology as well as specialists in the history of medicine.

Biswamoy Pati was Senior Fellow at the Nehru Memorial Museum and Library, New Delhi, and taught Modern Indian History at the Department of History, University of Delhi, India. His research is on the diversities of colonial South Asia and some of his books include *Resisting Domination: Peasants, Tribals and the National Movement on Orissa, 1920–1950* (1993) and *South Asia from the Margins: Echoes of Orissa, 1800–2000* (2012). He edited *The 1857 Rebellion* (2007); and co-edited (with Mark Harrison) *Health, Medicine and Empire* (2001) and *The Social History of Health and Medicine in Colonial India* (2009); and (with Waltraud Ernst) *India's Princely States: People, Princes and Colonialism* (2007).

Mark Harrison is Professor of the History of Medicine and Director of the Wellcome Unit for the History of Medicine, University of Oxford, UK. He has written widely on the history of medicine in relation to war, medicine and imperialism. His publications include *Public Health in British India* (1994); *Climates and Constitutions: Health, Race, Environment and British Imperialism in India 1600–1850* (1999); *Medicine in an Age of Commerce and Empire: Britain and Its Tropical Colonies 1660–1830* (2010); *Contagion* (2011); several edited volumes; and *Health, Medicine and Empire: Perspectives on Colonial India* (2001) and *The Social History of Health and Medicine in Colonial India* (2009) both co-edited with Biswamoy Pati.

The Social History of Health and Medicine in South Asia

Series editors: Biswamoy Pati

Department of History, University of Delhi, India

Mark Harrison

Director of the Wellcome Unit for the History of Medicine and Professor of the History of Medicine, University of Oxford, UK

Since the late 1990s, health and medicine have emerged as major concerns in South Asian history. The Social History of Health and Medicine in South Asia series aims to foster a new wave of inter-disciplinary research and scholarship that transcends conventional boundaries. It welcomes proposals for monographs, edited collections and anthologies which offer fresh perspectives, innovative analytical frameworks and comparative assessments. The series embraces diverse aspects of health and healing in colonial and postcolonial contexts.

Books in this series

Colonial Modernities: Midwifery in Bengal, c. 1860–1947
Ambalika Guha

Society, Medicine and Politics in Colonial India
Edited by Biswamoy Pati and Mark Harrison

For a full list of titles in this series, please visit www.routledge.com/The-Social-History-of-Health-and-Medicine-in-South-Asia/book-series/ SHHM

Society, Medicine and Politics in Colonial India

Edited by
Biswamoy Pati and
Mark Harrison

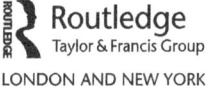

Routledge
Taylor & Francis Group

LONDON AND NEW YORK

First published 2018
by Routledge
2 Park Square, Milton Park, Abingdon, Oxon OX14 4RN

and by Routledge
605 Third Avenue, New York, NY 10017

First issued in paperback 2020

Routledge is an imprint of the Taylor & Francis Group, an informa business

British Library Cataloguing-in-Publication Data
A catalogue record for this book is available from the British Library

Library of Congress Cataloging-in-Publication Data
A catalog record for this book has been requested

ISBN 13: 978-0-367-73525-8 (pbk)
ISBN 13: 978-1-138-28633-7 (hbk)

Typeset in Sabon
by Apex CoVantage, LLC

This volume is dedicated to the memory of our esteemed and much-loved colleague Biswamoy Pati (1955–2017) who passed away unexpectedly during the final stages of editing. He will be remembered not only for his many fine contributions to scholarship but for his vibrant personality and his passion for truth and justice. Biswamoy was consistently a champion of people and of subjects which had been overlooked and we hope that his work will continue to inspire younger scholars, for whom he had an enormous affection. This book, and the series of which it is a part, would not have been possible without him. He will be sorely missed.

Contents

Figure and tables

Figure

Tables

Contributors

Jane Buckingham is Associate Professor of History at University of Canterbury, New Zealand. She specializes in the history of medicine, health, disability and law.

Burton Cleetus teaches Modern Indian History at the Centre for Historical Studies, Jawaharlal Nehru University, New Delhi, India. His research interest includes various aspects of the institutionalization and modernization of indigenous medical practices in India.

Debjani Das is Assistant Professor of History in Vidyasagar University, West Bengal, India. She is the author of *Houses of Madness: Insanity and Asylums of Bengal in Nineteenth Century India* (2015).

Achintya Kumar Dutta is Professor at the Department of History, The University of Burdwan, India. He has been a Post-Doctoral Commonwealth Fellow at the School of Oriental and African Studies, London, UK. His specialization is in the areas of economic history and the history of medicine. He is the author of *Economy and Ecology in a Bengal District Burdwan 1880–1947* (2002) and has co-edited *History of Medicine in India: The Medical Encounter* (2005; with Chittabrata Palit)

Amna Khalid is Assistant Professor of History at Carleton College, USA. She has co-edited *Public Health in the British Empire: Intermediaries, Subordinates, and the Practice of Public Health, 1850–1960* (2011; with R. Johnson). She is currently working on her forthcoming manuscript, *Pilgrimage, Place, & Public Health: The Sanitary Regulation of Sacred Space in British India*.

Saurabh Mishra is Lecturer in Modern History at the University of Sheffield, UK. He specializes in the history of medicine in the subcontinent, but is also interested in situating this within wider social history. His past monographs include *Beastly Encounters of the Raj: Livelihoods, Livestock and Veterinary Health in North India, 1890–1920* (2015) and *Pilgrimage, Politics and Pestilence: The Haj from the Indian Subcontinent, 1860–1920* (2011). His current project is on the history of birdwatching in colonial India.

Sujata Mukherjee is Professor at the Department of History, and former Dean of the Arts Faculty, Rabindra Bharati University, Kolkata, India. She has written extensively on the social history of medicine, environment and social reforms in modern India. Her latest authored book is *Gender, Medicine, and Society in Colonial India: Women's Health Care in Nineteenth- and Early Twentieth-Century Bengal* (2017).

Mridula Ramanna is author of *Western Medicine and Public Health in Colonial Bombay, 1845–1895*; *Health Care in Bombay Presidency, 1896–1930*; *Edward Moor*; and several chapters in edited volumes.

Barbara N. Ramusack is Charles Phelps Taft Professor of History Emerita at the University of Cincinnati, USA. Her current research focuses on maternal and infant health during late colonial Madras city and Mysore princely state.

Leela Sami completed her doctorate from the University of London, UK, in 2007. She currently lives in Providence, Rhode Island, and is pursuing a second career in elementary education.

Samiksha Sehrawat is Lecturer in History of Medicine and South Asia, Newcastle University, UK. She works on gender history with a focus on maternal health, development and women as colonial experts.

Acknowledgements

The editors would like to thank the contributors to this volume for their participation in this project and their timely cooperation with editing. We would also like to express our gratitude to Antara Ray Chaudhury, Shashank Sinha, Rimina Mohapatra, Avneet Kaur and others at Routledge for their help, guidance and encouragement.

Introduction

Mark Harrison and Biswamoy Pati

The meanings and consequences of modernity have been prominent in the historiography of colonial South Asia for many years. Indeed, it is from within this field of scholarship that the notion of modernity has received some of its most trenchant critiques, most famously in the work of Dipesh Chakrabarty.[1] This volume was not originally conceived as an engagement with the idea of modernity, yet the theme unites most of the essays collected here, whether in relation to the agenda of the colonial state or the deployment of 'modernity' (and its counterpoint, 'tradition') within the context of healing and health-care. In highlighting these themes we do not wish to detract from the specific aims the authors have set themselves, but modernity and modernization provide a useful framework in which to understand these essays and their relationship to other works on the history of medicine in colonial South Asia and beyond. Another reason for highlighting this theme is that relatively few historians of health and medicine in colonial India have reflected explicitly on the theme of modernity, notwithstanding the strong currents in South Asian historiography as a whole. In this sense, the literature on medicine lags behind that on some other Asian contexts (particularly East Asia) and, of course, the larger body of scholarship on health and medicine in the West.[2] However, things are beginning to change. Modernity looms large in Rachel Berger and Projit Mukharji's recent books on Ayurveda,[3] for example, and in William J. Glover's and Sandip Hazareesingh's monographs on urban reform.[4] Mukharji's earlier work *Nationalizing the Body* also tackles the issue of modernity through the lens of nationalism, while David Hardiman does so through that of missionary Christianity.[5]

A number of interpretative matters arise from these works, as well as from the literature on modernity and medicine in other colonies. One of these is whether modernity should be viewed as a thing in itself – as a process or form of organization – or as a rhetorical tool, frequently used to legitimate colonial rule. This relates closely to the question of whether a concept originating in the analysis of Western societies can or should be applied elsewhere. And, if modernity still has anything to recommend it, how far should the concept be adapted to meet the requirements of other contexts? In other words, is there a single modernity or many? Berger appears to accept that 'the modern' is applicable to colonial India and regards it as a distinct historical period, the main theme of her book being how Ayurveda came to terms with modernity in the early twentieth century. Her conception of modernity recognizes its specifically colonial dimensions, as well as shifts over time. Hazareesingh's approach is similar in some respects, steering a 'middle course' between grand narratives of modernity (such as Berman's[6]) and that of postcolonial critics for whom the very notion of modernity is suspect. He stresses the diverse forms through which modernity became manifest in the city of Bombay, just as Glover's work on Lahore acknowledges that old and new parts of the city became modern in their own ways.

Despite recognizing different facets of modernity, the authors mentioned above regard the concept as describing something concrete. Hardiman also sees modernity as implying a particular world view, evident in colonial and non-colonial contexts, but constrained in important respects by the racialized nature of colonial rule. He rejects, however, the notion that modernization inevitably brings secularization, coining the phrase 'Christian modernity' to describe the fusion of science and theology in missionary discourses.[7] Mukharji, however, sees modernity as more of a discursive formation than a political or social one. He adopts a position similar to many postcolonial scholars in seeing modernity as fluid and multifaceted. He appears to endorse the notion of 'alternative modernities', emphasizing the hybrid and indeterminate states produced by the process of 'vernacularization'. This insight builds on the work of Gyan Prakash and others who have highlighted the diverse ways in which Indians appropriated Western medicine and science.[8] However, it resembles even more the approach of postcolonial scholars such as Warwick Anderson, who have sought to challenge the assumption that Western knowledge is objective and universally applicable.[9]

We shall return to some specific aspects of these studies in a moment but before doing so it may be useful to reflect on the general positions they represent. As indicated above, some scholars of health and medicine have continued to see the notion of modernity as useful but seek a way of avoiding the hegemony that modernity represented. The notion of 'alternative modernities' has therefore proved attractive as it allows for the possibility that modernity can be understood in multiple ways, some of which may be subversive of dominant political or cultural forms. In the context of science and medicine, the use of this concept – as Anderson clearly intends – legitimates local adaptations and re-workings of Western knowledge, thereby frustrating the application of modernity as a normative concept.[10] And yet, the term 'alternative modernity' presupposes that modernity was or is a global phenomenon and implies a dominant modernity against which all 'alternatives' are defined. The term consequently offers not so much the possibility of escape but of entrapment. It succeeds not, as intended, in 'provincializing' the West but in reifying a standard modernity from which alternative versions differ. The concept of 'multiple modernities' might seem more serviceable in this respect, as it acknowledges that modernity took many forms depending on local political circumstances and cultural legacies.[11] But the notion of plural modernities obscures those features which make it possible to speak of modernity at all. 'Varieties *of* modernity' is arguably a more accurate description.[12]

A closely related problem, which applies particularly to the notion of alternative modernities, is that it implies that people were (or are) at liberty to shape modernity according to their preferences. This ignores the very real constraints that modernity imposes. As Frederic Jameson has argued, 'the "cultural" notion that you can fashion your own modernity differently' overlooks 'the other foundational meaning of modernity which is that of a worldwide capitalism'.[13] Jameson is alluding here to the tendency of postcolonial criticism to shift its analytical focus from capitalism to colonialism, and from political economy to culture. But modernity – including colonial modernity – has been powerfully shaped by capitalism, and the globalization of capital has led to the globalization of the values of European and American societies, even if these have encountered resistance and adaptation. Different forms of modernity (colonial and otherwise) can exist but only within the constraints of global capitalism. The fetishizing of cultural difference therefore detracts from the central features of modernity, through which much of the world has been forced to shape its destiny. As Arif Dirlik writes, 'The self-representations of Euromodernity may be self-serving, ideological or illusory, but there is no denying either the profound changes the world has gone through over the past three centuries, or the transformations in self-consciousness that these changes have brought about.'[14]

If the concept of modernity has any meaning beyond the purely rhetorical, then it is important to state clearly what it stands for and how it might help us to make sense of the history of health, medicine and disease. The term 'modernity' originated in the mid-nineteenth century in order to describe a sense of rupture – of disorientation but also delight in the making of society anew. Since then, modernity has acquired many layers of meaning. As one of the classical theorists of modernity, Weber attempted to describe the rapid changes of his own time – the expansion of industrial capitalism; bureaucratization; secularization and professionalization – but modernity has come to represent many things to many people. There are numerous typologies of modernity and a good deal of uncertainty as to whether it is a state we have transcended or remain within. These many different views of modernity are often obscured by the fact that it has become a kind of shorthand, used to describe a set of social forms and values. All that the historian can do is to determine which, if any, has explanatory potential.

Over the last few decades, it is Foucault's critique of modernity that has tended to dominate the historiography of colonial medicine, rather than the classical theorists; although by no means completely. As a result, it is the disciplinary aspects of medicine and hygiene which are emphasized most, the power of modern states, according to Foucault, lying primarily in populations (biopower) rather than territory. This modern regime of power was distinctive in that it operated on the mind (throughout the maintenance of norms) rather than directly on the body. Aspects of health and medicine under modernity, hitherto regarded as humane, liberating or progressive, have come to be seen as new modalities of power, which Foucault termed 'governmentality'. This entailed 'a form of surveillance and control as attentive as that of a head of a family over his household and his goods'.[15] Overall, the tendency of Foucault's work has been to question the teleological idealism of modernity and in this sense it differs fundamentally from most other theories of modernity (most obviously that of Marx). It also differs in its reluctance to ascribe modernity to any particular cause – such as capitalism – and in having an ambiguous attitude towards causality. However, Foucault's oeuvre shares some features with Weber's work, in that it shows a similar interest in 'the iron cage of rationality' (as Weber termed it) as well as recognizing the existence of multiple forms of domination.[16] Elements of all these theories are present in some recent interpretative syntheses, most notably that of Giddens, which holds that modern societies are characterized by several core attributes including capitalism, industrialization, bureaucracy, surveillance, and by the view that the world is open to transformation. According to Giddens, the essence of modernity is that it looks to the future rather than to the past, and that it has wrought radical changes in the experience of time and space.[17]

Although Giddens's concept of modernity remains fixed on key attributes, it takes account of cultural differences as well as the evolution of modernity over time. Unlike Foucault and classical theorists of modernity, Giddens cannot be so easily accused of generalizing from purely Western examples.[18] Indeed, there is no reason why any theory of modernity should be incompatible with non-Western contexts. Although Giddens has probably underestimated the continuing validity of 'tradition' in modern societies, the constellation of traits which he regards as intrinsic to modernity have long existed in South Asia and many other parts of the world. Medical modernity, for example, is as recognizable in *fin de siècle* Calcutta as in London or Paris. One can observe in all these contexts the bureaucratization of medicine; a significant role for medical and other experts in governance; the impact of commercialization and industrialization on health (physical and mental); an increasing degree of professionalization; and, to an increasing degree, the operation of biopower. One could analyze any of these dimensions independently of a larger conception of modernity and in many cases it would be desirable to do so. But one would lose sight of the complex interrelationship between them; the very thing which animated classical theorists and to which Giddens remains committed. It is difficult to understand the professionalization and 'technologization' of medicine separately from the process of industrialization which made possible the mass production of items as diverse as tabloids (pills) and stethoscopes. These and other aspects of modern medicine were closely associated with the process of urbanization and the advent of mass media, initially in the form of print. They were as apparent in Asian and African settings as they were in Europe or America.

To note these similarities is not to deny that there were differences in the ways in which modernity was experienced in colonial and non-colonial contexts. Indeed, the notion of 'colonial modernity' has become commonplace in scholarship on the European, American and Japanese empires. As with modernity in general, there is no universally agreed definition of colonial modernity or modernities. Some writers, such as Marian Aguiar, emphasize mobility, arguing that colonial modernity was expressed in narratives of progress which necessitated the movement of knowledge, materials and commodities, and of course, persons. These movements were essential to the viability of capitalism but also to the legitimacy of the colonial enterprise. The transformation of pre-modern cultures through technology, education, law and so forth was increasingly touted as a justification for imperialism. Colonial modernity has also been said to place more emphasis upon technology than other forms of modernity, especially the railways that enabled India and other colonies to be integrated within a global capitalist system.[19] Neither of these claims is particularly convincing. It is difficult to see that more emphasis was placed on technology in India than in Europe or perhaps even more decidedly in the USA.[20] Similarly, while the movement of peoples, commodities and knowledge was essential to the survival of an imperial system, it was a prominent feature of modernity everywhere and it seems inappropriate to distinguish it as unique to the colonies.

Another way of envisioning colonial modernity in India is to see it (like Gyan Prakash) as a form of 'belated' Enlightenment, in which modernity found expression through communities – rather than through civil society and voluntary institutions, as in Europe. According to Prakash, whereas bourgeois civil society treated its constituents as sovereign individuals whose relations were mediated by markets and laws, communities invoked primordial bonds of blood, religion, culture and territoriality. While many aspects of colonial modernization were embraced by Indian elites, some – particularly the education of women – proved threatening to males. Some did accept and even champion female education but they attempted to create a boundary that would prevent education from giving too much freedom to women, deploying notions of community (culture, traditions and social memories) to prevent the intrusion of Western morals and liberties. While dressed in traditional garb, the idea of community was still capable of expressing modern collective identities such as the nation and the nation-state. Thus, while colonial India cannot be placed within any standard trajectory of modernity, many Western values were adapted in modified form. Indeed, the idea of community was formed in the image of the state.[21]

Prakash's carefully explicated idea of colonial modernity has much to recommend it. Too often, the concept is poorly defined and simply reflects the recent fashion for stressing the plurality of experience.[22] Modernity certainly appeared in many guises and we can sometimes find evidence of local currents of change and reform alongside those initiated by colonial regimes.[23] Indigenous elites also participated in the making of Western science.[24] And those technologies and ideas that were imported from the West were often adapted by local elites.[25] But those not in a strong position to reshape modernity in their own image – in other words, the vast majority of colonial subjects – were compelled either to resist (often fruitlessly) or merely to acquiesce.

If we are looking to make generalizations about colonial modernity, then perhaps the clearest contrast with modernity elsewhere is in the ways in which it was managed. We can see this at multiple levels: for example, in spatial ordering (e.g. the separation of racial groups), the management of flows (e.g. racial filtering), state governance (policy bias), (restricted) opportunities to participate in the professions, (unequal) opportunity of access to services and so forth. Modernity never promised to erase all inequalities but in Europe and America it was at least tempered by democratic institutions and an ethos of collective good. Equality of opportunity was strongly emphasized, in accordance with the rational allocation of talent and resources. This was never perfectly realized, even in the West, but when expressed in a colonial context such aspirations sounded hollow or raised expectations that could never be met. This fundamental tension – between the promise of modernity and the impossibility of realizing it – is what most strongly characterized modernity in the colonies. That said; one has to acknowledge some change in the parameters of colonial modernity over time, as well as important differences between contexts. There was far greater opportunity to succeed professionally in India or Ceylon, for example, than in tropical Africa. After the First World War, the professions – especially medicine – became increasingly open to colonial subjects, including access to some of the top government positions. This began subtly to influence the ways in which medicine and public health were undertaken. A similar trajectory can be seen in governance, with an increasing number of government departments – as well as municipal and local bodies – being brought under indigenous control. Ultimately, however, the direction and management of modernity was in the hands of foreign elites. On an international level, too, the management of modernity exhibited definite inconsistencies and biases. This was clearly the case when it came to the movement of colonized peoples, whose liberty was often bounded by contract (as in the case of indentured or slave labourers) or subject to unequal controls because of their presumed threats to health and political stability.[26] The international management of disease through agencies in the Middle East provides a perfect example of this, the screening process differing markedly for European or Asian and African travellers.[27] The same is true of populations moving through the Japanese empire.[28]

Colonial modernity appeared in different guises but was modernity nonetheless. The social formations which developed under imperial rule were much the same as in the West, albeit more rudimentary and mediated by local cultures and other circumstances. The same can be said of the ways in which modernity was experienced. Economic and social transformations wrought by capital were typically more rapid and brutal in colonial contexts but the long-term mental and physical consequences of change exhibit many similarities. On the one hand, modernity offered the prospect of liberation from tradition, of remaking oneself anew. On the other, there were new anxieties and tensions and an enhanced individuality experienced as anomie, alienation and disenchantment. The 'diseases of modern' life, as they were sometimes termed, knew no boundaries.[29] In many countries and colonies, the idea of the nation became a refuge for those looking to recreate social identity.[30] Another common reaction to the disorienting and isolating tendencies of modernity was the revitalization or invention of 'tradition'.[31] While it seems paradoxical, 'tradition' was often put to the service of modernity, normalizing and legitimating new values and formations. In the colonies, this had distinctive dimensions – the invention of 'national', ethnic or racial histories which were intended to restore pride and bolster movements for reform and liberation. This had important implications for health and medicine, as the restoration of health was linked in many countries with moral and physical renewal.

The politics of the body differed as much between colonial contexts as between countries in the West or in imperial Japan, where it came to express distinctive fascist, democratic and socialist ethics. But in all cases, the worth of the individual came to be evaluated in terms of his or her ability to contribute to collective goals – the ability to work, fight or reproduce. Historians of health and medicine have explored many aspects of this body politics, including in colonial settings or quasi-colonial settings. Perhaps the most influential of these works is Ruth Rogaski's *Hygienic Modernity*, which examines the changing constellation of ideas around bodily regimens at the onset of imperial intervention in China. Rogaski shows how the meanings of bodily practices gradually changed to incorporate Western ideas of hygiene and national sovereignty.[32] Scholarship on colonial India has shown how similar concerns with health and national regeneration featured in literature produced by and for various communities, reflected too in advertisements for tonics and other products said to promote health, longevity and fecundity.[33] In the present volume, such concerns feature particularly in the chapter by Amna Khalid, in which we see how colonial sanitary agendas were absorbed and then deployed in disputes over the sanitary regulation of the *kumbh mela*. Whereas ideological and national goals often coalesced, modernity brought with it the opportunity for self-definition on a larger scale. Bodily and spiritual cultivation might be undertaken for the good of humanity as a whole, as opposed to that of the nation. Dietary habits such as vegetarianism were cultivated globally, not simply for ethical reasons, or for purposes of health, but in the hope that they would foster non-violence.[34]

Other forms of bodily discipline, including fasting, were used by Gandhi and his followers to achieve similar objectives.[35] These trends were often conceived as alternatives to modernity but would have been impossible without the information revolution and disciplinary tendencies which modernity inaugurated. More obviously modern were those who espoused violent revolution internationally; they too had a distinctive body politics which took different forms as revolutionary politics developed.[36]

One area in which modernity posed a challenge to nationalism in India was in the attempts to revitalize what were increasingly presented as indigenous medical traditions, most obviously Ayurveda and Unani. Although these were presented as authentic expressions of community or nation, they faced a stiff challenge from Western medicine, which was not only championed by the colonial regime but practised by a growing number of Indians. Ayurveda, Unani and some other forms of medicine attempted to meet this challenge by incorporating elements of Western science and standardizing their teaching and practice.[37] In some cases, this was done explicitly in the name of modernity but also justified, as Burton Cleetus shows in this volume, in the name of tradition. This normally entailed the homogenization of diverse practices and the idealization of a classical past. In such cases, it is evident that both 'modernity' and 'tradition' did important rhetorical work and, in this sense, it is difficult to distinguish between them. But the legitimation of reform as in accordance with tradition ought not to detract from what was essentially a global phenomenon – the attempt to impose system on diverse practices and to acquire the same scientific status as Western medicine itself. As Ayurveda and other Indian medical 'traditions' underwent these changes, they also acquired the capacity to globalize themselves – their claims to validity becoming increasingly universal (like Western medicine) rather than confined to particular places or constitutions. Like Western medicine, they were able to utilize print media and other modern technologies to create a market that transcended not only locality but nation.[38]

However, as Saurabh Mishra points out in his chapter, one should not overstate the pressure for change. Although practitioners of Tibb began to incorporate elements of Western medicine, including the germ theory, at the turn of the twentieth century, it would appear that medical writings on cholera (*haiza*) were little affected by the concerns of either Western medical practitioners or the colonial state. One last point that needs to be emphasized when considering medical plurality is that the vast majority of Indians would have encountered neither Western or nor classical Indian practitioners on a regular basis. Unlike in the West, modernity created space for a multiplicity of blended practices to develop, which were neither licensed by the state nor regulated by custom and tradition.[39]

Several of the chapters in the current volume are concerned with gender, which, as we highlighted in our previous collection, has been one of the major growth areas in the historiography of health and medicine in colonial India. When considering how this relates to modernity, it is worth considering the remarks made by Prakash about the centrality of gender to the notion of community in India, and of the special role it played in mediating and defining the modern. As Jane Buckingham shows, interventions by the colonial state were sometimes predicated on the defence of Indian women against superstition and barbarism. Shifts in colonial discourse in relation to gender are highlighted in Samiksha Sehrawat's chapter on the Association of Medical Women in India, reflecting a broader change of emphasis from traditional motherhood to feminization. In Sujata Mukherjee's chapter, we can see how the idea of community (and nation) came to be policed in the context of the family, through medical discourses on sexuality. In both instances, the regulation of gender, while bearing some relation to Western contexts, was distinctively colonial and Indian. As in most colonies, regulation of sexuality was regarded as crucial to the articulation of national and cultural differences.[40] However, as we read in Dagbani Dais's chapter on the management of the insane, it seems that gender discrimination trumped that of race; there being distinct similarities in the ways in which female insanity was portrayed among Europeans and Indians.

Another subtheme reflecting modernity in this collection is the expanding role of medical expertise and the growth of medical institutions. Leela Sami shows how medical experts began to carve out a role for themselves in the management of famine, for instance. Mark Harrison's chapter similarly demonstrates the opportunities that existed for medical experts in the political field but also the constraints in which they operated. Medical expertise was utilized selectively according to power struggles within India and between British Indian administrators and the government in London. This alerts us to the fact that colonial modernity was never uniquely Indian. What happened in India was conditioned by imperial and international expectations, especially as regards the sanitary management of India and its contact with the West. Within India, however, there were distinct differences in the ways in which the colonial state envisaged its medical responsibilities.[41] Biswamoy Pati shows that treatment was accorded a far lower priority in institutions for the Indian insane than in their British equivalents. Similarly, as Achintya Dutta argues, in the case of *kala-azar*, the state was not unresponsive but there was a lack of urgency and consistency that was typical of colonial situations. The obvious exception was in emergencies like epidemics. When it came to the latter, as Mridula Ramanna demonstrates in her chapter, the agency of Indian doctors was often crucial in making measures intelligible and acceptable to the population at large.

Barbara Ramusack's chapter raises the interesting question of missionary modernity. Concepts of health and hygiene were central to missionary teachings in most colonial contexts, while medical treatment was typically accompanied by some degree of evangelizing. Science underpinned strictures on bodily and spiritual discipline and this ensured that missionary medical discourses were distinctively modern.[42] In this sense, there was little difference between missionary activity in India and in the slums of London or Glasgow. However, Christian modernity did exhibit different characteristics in colonial contexts. While the possibility of redemption and transformation was theoretically open to anyone who accepted the gospels and strictures on hygiene, there was considerable ambiguity about how far colonized peoples could become modern.[43] The 'rule of colonial difference', as Dipesh Chakrabarty has termed it, was often applied.

Medical modernity in the colonies was clearly different from that in most Western contexts and its manifestations in India differed, in turn, from those in other colonies. But these differences are outweighed by the similarities. In most states, medicine was being employed as a technology of governance and population management. Its status was rising as it became crucial in dealing with the manifold consequences of social and economic change, whether in the form of disease and urban squalor, alienation and social tension. For all these problems medicine appeared to offer solutions. These varied greatly from one context to another but the general trend towards medicalization was evident in the colonies as well as in imperial capitals. It could hardly have been otherwise, for the political and economic context in which India and other colonies existed was a distinctly international one. The disease ecology of India – in rural and urban areas – was transformed by the incorporation of the subcontinent into what was becoming a world market.[44] This momentous shift was enabled by the application of industrial technologies like steam power, most obviously in the form of railways, steamships and factories. The linking together of the world by electric telegraphy enabled imperial assemblages to work as systems and ultimately enabled the formation of an international order that would take shape in bodies such as the League of Nations after the First World War. These developments not only encouraged the movement of ideas and expertise but also, increasingly, of expectations. The idea that the modern state should be able to care for the health of its subjects, and even colonial citizens, had become commonplace by the 1930s.[45] Imperial territories everywhere – including the administration in India – responded to these expectations, which, at the same time, were increasingly articulated by movements of national liberation. This was a self-consciously modern world and British India, despite all its contradictions, was a part of it.

Notes

1 Dipesh Chakrabarty, *Provincializing Europe: Postcolonial Thought and Historical Difference*, Princeton, NJ: Princeton University Press, 2000.
2 Even in Western contexts, the engagement of historians of medicine with modernity has been rather superficial: see Roger Cooter, 'Medicine and Modernity', in Mark Jackson (ed.), *The Oxford Handbook of the History of Medicine*, Oxford: Oxford University Press, 2011, 100–17.
3 Projit Bihari Mukharji, *Doctoring Traditions: Ayurveda, Small Technologies, and Braided Sciences*, Chicago: University of Chicago Press, 2016; Rachel Berger, *Ayurveda Made Modern: Political Histories of Indigenous Medicine in North India, 1900–1955*, Basingstoke & New York: Palgrave Macmillan, 2013.
4 Sandip Hazareesingh, *The Colonial City and the Challenge of Modernity: Urban Hegemonies and Civic Contestations in Bombay (1900–1925)*, Hyderabad: Orient Longman, 2007; William J. Glover, *Making Lahore Modern: Constructing and Imagining a Colonial City*, Minneapolis: University of Minnesota Press, 2007.
5 Projit Bihari Mukharji, *Nationalizing the Body: The Medical Market, Print and Daktari Medicine*, London: Anthem Press, 2009.
6 Marshall Berman, *All That Is Solid Mets into Air: The Experience of Modernity*, London: Verso, 1983.
7 David Hardiman, *Missionaries and Their Medicine: A Christian Modernity for Tribal India*, Manchester: Manchester University Press, 2008, 6–7.
8 Gyan Prakash, *Another Reason: Science and the Imagination of Modern India*, Princeton, NJ: Princeton University Press, 1999.
9 Warwick Anderson, 'Introduction: Postcolonial Technoscience', *Social Studies of Science*, 32, 5–6 (2002), 643–58.
10 Anderson, 'Postcolonial Technoscience'; see also his 'Making Global Health History: The Postcolonial Worldliness of Biomedicine', *Social History of Medicine*, 27, 2 (2014), 372–84.
11 S.N. Eisenstadt, 'Multiple Modernities', *Daedalus*, 129, 1 (2000), 1–29.
12 Volker H. Schmidt, 'Multiple Modernities or Varieties of Modernity?' *Current Sociology*, 54 (2006), 77–97.
13 Frederic Jameson, *A Singular Modernity: Essays on the Ontology of the Present*, London: Verso, 2002, 13.
14 Arif Dirlik, 'Thinking Modernity Historically: Is "Alternative Modernity" the Answer?' *Asian Review of World Histories*, 1, 1 (2013), 5–44, 37.

15 Michel Foucault, 'Governmentality', in Graham Burchell et al. (eds.), *The Foucault Effect: Studies in Governmentality*, Chicago: University of Chicago Press, 1991, 92.

16 C. Koopman, 'Revising Foucault: The History and Critique of Modernity', *Philosophy & Social Criticism*, 36 (2010), 545–65.

17 Anthony Giddens, *Conversations with Anthony Giddens: Making Sense of Modernity*, Stanford: Stanford University Press, 1998; idem, *The Consequences of Modernity*, Cambridge: Polity Press, 1990.

18 Timothy Mitchell, *Questions of Modernity*, Minneapolis: University of Minnesota Press, 2000.

19 Marian Aguiar, *Tracking Modernity: India's Railway and the Culture of Mobility*, Minneapolis: University of Minnesota Press, 2011.

20 Michael Adas, *Dominance by Design: Technological Imperatives and America's Civilizing Mission*, Cambridge, MA: Harvard University Press, 2006.

21 Gyan Prakash, 'Civil Society, Community, and the Nation in Colonial India', *Etnográfica*, 6, 1 (2002), 27–39.

22 Pradip Basu (ed.), *Colonial Modernity: Indian Perspectives*, Kolkata: Setu Prakashani, 2011; Gi-Wook Shin and Michael E. Robinson (eds.), *Colonial Modernity in Korea*, Cambridge, MA: Harvard University Press, 1999; Tani E. Barlow (ed.), *Formations of Colonial Modernity in East Asia*, Durham, NC: Duke University Press, 1997.

23 E.g. The shift from Persian to Arabic and the 'scientization' of Unani Tibb: see Seema Alavi, *Islam and Healing: Loss and Recovery of an Indo-Muslim Medical Tradition, 1600–1900*, Basingstoke: Palgrave Macmillan, 2008.

24 Kapil Raj, *Relocating Modern Science: Circulation and the Construction of Knowledge in South Asia and Europe, 1650–1900*, Basingstoke: Palgrave Macmillan, 2007.

25 E.g. Prakash, *Another Reason*; Roy MacLeod and Deepak Kumar (eds.), *Technology and the Raj: Western Technology and Technical Transfers to India, 1700–1947*, New Delhi: Sage, 1995.

26 Laurence Brown and Radica Mahase, 'Medical Encounters on the *Kala Pani*: Regulation and Resistance in the Passages of Indentured Indian Migrants', in D.B. Haycock and S. Archer (eds.), *Health and Medicine at Sea 1700–1900*, Woodbridge: The Boydell Press, 2009, 195–212.

27 See for example: Saurabh Mishra, *Pilgrimage, Politics and Pestilence: The Haj from the Indian Subcontinent 1860–1920*, New Delhi: Oxford University Press, 2011.

28 Jeongran Kim, 'The Borderline of "Empire": Japanese Maritime Quarantine in Busan c.1876–1910', *Medical History*, 57 (2013), 226–48.

29 Benjamin W. Richardson, *Diseases of Modern Life*, New York: D. Appleton & Co, 1876.

30 Alexander Motyl (ed.), *Encyclopedia of Nationalism*, Vol. 1, San Diego: Academic Press, 2001, 262, 510.

31 Eric Hobsbawm and Terence Ranger (eds.), *The Invention of Tradition*, Cambridge: Cambridge University Press, 1983.

32 Ruth Rogaski, *Hygienic Modernity: Meanings of Health and Disease in Treaty-Port China*, Berkeley: University of California Press, 2004.

33 See for example: Madhrui Sharma, *Indigenous and Western Medicine in Colonial India*, New Delhi: Foundation Books, 2012; Ishita Pande,

Medicine, Race and Liberalism in British Bengal: Symptoms of Empire, London: Routledge, 2010; Guy Attewell, *Refiguring Unani Tibb: Plural Healing in Late Colonial India*, Hyderabad: Orient Longman, 2007, chap.6; David Arnold, ' "An Ancient Race Outworn": Malaria and Race in Colonial India, 1860–1930', in W. Ernst and B. Harris (eds.), *Race, Science and Medicine, 1700–1960*, London: Routledge, 1999, 123–43.

34 Tristram Stuart, *The Bloodless Revolution: A Cultural History of Vegetarianism from 1600 to Modern Times*, New York: Norton, 2007, 423–30.

35 Srirupa Prasad, *Cultural Politics of Hygiene in India, 1890–1940*, Basingstoke: Palgrave Macmillan, 2015, chap.3; M.K. Gandhi, *Non-Violent Resistance (Satyagraha)*, Mineola, NY: Dover Publications, 2001.

36 Antoine de Baeque, *The Body Politic: Corporeal Metaphors in Revolutionary France, 1770–1800*, Stanford: Stanford University Press, 1997; Rolf Hellebust, 'Aleksei Gastev and the Metallization of the Revolutionary Body', *Slavic Review*, 56, 3 (1997), 500–18.

37 Mukharji, *Doctoring Traditions*; Berger, *Ayurveda Made Modern*; Attewell, *Refiguring Unani Tibb*; D. Kumar and R.S. Basu (eds.), *Medical Encounters in British India*, New Delhi: Oxford University Press, 2013; P. Bala (ed.), *Contesting Colonial Authority: Medicine and Indigenous Responses in Nineteenth-and Twentieth-Century India*, Plymouth: Lexington Books, 2012; Kavita Sivaramakrishnan, *Old Potions, New Bottles: Recasting Indigenous Medicine in Colonial Punjab 1850–1945*, Hyderabad: Orient Longman, 2006.

38 Madhulika Banerjee, *Power, Knowledge, Medicine: Ayurvedic Pharmaceuticals at Home and in the World*, Hyderabad: Orient BlackSwan, 2009; Maarten Bode, *Taking Traditional Knowledge to Market: The Modern Image of the Ayurvedic and Unani Industry 1980–2000*, Hyderabad: Orient BlackSwan, 2008; D. Wujastyk and F.M. Smith (eds.), *Modern and Global Ayurveda: Perspectives and Paradigms*, Albany, NY: SUNY Press, 2008.

39 D. Hardiman and P.B. Mukharji (eds.), *Medical Marginality in South Asia: Situating Subaltern Therapeutics*, Abingdon: Oxford, 2012.

40 Antoinette Burton (ed.), *Gender, Sexuality and Colonial Modernities*, London & New York: Routledge, 1999.

41 The literature on this subject is vast but for a range of perspectives, see the introductions to B. Pati and M. Harrison (eds.), *The Social History of Health and Medicine in Colonial India*, Abingdon: Routledge, 2009; idem (eds.), *Health, Medicine and Empire: Perspectives on Colonial India*, Hyderabad: Orient Longman, 2001. See also Samiksha Sehrawat, *Colonial Medical Care in North India: Gender, State, and Society c.1840–1920*, New Delhi: Oxford University Press, 2013; Sanjoy Bhattacharya, Mark Harrison and Michael Worboys, *Fractured States: Smallpox, Public Health and Vaccination Policy in British India 1800–1947*, Hyderabad: Orient Longman, 2005; Mark Harrison, *Public Health in British India: Anglo-Indian Preventive Medicine 1859–1914*, Cambridge: Cambridge University Press, 1994; David Arnold, *Colonizing the Body: State Medicine and Epidemic Disease in Nineteenth-Century India*, Berkeley: University of California Press, 1993.

42 David Hardiman (ed.), *Healing Bodies, Saving Souls: Medical Missions in Asia and Africa*, Amsterdam & New York: Rodolpi, 2006.

43 Hardiman, *Missionaries and Their Medicine*.
44 For a general discussion of this, see Mark Harrison, 'A Global Perspective: Reframing the History of Health, Medicine, and Disease', *Bulletin of the History of Medicine*, 89, 4 (2015), 639–89; idem, 'Disease and World History from 1750', in J.R. McNeill and K. Pomeranz (eds.), *The Cambridge World History: Volume VII. Production, Destruction, and Connection, 1750-Present. Part 1: Structures, Spaces, and Boundary Making*, Cambridge: Cambridge University Press, 2015, 237–57.
45 Harrison, 'A Global Perspective', 671–2.

1 The sentencing of assisted suicide in the Nizamut Adawlut, 1810–1829

Religion, health and gender in the formation of British Indian criminal law

Jane Buckingham

In early nineteenth-century north India, suicide offered a culturally legitimate alternative to a life of social and ritual abandonment for those marginalized by widowhood or illness. In such cases suicide, typically by burning or burial alive, was resorted to both as a way of ending present suffering and a response to the ritual consequences of their condition. Such forms of suicide typically required the help of others and this chapter focuses on the differences in British approaches to sentencing of those who assisted at such traditional forms of suicide. In Hindu textual shastric tradition the suicide of leprosy sufferers and of widows was linked, and this connection between these forms of suicide became a key legal reference point for British understanding of the Hindu law of suicide. However, differences in sentencing show that while assistance at the suicide of the Hindu widow was typically perceived in cases brought before the Nizamut Adawlut (the superior criminal court in Bengal) as approximating homicide, assisting the leprosy sufferer to die was more often understood as euthanasia. This chapter argues that sentencing of assistants at suicides exemplified the tension between Islamic, Hindu and British legal traditions embedded in British legal practice in India and that the religious associations of both those committing suicide and their assistants contributed substantially to the sentences received. Further, this chapter suggests that the health and gender of the person committing suicide contributed to the development of a differential British legal response to forms of suicide by widows and the infirm despite reference to their linkage in shastric tradition as a precedent in judgement.

The culpability of those who assist others to commit suicide is still a point of debate in the Indian Penal Code,[1] and this chapter contributes to contextualization of contemporary Indian discussion on the decriminalization of suicide and the ethics and law of euthanasia[2] within the historical framework of British legal intervention in India. Foundational work on the complex nature of colonial Indian law by Derrett, Fisch, the Rudolphs and Cohn[3] has been augmented by specific work on criminal law including Yang's edited volume on crime and criminality and, more recently, Sen's study of convict society and Radhakrishna's analysis of criminalization of communities under the Criminal Tribes Act.[4] The gendering of crime is a relatively recent investigation with Singha considering the colonial construction of legal capacity in female children and Anagol the nexus of early widowhood and the colonial development of the 'infanticidal woman' as 'female criminal'.[5] The focus of historiographical work on women and crime has previously been on the figure of the *sati*, the widow as victim and site of tradition and on the event of sati as negotiated territory for the expression of gendered power relations.[6] The focus of this chapter on the sentencing of those assisting a widow to commit suicide marks a new contribution to the already voluminous literature on the practice and its attempted abolition during the British colonial period.[7]

The suicide of leprosy sufferers, by contrast, has attracted little attention from contemporaries or historians, even though the practice is positioned in the British Parliamentary Papers alongside sati as an equivalent legal dilemma for British colonial authorities. The most substantial recent work on leprosy suicide is Shubhada Pandya's 'Very savage rites' which records instances of suicides by leprosy sufferers and analyzes them as examples of traditional forms of suicide 'tolerated' by the British colonial legislators.[8] It does not, however, develop an analysis of the sentencing of assistants at the suicides. Nor does it develop the relationship between these forms of suicide and sati as contributing to the development of British law in India. Similarly, in comparison with the massive current historiography on British ideas of and legal intervention in the practice of sati by Hindu widows, there is little published on colonial legal engagement with leprosy in India.[9] Although cases of assisted suicide by both widows and leprosy sufferers were often discussed concurrently in British debates on legal regulation, this chapter is the first to employ this juxtaposition as a means of investigating early nineteenth-century colonial legal engagement with India.

Forms of assisted suicide

Both the suicide of leprosy sufferers and of widows could be performed by fire or by burial alive, though immolation was more commonly performed by widows and burial alive by leprosy sufferers. In the cases of suicide by leprosy sufferers brought before the Nizamut Adawlut in the first part of the nineteenth century, only that of Government *vs* Sohawun combined burial alive with burning. In this instance the fire was lit in a pit into which the leprosy sufferer threw himself, later being covered over by his son. The case of Government *vs* Sohawun cites extensively Hindu legal opinion and textual authorities representing the entering of fire as a means of 'promoting . . . spiritual welfare'.[10]

In practice, however, most instances of leprosy suicide were by burial alive and more consistent with the model of death for the out-caste leprosy sufferer offered by the *Bhawishya Purana* than that of purification by fire. Widows of the *jogee* community similarly practised burial alive which strengthens the association of burial with being outside caste.[11] Out-casting of leprosy sufferers from family and community depended more on their economic status than on their illness.[12] However, the *Bhawishya Purana* stipulates a certain level of physical degradation as grounds for limiting the funeral rights for the leprosy sufferer, in particular refusing cremation of the body:

> that leper is most vile in respect of all religious acts, who is afflicted with ulcers on all his limbs, *especially* on his temples, forehead and nose;
> When he dies, let his corpse be cast near a sacred river or other holy place, or at the root of a sacred tree; let not a funeral cake or libation of water be offered, nor his corpse be burnt, nor obsequies be celebrated:[13]

The *Bhawishya Purana* cautions that even assistance at the cremation of a leprosy sufferer caused ritual pollution which had to be removed by the appropriate actions.

> Should a man, through affection burn the corpse of a leper, who has been six or even three months, infected with the disease, that man must perform the lunar penance of an anchoret.[14]

In judging cases of assisted suicide of leprosy sufferers, the British gave considerable weight to the shastric endorsement of such suicides and the belief in their efficacy in removing the taint of leprosy from the family. The Judge of the Circuit Court in the Goruckpore sessions noted in his recommendation for the unconditional release of Sohawan, charged with homicide for assisting his father Akbar to burn himself alive:

> It is supposed that the leprosy is a visitation of Providence for some offence or other, and that the souls of the victims are purified by fire from the taint of the disease, and exempted from passing into impure bodies after death. There is also a popular notion that by this self-devotion the disease is rooted out of the family.[15]

However, the *karmic* benefits to the family of association with the leprosy sufferer's suicide could not outweigh the shame of the disease. By contrast the act of burning alive by a sati and assistance at her death were propitious events bringing karmic benefits to all involved. The woman who became a 'sati' was elevated in status, saved her husband's spirit from the underworld and lived with him in bliss. As the Hindu law giver Brihispati explained: 'In the same manner as a snake-catcher drags a snake from his hole, so does a woman who burns herself draw her husband out of hell; and she afterwards resides with him in heaven.'[16] Unlike the leprosy sufferer, the sati was venerated as one touched with divine power.[17]

The changing position of assisted suicide in British Indian criminal law

In their conceptualization of criminal law in India, the British recognized a relationship between assisted suicide by widows and leprosy sufferers far beyond the occasional parallel in technique of immolation or burial alive practised by widow and leprosy sufferer alike.[18] In early cases brought before the Nizamut Adawlut, 'the ceremony of Suttee' and 'suicide committed by Hindoos in cases of extreme sickness' were linked as specific forms of assisted suicide under Resolution 25 June 1817.[19] Though regarded with abhorrence as contrary to both British law and Christian culture,[20] colonial legislators identified suicide by widows and leprosy sufferers as forms of suicide permitted, though not enjoined, by shastric tradition.[21] Since the Brahmanic legal textual tradition provided the dominant model for British legal identification, appropriation and interpretation of Indian 'traditional' legal ideas and practice,[22] the sanction of these forms of suicide in the *shastra* had the force of precedent in the early British efforts to develop a new criminal law for India.[23] Consequently, such forms of suicide were to be tolerated and those participating in the practice were not necessarily to be subject to the law of homicide as it existed at the time. A further ground for viewing assistance at such suicides with lenience was that these particular forms of suicide were regarded by British legal and government authorities as having some dimension of honour and self-sacrifice and thus were seen as possessing a moral and ethical value. Despite official revulsion for suicide, the judges of the Nizamut Adawlut, Harrington, Rees and Turnbull recorded the court's opinion that both the suicide of a widow and a leprosy sufferer represented forms of sacrificial devotion, the former to her husband and the latter to the family which was popularly believed to be freed from the disease by the sufferer's suicide.[24]

The legal position on assisted suicide shifted considerably from the late eighteenth to the early nineteenth centuries and reflected an increasing dependence on the Hindu textual tradition in framing and legitimizing British legal policy and practice in India. In 1799, the Bengal Regulations ordered the sentence of death to those assisting in suicides but allowed some scope for discretion in ordering capital punishment. The Bengal Regulation, Nizamut Adawlut Section 3, Regulation VIII, 1799, directed the sentence of death in cases 'where one puts to death another at the desire of the sufferer' but only where the Nizamut Adawlut could find no circumstances to ask for mercy.[25] By 1817, however, the position had changed to accommodate the forms of suicide supported in Brahmanic tradition. On 22 June 1817, the Nizamut Adawlut stated that Section 3 did not apply to sati or to the suicide of leprosy sufferers, because these acts were sanctioned in the *sastras*. The position was confirmed by a resolution of the Nizamut Adawlut under the date of 25 June 1817. Elaborating this position, the bench of the Nizamut Adawlut, in correspondence with Mr. Watson, the Calcutta Circuit judge, made an express distinction between Indian customary forms of slaying such as the 'raujkoomar's destroying his daughter' and child sacrifice, which were not sanctioned in the *sastras*, and the assistance given to a sati or a leprosy sufferer wishing to die. Only the former which lacked *shastric* endorsement were deemed to be murder.[26]

The 1817 decision was not a new regulation but an interpretation of the 1799 regulation regarding the law of homicide.[27] Consistent with the British inclination in the early formulation of criminal law to use Brahmanic precedent in legitimizing their own legal pronouncements,[28] the 1817 decision was based in part on the opinion of Hindu pundits given in the Nizamut Adawlut's hearing of Government *vs* Sohawun on 7 August 1810. The Nizamut Adawlut ruled that 'no culpability attaches to the son', Sohawun, because his assistance of his father, who was severely afflicted with leprosy, in burning and burying himself alive was consistent with the shastric tradition. The notes to this case make an explicit link between the judgement of Government *vs* Sohawum and the formulation of the resolution of 25 June 1817. The notes confirm the relationship, in both shastric and the emerging British criminal law, between 'the ceremony of Suttee' and 'the suicide committed by Hindoos in cases of extreme sickness'. Since the Nizamut Adawlut considered such suicide of leprosy sufferers 'to resemble, in principle, the female sacrifice of Suttee', the revised colonial regulation was to cover both. The court observed that:

> although both are within the letter of Section 3, Regulation VIII. 1799, which declares, 'it shall not justify any prisoner convicted of wilful homicide, that he or she was desired by the party slain to put him or her to death,' yet neither has been considered within the intention of that section; which, as expressly stated in it, was 'to preserve the lives of many from the effects of passion or revenge, aided by the enormous prejudices of superstition.'[29]

Negotiation between legal traditions

British efforts to regulate homicide and draw on shastric precedent functioned not only in relationship with Brahmanic tradition but within the existing Islamic frameworks of criminal law inherited from the Mughal state. The 1810 case, Government *vs* Sohawun, indicates the complex of legal systems engaging British efforts to practice law. As the case progressed from circuit to High Court, the efforts of the British law officers to negotiate between the different parameters of the Islamic criminal law and the Hindu shastric tradition in order to reconcile assisted suicide with their own expectations of the law of homicide are evident. In the charge of homicide brought before the Circuit Court against Sohawun the principal legal framework for the Circuit judge's response was Indian Islamic criminal law. The *futwa* (opinion) of the law officers attached to the Court of Circuit declared that a sentence of *kissas* (retaliation)[30] against Sohawun was barred because it was not a case of wilful murder and the deceased had voluntarily flung himself into the fire where he died. However, the *futwa* continued, the prisoner Sohawun was 'liable to discretionary punishment,[31] for having, in pursuance of his father's directions, prepared the pit and set fire to the fuel with which he had filled it'.[32]

Revealing tension between Islamic and Hindu tradition in those areas which interposed criminal law into personal religious practice, the Circuit judge disagreed with the *futwa*, arguing rather that suicide was countenanced by Hindu religious tradition in the case of severe leprosy and that this sanction and the religious and ritual significance of the act removed the taint of homicide from the suicide's assistant. The Circuit judge advocated unconditional release of the prisoner Sohawun on the grounds that the leprosy sufferer's action was consistent with Hindu belief that by such self-sacrifice the sufferer would purge his spirit from the taint of the disease, freeing him from rebirth into an impure body and freeing his family from a recurrence of leprosy. He continued, that since at the time the custom of sati was being tolerated,

> it would be quite inconsistent with that spirit of toleration to punish persons, who, from the strongest motives of piety, have complied with the earnest entreaties of their parents, and have relieved them from an existence which has become painful to them, disgusting to their friends, and useless to society.[33]

When the case came before the Nizamut Adawlut, on appeal against the Circuit Court's *futwa*, the Nizamut Adawlut's Islamic law officers declared that since the father had thrown himself on the pyre the prisoner was not guilty of burning his father alive, and thus ordered his release. Despite the power of the *futwa*,[34] the judges of the Nizamut Adawlut referred the matter to the Hindu pundits before bringing down their decision. The pundits concurred with the opinion of the Circuit Court that the *shastric* literature sanctioned self-immolation for ritual benefit by those with a severe and incurable form of leprosy and that the son, in assisting his father, bore no culpability for murder. The Nizamut Adawlut concurred with both the Hindu justification for assisting in the suicide and the Nizamut Adawlut's *futwa* acquitting the son, and discharged the prisoner without sentence.[35]

The recourse to Hindu pundits in the case and both the Circuit judge and the Nizamut Adawlut's privileging of the pundits' opinion reflect British caution in developing an aspect of criminal law which might prove contrary to the religion and custom of the Hindu majority in India. British rejection of the *futwa* in the Circuit Court also emphasized the increasing tendency for British legal authorities to construct and legitimate their authority in criminal law, and particularly their assumption of the right over the life and death of their subjects, according to the frameworks of Brahmanic tradition rather than in Islamic legal terms. Bengal Regulation 14, 1810, increased the authority of the Nizamut Adawlut allowing the judges to mitigate or even to pardon a sentence given by *futwa*. However, the Circuit Court judges had to appeal to the Nizamut Adawlut to uphold decisions against their Islamic law officers. Although the Circuit judges remained bound to the *futwas* of the Circuit Court unless successfully appealed to the Nizamut Adawlut, Regulation 17, 1817, increased the Nizamut Adawlut's powers allowing the court to alter and even increase any sentence declared by the *futwa*.[36] The sentencing of assistants at a sati in 1821 reflected this movement away from the authority of the Islamic criminal law in practice. As the second judge of the Nizamut Adawlut made clear in the discussion of the law governing sati in the 1821 case, Government *vs* Bhuraichee and others:

> The essence of the – is, that if the suttee be according to the shaster, it is lawful; if not, criminal. With this declaration from the supreme authority, I can not see how a Hindu can, in common sense or common equity, be made amenable to the Moohummudan law for the offence.[37]

The British were moving away from Mughal precedent embedding their claims to legal sovereignty in Brahmanic Hindu tradition rather than in the remnants of Islamic Nizamut authority.[38]

Not that British legal authority had much respect for the Brahmanic legal tradition which they were endeavouring to administer. Cruso's 1786 eye witness account of sati at Pune which opens the records on sati collected in the 1821 Parliamentary Papers dwells in detail on the widow Tooselboy as the centre of a publicly celebrated auspicious event sanctioned by Brahmanic tradition. As Cruso describes, her path was 'marked by the goolol and betel leaf, which she had scattered as she went along' and she was attended by relatives, the public kept back by a government guard. Brahmins not only endorsed the event by their presence but directly benefited since Toolseboy 'distributed among the Brahmins two thousand rupees, and the jewels with which she came decorated'.[39] In Government *vs* Sohawun the judge of the Circuit Court commented on the inconsistency of punishing assistants at the discreet suicide of a leprosy sufferer while 'young widows are suffered to devote themselves every day in the province of Benares, on the funeral piles [sic] of their husbands, in the midst of Brahmins, and a train of attendants'.[40]

Participation of Brahmins in sati confirmed British ambivalence about the role of Brahmanic tradition in developing criminal law in India. On the one hand the law sought to function in accordance with Brahmanic tradition; on the other, Brahmins were seen as direct beneficiaries and supporters of 'barbaric' and 'superstitious' customs.

Although the colonial law officers of the Nizamut Adawlut asserted the shastric precedent and equivalence of suicide by leprosy sufferers and Hindu widows, sati was seen as a ritual act, qualitatively different from the suicide of the infirm. Sati was perceived by British observers in India and at home as essentially a public performance, replete with elements of ritual and superstition, deeply offensive to the British Evangelical Protestantism which, from the early 1800s, increasingly sought to influence the ideology of British colonialism in India.[41] British engagement with sati can certainly be critiqued in terms of the intervention of a foreign and colonizing culture.[42] But as a public event, sati exposed the vulnerability of British authority and sovereignty in the face of Indian legal and cultural tradition.

Religious community and criminal 'intent'

Despite aversion to sati, reluctance to sentence those assisting in the suicide of widows on charges of murder reflected the broader British understanding of culpability as related to full cognizance of the crime committed. Linked to this was the British concept of 'intention' as the basis of culpability. Part of the logic for lenience in sentencing assistants at suicides was the idea that Hindu culture was essentially flawed in its understanding of suicide and assisted suicide because it lacked the ethical insight of the British legal tradition which perceived suicide and homicide as essentially both 'sinful' and unlawful. Since, from a Hindu point of view, assisting a leprosy sufferer to commit suicide was often understood as an act of familial duty the Courts argued that those accused were ignorant of the homicidal nature of their crime.[43] Ignorance of crime meant that the assistant at a suicide sanctioned in Hindu tradition could not have acted with the intent to commit a crime.

The precedent set in 1810 by Government *vs* Sohawun was followed in subsequent cases. In Government *vs* Sheoo Suhaee and Chotoo, for example, the prisoners were charged with assisting the leprosy sufferer, Anoopun Tewaree, a Brahmin, to 'decease himself by drowning'. The Benares Circuit Court's law officer delivered the *futwa* that since 'self-destruction is prohibited by law' both prisoners were to be considered 'criminal' and were liable for discretionary punishment by *acuboot*.[44] However, the Circuit judge, citing the prisoners' motives, recommended that they be released unconditionally. When the case came before the Nizamut Adawlut the *futwa* followed the same principle as in the Circuit Court but again the Islamic law was overthrown by the British legal authorities who upheld Hindu custom supported by the British legal principle of intent against Islamic criminal law. The judgement brought down by H.T. Colebrooke and J. Fombelle drew specifically on the precedent of Government *vs* Sohawun, 7 August 1810, and declared that the prisoners 'were justified by the tenets of their superstition' and so the judges 'did not consider them proper objects of punishment' directing rather that they 'should be immediately set at liberty'.[45] Similarly, in the case of Government *vs* Ramdut and Balgobind, the fourth judge of the Nizamut Adawlut, W. Dorin argued for a lenient sentence of two years' imprisonment for the assistants in the sati of Gunshea partly on the grounds that: 'The defendants, in their share of the transaction, seem to have acted under the decided influence of superstition, and from no discoverable motive of private malice'.[46]

Complicating further British efforts to standardize a legal response to assisted suicide within a framework of both Islamic and personal law was the colonial notion that only 'Hindus' were eligible to participate in aspects of 'Hindu' law. Despite British essentialist conceptualizations of personal law as religiously exclusive, people of non-Hindu background did follow practices of assisted suicide identified by British legal authorities as 'Hindu'. In practice there was little to separate the experience and actions of the assistant at the suicide of a Muslim leprosy sufferer from that at the death of a Hindu. In the 1810 case, Government *vs* Badul Khan and four others, the deceased, Mussummaut Dhuna, was so badly afflicted with leprosy that 'her toes and fingers were falling to pieces, and worms had got into her feet and body'. The deceased urged her son-in-law, Badul Khan, to bury her and 'thereby put an end to her sufferings, and redeem her from the torments and misery which are supposed to be reserved for persons dying of that loathsome complaint'. This belief that burial would free the leprosy sufferer in the afterlife, cited by court pundits as part of shastric tradition, was clearly held by the deceased. Mussummaut Dhuna was so desperate that she threatened Badul Khan 'that if he did not comply on the day of judgement she would appear against him'.[47] Despite her threats the prisoner did not comply with her wishes but prepared a grave only when the signs of approaching death became clear, carrying her to the graveside when she was all but dead. The physical degradation of the deceased, the desire for relief from suffering and the reluctance of the assistant to bring about a death are just as in the cases where Hindus assisted at the suicide of leprosy sufferers.

However, the British justices of the Nizamut Adawlut did not extend their tolerance and appreciation of the 'pious duty' of the Hindu who assisted a severely ill family member to their death to the Muslim who took the same action. In Government *vs* Badul Khan and four others the Circuit judge argued that those accused of assisting the suicide were guilty 'on the grounds of ignorance of the creed which they profess' and that '[t]here was a clear and manifest intention of putting an end to the existence of the sufferer'. Being Muslim did not allow the mitigation of culpability on the basis of ignorance of the true nature of their crime, a position allowed to the Hindus. Rather, the Circuit Court judge ordered that 'the prisoners, being Moosulmauns, are proper objects of punishment' since assistance at suicide was a crime under Islamic law. Intent on a prosecution, the *futwa* excusing the prisoners on the grounds that they were not certain that the deceased was dead before burial was rejected by the Circuit Court.

When Government *vs* Badul Khan came before the Nizamut Adawlut the Circuit Court's position was upheld. The lenience towards assisted suicide in the shastric literature, while broadly acceptable as a legitimizing component to incorporate into colonial criminal law, was not to apply in Muslim cases. The law officers of the Nizamut Adawlut broadly concurred with the *futwa* of the Circuit Court but declared the prisoner Badul Khan liable for discretionary punishment 'being convicted, on his own confession, of having committed an unlawful and culpable act, in burying his mother-in-law, without ascertaining that she was dead'. The Nizamut Adawlut upheld the *futwa* for discretionary punishment on the basis that the 'offence . . . derived no countenance from the Moosulmaun law', though since the prisoner had already been confined for six months the Court did not extend the sentence.[48] Colonial legal authorities in constructing a new Indian criminal law insisted on the compartmentalization of personal law strictly on community lines even where the fluidity of Indian religious culture was evident in the case presented. In the developing colonial law the shastric lineage of the practice and its status as Hindu custom did not make assisting at the suicide of a leprosy sufferer or of a widow acceptable among non-Hindus no matter what they believed. The difference between the sentencing of the Muslim and Hindu assistants at the suicide of a leprosy sufferer did not derive from the circumstances of their cases, which tended to be similar, but from British privileging of a very limited concept of religious adherence and identity in the development of a new criminal law for India.

The case of Government *vs* Badul Khan and four others proved as important as Government *vs* Sohawun in setting in place the principles of sentencing cases of assisted suicide. The notes to the case in the Nizamut Adawlut confirmed the opinion of the Circuit judge that assisting at such suicides was inappropriate for Muslims since the practice was essentially Hindu not Muslim. Muslim assistance at assisted suicide was condemned at both Circuit and Superior Court levels on the basis that it was 'practised under the influence of one of the many superstitious ideas which the Moohummudans have adopted from the Hindoos'.[49] In an effort to enforce the British conception of personal law as exclusive, and to reduce the incidence of assisted suicide the case of Government *vs* Badul Khan prompted the Nizamut Adawlut judges, J.H. Harington and J. Fombelle, to recommend that:

> With a view of checking the barbarous custom under the influence of which Badul Khan had committed his offence, and which was thus declared to derive no countenance from the Moosulmaun law, . . . proclamations should be issued in those provinces where the custom was prevalent, warning the Moosulmaun community of the punishment to which they would subject themselves by being guilty of such a practice.[50]

Cases of assisted suicide by widows also occasionally involved Muslim assistants and, as with cases of suicide by leprosy sufferers, sentencing was more rigorous for Muslim participants on the grounds that there was no Muslim precedent for the practice of sati and no mitigation except ignorance of their own law. The 1821 case of homicide, Government *vs* Bhuraichee and others, was a complex case of sati, including forceful return of the 14-year-old Brahmin widow Hoomuleea to the funeral pyre of her absent husband. The death blow was struck with a sword by the Muslim, Bhuraichee. This case clearly did not conform with the shastric prohibition against women being drugged or coerced into suicide. Further, it involved a Brahmin woman committing sati without her husband's body. On both grounds it was 'illegal' under the terms of the British regulation of the practice.[51] However, in sentencing, the Nizamut Adawlut declared that the religious beliefs of the participants were a key factor.[52]

Sentencing was vigorously debated between the judges of the Nizamut Adawlut. While the direct attack on the victim with a sword gave the case elements of murder, the case was ultimately tried as a form of assisted suicide complicated by forceful intervention. This case occurred at the time that the British were endeavouring to reduce incidents of sati by claiming that only those practised according to shastric tradition could be allowed. In an effort to use what were mistakenly understood as 'prescriptive and normative' Hindu legal texts to contain the practice, shastric injunctions regarding sati were sought by the British from the pundits of the Nizamut Adawlut.[53] As that tradition was interpreted in the Nizamut Adawlut, any woman of caste was permitted to burn on her husband's funeral pyre. However, if she was responsible for infant children, was pregnant or under the age of puberty she was prohibited from burning.[54]

Included in this concept of a 'legal' sati was the notion that only voluntary sati was a legitimate practice without legal penalty. Compared with cases heard before the Nizamut Adawlut from 1820 to the abolition of sati in 1828, where compulsion was not emphasized, the sentencing of Bhuraichee and others was generally more severe. Occasionally a sati practised in full compliance with the principles of shastric tradition and so identified by the British as 'legal' came before the Nizamut Adawlut and resulted in acquittal.[55] More common were sentences of six months to one year without labour.[56] Though no direct compulsion was involved, the more severe sentence of two years' imprisonment on both defendants in the 1823 case, Government *vs* Ramdut and Balgobind, was given because the widow had no information of her husband's death other than having seen his ghost.[57] Instances of coercion attracted the most severe sentencing as not only 'illegal' in the sense of not concurring with British efforts to make sati comply with Brahmanic tradition but as inhumane.[58]

According to the emerging British legal culture the culpability of the Hindu assistants was reduced by their belief that sati was a legitimate practice despite the 'illegality' of coercion. At the same time, the British insistence on the exclusivity of religious law contributed to the more severe sentencing of the Muslim participants. Bhuraichee, who at the instigation of the onlookers, struck the death blow with his sword, was imprisoned with labour for five years. The other Muslim participant, Roosa, who was arraigned as 'accessory before the fact' was similarly heavily sentenced with three years' imprisonment with labour though his role was limited to 'abetting' Bhuraichee. By contrast, Sheolal and Bhichook, Hoomuleea's uncles who forced her back into the fire and shared with Bhuraichee the original charge of murder, reduced to culpable homicide, were sentenced to one year's imprisonment without labour. In this case British sentencing confirmed the idea that religious community affects intention and thus legal culpability. Unlike Government *vs* Badul Khan and four others, in this case 'ignorance' is seen as a mitigating factor reducing the culpability of the Muslim participants from murder to culpable homicide. Even so, despite the 'illegality' of the sati the sentencing of the Hindus involved is lenient compared to that of the Muslims. This case points to the inconsistency within principles of sentencing in the Nizamut Adawlut despite the precedents of the 1810 cases. Further, it suggests that the courts used these opportunities to emphasize the notion of adherence to particular religious tradition as exclusive in law and as essential elements in the assessment of criminality.

Religion, gender and agency

Mani argues that both sati and leprosy sufferers were perceived by the British as entirely surrendering their agency to religion.[59] However, in British recording of cases of assisted suicide by leprosy sufferers the emphasis is rather on the agency of the victim who wished for death and, as in Government *vs* Sohawun, was empowered by the expectation that their actions would be of ritual and religious benefit to the family. On 24 August 1812, the Nizamut Adawlut released Mussummaut Hunsoo, the widow and Mooktaran, the son of a Hindu leprosy sufferer Rutna whom they had buried alive on his request. Despite the charge of homicide, Mr. Kerr, the Circuit judge who referred the trial, commented that since Rutna had requested to be buried alive such a suicide was a 'self-sacrifice, made with the hope of guarding the progeny from so terrible a visitation'.[60]

By contrast, female vulnerability to coercion, which increased the severity of sentencing in Government *vs* Bhuraichee and others, was a significant factor in the representation of the sati in British government and legal proceedings as 'the victim', the 'poor creature' and the 'infatuated victim'. The woman was constructed as unable to act autonomously, as conditioned from birth to prefer the meritorious self-sacrifice of sati to the ignoble life of a widow. Evidence brought before the courts of women insisting on being burnt despite efforts to prevent them, and of calm fortitude before their deaths, did little to dispel the British conceptualization of the sati as victim.[61] The strength of the impression that 'voluntary sati' was not possible was heightened by the emphasis on forced sati in missionary and newspaper accounts[62] and was frequently confirmed by cases of compulsion coming before the courts as cases of 'illegal' sati. According to the traditions referenced by the British legal authorities, a woman who had resolved to burn and had performed the appropriate ceremonies but could not face the pyre could be returned to society and her family after the performance of the appropriate rituals and austerities.[63] However, as the cases before the courts indicated, suicide of widows was not always performed according to such prescriptions. Not only was there variation between interpretations of the shastric tradition but considerable customary and regional variation in the practice.[64] Further, as Mr. Law, third judge of the Nizamut Adawlut, noted in

Government *vs* Bhuraichee and others, there was a strong belief that a family would suffer 'indelible disgrace' if a sati was not completed once it had begun.[65]

Of greatest concern to those pronouncing sentence on the assistants at sati were the violent breaches of shastric injunction, the cases of forced sati and of sati by girls as young as nine and twelve.[66] Before the British attempts to abolish sati,[67] G. Dowdeswell, Secretary to Government, Judicial Department, wrote to the Register of the Nizamut Adawlut in 1805 requesting that 'means may be adopted to prevent the illegal and unwarrantable practice of administering intoxicating medicines to women . . . and to rescue from destruction such females, as, from immaturity of years, or other circumstances, cannot be considered capable of judging for themselves, in a case of so serious and awful a nature, as that to which these remarks refer'.[68]

Unlike occurrences of sati, in no case of assisted suicide by leprosy sufferers which came before the Nizamut Adawlut between 1810 and 1829 was coercion a factor. Further, the sufferer's desire to die was construed by the British legal authorities as completely reasonable given their wretched state of health. The judgement in Government *vs* Sheoo Suhaee and Chotoo, for example, notes:

> It appeared in evidence that the deceased had been long afflicted with a grievous leprosy; that the disease was so violent as to cause his members to drop off, and to reduce his body to a state of putrefaction: that in this deplorable condition, he had for some time formed the resolution of terminating existence; but that he was prevented from attaining his object,. . which he himself was incapacitated by extreme helplessness from performing.[69]

The Nizamut Adawlut was reluctant to sentence those assisting the gravely ill to their death on the basis that their actions were reluctantly performed and motivated by compassion rather than malice. As in the 1812 case of Government *vs* Mussummaut Hunsoo and Mooktara, both the Circuit judge and Nizamut Adawlut were reluctant to prosecute the deceased's widow and son, who had buried him alive at his request. As the Circuit judge noted: 'in my opinion, it would rather be cruel than humane to bereave the miserable parent of his last and only consolation'.[70] As such, the Nizamut Adawlut was inclined to acquit such assistants as on the basis that 'they were not fit objects of punishment'.[71] Implicit in the reluctance to sentence those assisting in the suicide of leprosy sufferers was a judicial sense that without health and youth the life of the leprosy sufferer was of little value and their desire to die a legitimate response to circumstances. While pity and disgust characterize British judicial representations of the leprosy sufferer, they are not represented, like the sati, as victims without agency.

The suicide of a young and healthy woman on her husband's funeral pyre captured the British heroic imagination in a way that the suicide of a leprosy sufferer could not.[72] Cruso's account which sets the tone for the tabled Parliamentary Papers on Sati lingers over the physical features of the 19-year-old widow, Toolseboy: 'her stature above the middle standard, her form elegant, and her features interesting and expressive; her eyes, in particular, large, bold and commanding'. To Cruso, 'these beauties were eminently conspicuous, notwithstanding her face was discoloured with turmeric, her hair dishevelled and wildly ornamented with flowers'.[73] Explicit in this description is the valuing of youth, beauty and health. Later reports of cases recorded in both the Nizamut Adawlut and British Parliamentary Papers tend simply to note the age of the widow committing sati, which varied from girls to relatively elderly women.[74] However, British legislators clearly ascribed particular value to youth and health, remarking on the 22-year-old widow 'in the full vigour of health and strength'[75] and children such as the 9-year-old Kumly from Midnapore as causes for intervention.[76] Cruso describes Toolseboy as a ritual sacrifice who 'gave herself, in the meridian of life and beauty, a victim to a barbarous and cruelly consecrated error of misguided faith'.[77]

Conclusion

The sentencing of assistants in the suicide of widows and those afflicted with leprosy demonstrates something of the complexity of legal and cultural factors affecting the formation of British criminal law in India. Both Brahmanic and Islamic legal and religious opinions were used together with case law to develop precedents in sentencing of assistants at suicides which released them from the penalties typically associated with homicide and murder. The application of legal and religious precedent in judging cases of assisted suicide was, however, further mitigated by the health and gender of the person seeking suicide. Although both sati and suicide by leprosy sufferers were identified by the British law givers as religious rites,[78] suicide by leprosy sufferers was in addition perceived as a form of euthanasia. In British thinking, compassion for the sick was a legitimate motive for assisting in a suicide but fear born of 'superstition' was not. The entreaty which gave the leprosy sufferer agency also freed their assistants from severity of sentencing under the charge of homicide. While the leprosy afflicted were understood as possessing greater agency in choosing death than the widow, their lives were judged to be less worth living. By the time of the abolition of sati, compassion was established in British legal practice as a justification for assisting the severely ill to their death.

Notes

1 Government of India, Law Commission of India, 'Humanization and Decriminalization of Attempt to Suicide', Report No. 210, October 2008, New Delhi, 10, 22–4. www.lawcommissionofindia.nic.in.

2 Purushottama Bilimoria, 'Legal Rulings on Suicide in India and Implications for the Right to Die', *Asian Philosophy*, 5–2 (1995), 159–80; Law Commission of India, 'Humanization and Decriminalization of Attempt to Suicide', Report No. 210, October 2008, 38–9.

3 Principal works include: J. Duncan M. Derrett, *Religion, Law and the State in India*, New Delhi: Oxford University Press, 1988; Jörg Fisch, *Cheap Lives and Dear Limbs: The British Transformation of the Bengal Criminal Law 1769–1817*, Wiesbaden: Franz Steiner Verlag, 1983; Lloyd I. Rudolph and Susanne Hoeber Rudolph, *The Modernity of Tradition: Political Development in India*, Chicago: University of Chicago Press, 1969, 251–93; B.S. Cohn, 'From Indian Status to British Contract', *Journal of Economic History*, 21–4 (1961), 613–28; B.S. Cohn, 'Some Notes on Law and Change in North India', *Economic Development and Cultural Change*, 8–1 (October 1959), 79–93.

4 Anand A. Yang (ed.), *Crime and Criminality in British India*, Tucson, Arizona: The University of Arizona Press, 1985; Satadru Sen, *Disciplining Punishment: Colonialism and Convict Society in the Andaman Islands*, New Delhi: Oxford University Press, 2000; Meena Radhakrishna, 'Surveillance and Settlements Under the Criminal Tribes Act in Madras', *The Indian Economic and Social History Review*, 29–2 (1992), 171–98.

5 For Example: R. Singha, *A Despotism of Law: Crime and Justice in Early Colonial India*, New York: Oxford University Press, 1998; Radhika Singha, 'Colonial Law and Infrastructural Power: Reconstructing Community, Locating the Female Subject', *Studies in History*, 19 (2003), 87–126; Padma Anagol, 'The Emergence of the Female Criminal in India: Infanticide and Survival Under the Raj', *History Workshop Journal*, 53 (2002), 73–93.

6 Werner Menski critiques some of these themes in his review of John Stratton Hawley (ed.), *Sati, the Blessing and the Curse: The Burning of Wives in India*, New York: Oxford University Press, 1994. Werner Menski, 'Sati: A Review Article', *Bulletin of the School of Oriental and African Studies*, 61 (1998), 74–81. In addition to Lata Mani's ground-breaking study *Contentious Traditions: The Debate on Sati in Colonial India*, Berkeley: University of California Press, 1998, and Catherine Weinberger-Thomas, *Ashes of Immortality: Widow-Burning in India*, trans. Jeffrey Mehlman and David Gordon White, Chicago: University of Chicago Press, 1999, recent substantial works include: Jörg Fisch, *Immolating Women:*

A Global History of Widow-Burning from Ancient Times to the Present, trans. Rekha Kamath Rajan, New Delhi: Permanent Black, 2005 and Andrea Major, *Pious Flames: European Encounters with Sati*, New Delhi: Oxford University Press, 2006.

7 Discussions of the opposition to sati and British efforts at abolition include Ajit Kumar Ray, *Widows Are Not for Burning: Actions and Attitudes of the Christian Missionaries, and Native Hindus and Lord William Bentinck*, New Delhi: ABC Publishing House, 1985; Lata Mani, 'Production of an Official Discourse on "Sati" in Early Nineteenth Century Bengal', *Economic and Political Weekly*, 21–17 (26 April 1986), WS32–WS40.

8 Shubhada S. Pandya, ' "Very Savage Rites": Suicide and the Leprosy Sufferer in Nineteenth Century India', *Indian Journal of Leprosy* 73 (2001), 29–38.

9 Jane Buckingham, 'The "Morbid Mark": The Place of the Leprosy Sufferer in Nineteenth Century Hindu Law', *South Asia* XX–I (1997), 57–80; Jane Buckingham, *Leprosy in Colonial South India: Medicine and Confinement*, Basingstoke: Palgrave Macmillan, 2002, esp. Chapter 7.

10 Gvt *vs* Sohawun, 7 August, 1810, in W.H. MacNaghten, *Reports of Cases Determined in the Court of Nizamut Adawlut*, Vol I (New Edition), Calcutta: Baptist Mission Press,1827, [Hereafter NA, Vol. I], 221.

11 *Papers Relating to East India Affairs viz Hindoo Widows and Voluntary Immolations*, 10 July 1821, *British Parliamentary Papers* (749) XVIII, [Hereafter PP 10 July 1821, (749) XVIII], 395, 398–9.

12 Buckingham, *Leprosy in Colonial South India*, 163–4, 170–1.

13 H.T. Colebrooke, *A Digest of Hindu Law on Contracts and Successions*, 4 Vols, Calcutta, Printed at the Honourable Company's Press, 1797, [Hereafter Jagannatha's *Digest*] CCCXXII, 12.

14 Jagannatha's *Digest*, CCCXXII, 12.

15 Gvt *vs* Sohawun, 7 August 1810, NA, Vol. I, 220. See also *Proceedings of the Nizamut Adawlut*, 25 June 1817 in PP 10 July 1821, (749) XVIII, 403.

16 Bewasta of Pundits of Sudder Dewanny Adawlut, PP 10 July 1821, (749) XVIII, 336. See also Bayly, 'From Ritual to Ceremony', 172.

17 Radhika Singha, 'The Privilege of Taking Life: Some "Anomalies" in the Law of Homicide in the Bengal Presidency', *The Indian Economic and Social History Review*, 30–2, (1993), 205–6.

18 Archibald Campbell, 'On the Custom of Burying and Burning Alive of Lepers in India', *Transactions of the Ethnological Society of London* 7 (1869), 195–6.

19 Gvt *vs* Sohawun, 7 August, 1810, NA, Vol. I, 221, note.

20 Letter from the Court of Directors to the Governor General in Council, in the Judicial Department (Lower provinces), 17 June 1823 in *Papers Relating to East Indian Affairs: viz. Copies or Extracts of all Correspondence relative to the Burning of Widows on the Funeral Piles of their Husbands, since 23 March 1823. British Parliamentary Papers*, 18 June 1824 (443) XXIII, [Hereafter PP 18 June 1824 (443) XXIII], 355.

21 J.H. Harrington, W.E. Rees and M.H. Turnbull, Register, Extract from *the Proceedings of the Nizamut Adawlut*, 25 June 1817, PP 10 July 1821, (749) XVIII 403.

22 Derrett, *Religion, Law and the State in India*, Chapters 8–10; Nandini Bhattacharyya-Panda, *Appropriation and Invention of Tradition: The*

East India Company and Hindu Law in Early Colonial Bengal, New Delhi: Oxford University Press, 2008.

23 Jane Buckingham, 'To Make the Precedent Fit the Crime': British Legal Responses to Sati in Early Nineteenth-Century North India' in Barry Godfrey and Graeme Dunstall (eds.), *Crime and Empire 1840–1940: Criminal Justice in Local and Global Context*, Cullompton, Devon: Willan Publishing, 2005, 196–7.

24 J.H. Harrington, W.E. Rees and M.H. Turnbull, Register, Extract from the *Proceedings of the Nizamut Adawlut*, 25 June 1817, PP 10 July 1821, (749) XVIII, 402–3.

25 Gvt *vs* Degumber Pande, March 31, 1823, in W.H. MacNaghten, *Cases Determined in the Court of Nizamut Adawlut* (New Edition), Calcutta: Baptist Mission Press, 1827 [Hereafter NA, Vol. II], 247–8.

26 J Gvt *vs* Sohawum, 7 August, 1810, NA, Vol. I, 221, note; J.H. Harrington, W.E. Rees and M.H. Turnbull, Register, Extract from the *Proceedings of the Nizamut Adawlut*, 25 June 1817, PP 10 July 1821, (749) XVIII, 403.

27 Singha, 'The Privilege of Taking Life', 184–5.

28 Buckingham, 'To Make the Precedent Fit the Crime', 196–8; 'A Regulation for maintaining an observance of the Restrictions prescribed by the Shaster in the burning of Hindoo Widows on the Funeral Piles of their Husbands, or otherwise', PP 1821, (749) XVIII, 420–5. See also Singha, 'The Privilege of Taking Life', 185 note 18.

29 Gvt *vs* Sohawum, 7 August, 1810, NA, Vol. I, 221, note.

30 On *futwa* (*fatwa*) see Fisch, *Cheap Lives and Dear Limbs*, 44–7.
     Kisas: The sentence of *kisas* meaning retaliation – life for life, limb for limb – was applied only in cases of wilful murder and there were many restrictions in its application. A sentence of *kisas* was often commuted to *diya* – blood money. Often in cases where payment was not possible, imprisonment was substituted though it was not part of traditional Islamic law. Fisch, *Cheap Lives and Dear Limbs*, 13–6.

31 A range of categories of discretionary punishment established in Islamic law was applied in the Nizamut Adawlut. *Tazeer* was by its nature discretionary, being left to the judge to decide. It was a milder punishment than *kisas* and though it could, was not meant to include capital punishment or mutilation. It was often used as a means of sentencing imprisonment, an introduced punishment which fitted the more settled mughal world rather than the nomadic-based Islamic law from which mughal law had developed. *Acoobut*, though never defined in the Nizamut Adawlut and not part of the Bengal Islamic tradition's theory of discretionary punishment, was frequently cited in the Bengal regulations, in *futwas* and in Harrington's decisions as judge of the Nizamut Adawlut. The term as used in *futwas* approximated that of *siyasa* understood as 'the right of the ruler to interfere in the interest of the state and of public peace'. Typically it resulted in a similar or milder form of punishment than would be recommended under *siyasa*. In practice *acoobut* described discretionary punishment falling between the sharia tradition of *tazeer* and the 'extraordinary justice' of *siyasa*. Fisch, *Cheap Lives and Dear Limbs*, 18, 23, 112 and 66 note 174.

32 Gvt *vs* Sohawum, 7 August, 1810, NA, Vol. I, 220.

33 Ibid.
34 Fisch, *Cheap Lives and Dear Limbs*, 110–11.
35 Gvt *vs* Sohawum, 7 August, 1810, NA, Vol. I, 220–1.
36 Fisch, *Cheap Lives and Dear Limbs*, 110–11.
37 Gvt *vs* Bhuraichee et al., 7 August, 1821, NA, Vol. II, 93.
38 Vasudha Dalmia-Lüderitz, ' "Sati" as a Religious Rite, Parliamentary Papers on Widow Immolation, 1821–30', *Economic and Political Weekly*, 25 (January 1992), 59; Buckingham, 'To Make the Precedent Fit the Crime'; Lloyd I. Rudolph and Susanne Hoeber Rudolph, 'Barristers and Brahmans in India: Legal Cultures and Social Change', *Comparative Studies in Society and History* 8 (1965), 25, 35–6 and 25 note 5.
39 Extract from a letter from Sir Charles Ware Malet, Resident at Poona, 18 June 1787, Extract of Bengal Secret Consultations, 27 July 1787, PP 10 July 1821, (749) XVIII, 296.
40 Gvt *vs* Sohawun, 7 August, 1810, NA, Vol. I, 220.
41 Ray, *Widows Are Not For Burning*, 29–33; Andrew Porter, 'Religion, Missionary Enthusiasm, and Empire', in Andrew Porter (ed.), *The Oxford History of the British Empire: The Nineteenth Century*, Oxford: Oxford University Press, 1999, 222–23, 230–2.
42 For different approaches see: Mukopadhyay, Amitabha, 'Movement for the Abolition of Sati in Bengal', *Bengal: Past and Present*, 77 (Jan–June 1958), 20–41 and Mani, 'Production of an Official Discourse on *Sati*'.
43 Gvt *vs* Teeluk and Mohun, 12 April, 1828 in W.H. MacNaghten, *Cases Determined in the Court of Nizamut Adawlut* (New Edition), Calcutta: Baptist Mission Press, 1827–1828 [Hereafter NA, Vol. III] NA, Vol. III, 12 April, 1828, 127.
44 See note 32 above.
45 Gvt *vs* Sheoo Suhaee and Chotoo, 18 March, 1814, NA, Vol. I, 292–3.
46 Gvt *vs* Ramdut and Balgobind, 20 June, 1823, NA, Vol. II, 276.
47 Gvt *vs* Badul Khan and four others, 7 August, 1810, NA, Vol. I, 218–9.
48 Ibid., 218–20.
49 Ibid., 219–20, note.
50 Ibid., 219.
51 Dalmia-Luderitz, ' "Sati" as a Religious Rite', PE–59.
52 Gvt *vs* Bhuraichee and others, 7 August, 1821, NA, Vol. II, 94.
53 Mani, *Contentious Traditions*, 36–7.
54 Dalmia-Lüderitz, " "Sati" as a Religious Rite', 59.
55 See, for example, Gvt *vs* Mungal Rai and three others, 5 June, 1822, NA Vol. II, 179–80; Gvt *vs* Hurdial Singh, April 30, 1829, NA, Vol. III, 229–30.
56 Gvt *vs* Surnam Tewarry, July 1823, NA, Vol. II, 279–81; Gvt *vs* Juddoonath and two others, 29 March, 1824, NA, Vol. II, 320–1; Gvt *vs* Ajoodia Misser, 9 May, 1825, NA Vol. II, 391–2.
57 See, for example, Gvt *vs* Ramdut and Balgobind, 20 June, 1823, NA, Vol. II, 274–7.
58 Extract from the *Proceedings of the Nizamut Adawlut*, 25 June, 1817, PP 10 July 1821, (749) XVIII, 395–403; 'Regulation XVII, 1829', Bengal Regulations, 1826–1834, Vol. 6. India Office Records [Hereafter IOR].
59 Mani, *Contentious Traditions*, 36.

60 Extract from the *Proceedings of the Nizamut Adawlut*, 25 June 1817, PP 10 July 1821, (749) XVIII, 404–5.
61 Dalmia-Luderitz, ' "Sati" as a Religious Rite', 60.
62 Major, *Pious Flames*, 146–52; See also, for example, *The Times*, 28 December, 1808, 4; 11 June, 1810, 3; 21 June, 1821, 2.
63 Mukhopadhyay, 'Movement for the Abolition of Sati', 21–3.
64 Mani, *Contentious Traditions*, 36.
65 Gvt *vs* Bhuraichee and others, 7 August, 1821, NA, Vol. II, 93.
66 Mani, *Contentious Traditions*, 33.
67 Extract from the *Proceedings of the Nizamut Adawlut*, 25 June 1817, PP 10 July 1821, (749) XVIII, 395–403; 'Regulation XVII, 1829', Bengal Regulations, 1826–1834, Vol. 6. IOR.
68 G. Dowdeswell, Secretary to Government, Judicial Department, to S.T. Goad, Register, Nizamut Adawlut, PP 10 July, 1821, (749) XVIII, 317.
69 Gvt *vs* Sheoo Suhaee and Chotoo, 18 March, 1814, NA, Vol. I, 292.
70 Extract from the *Proceedings of the Nizamut Adawlut*, 25 June, 1817, PP 10 July 1821, (749) XVIII, 404–5.
71 Gvt *vs* Sohawum, 7 August, 1810, NA, Vol. I, 221 note.
72 Major, *Pious Flames*, 28–9, 95–8; A range of British and European romantic literatures both fiction and non-fiction were inspired by the event of sati. Fisch, 'Dying for the Dead', 293–4 and Major, *Pious Flames*, 100–2.
73 Extract from a letter from Sir Charles Ware Malet, Resident at Poona, 18 June 1787, Extract of Bengal Secret Consultations, 27 July 1787, PP 10 July 1821, (749) XVIII, 297.
74 See, for example, 'Detailed Statement of Suttees of Hindoo Widows Who Were Burnt or Buried with Their Deceased Husbands, in the Several Zillahs and Cities, During the Year 1815: Compiled from the Report of the Magistrates', *PP*, 749, XVIII (10 July 1821), 361–92.
75 Extract from the Bengal Courier, 16 October 1824, *Copies or Extracts of All Communications and Correspondence Relative to the Burning of Widows, on the Funeral Piles of Their Husbands, Since the 16th June 1824: With Such Proceedings as May Have Been had Thereon in the Court of Directors*, 5 July 1825 British Parliamentary Papers (518) XXIV, [Hereafter PP 5 July 1825, (518) XXIV], 443 cited in Dalmia-Lüderitz, ' "Sati" as a Religious Rite', 61.
76 Acting Magistrate of Midnapore to John Shore, Governor General in Council, Fort William, 17 May 1797, Extract Bengal Judicial Consultations, 19 May 1797 PP 10 July 1821, (749) XVIII, 316.
77 Extract from a letter from Sir Charles Ware Malet, Resident at Poona, 18 June 1787, Extract of Bengal Secret Consultations, 27 July 1787, PP 10 July 1821, (749) XVIII, 297.
78 Singha, 'The Privilege of Taking Life', 205.

2 The great shift
Cholera theory and sanitary policy in British India, 1867–1879

Mark Harrison

In 1866 an International Sanitary Conference met at Constantinople to consider the cholera epidemics which had ravaged Europe after the disease broke out at Mecca, the previous year. There had been several pandemic waves of cholera since the disease first became widespread in India, in 1817, but in an age of steam navigation, with journey times growing ever shorter, it seemed that cholera could now reach the Mediterranean within weeks of its passage from India. This realization posed formidable challenges to all Western governments, as well as to the Ottoman Empire, which agreed to host a sanitary conference convened at the request of Napoleon III of France. Fear of cholera was such that the Constantinople gathering lasted seven months, making it by far the longest of the international sanitary conferences held during the nineteenth century. This, the third of these conferences, was also the first to be devoted to cholera, with other important pandemic diseases, such as plague and yellow fever, taking a back-seat. It marked a turning point in sanitary diplomacy and ushered in a new concept of disease prevention in which the Middle East would become a kind of sanitary filter, protecting the West against Asiatic diseases. To this end, international boards of health were established within the Ottoman Empire, their purpose being to determine whether reports of disease further east necessitated the imposition of quarantine and the duration of its operation.[1]

The conference was not the first to identify either the Haj or India as the source of cholera epidemics in the Middle East but it was the first to place them firmly under the spotlight. Most states represented at the conference resolved to take preventative action against shipping from India, emphasizing the need to combat disease in countries close to the source of infection. In practice, these duties devolved upon the new boards of health established at Alexandria and Constantinople.[2] But attention was also directed to India itself, and the conditions which were regarded as propagating the disease. While the governments in London and Calcutta were pondering these issues, and awaiting details of the rules and regulations being drawn up by other states, India was afflicted by another severe epidemic (in 1867), seemingly radiating outwards from the pilgrimage site of Hardwar on the Ganges.[3] This outbreak gave urgency to long-running debates over how best to control the disease; especially, when, where and how to intervene in the internal pilgrimages made by Hindus.

The late 1860s and the early 1870s were crucial years as far as sanitary policy in British India was concerned. In the wake of the 1867 epidemic, there appears to have been a loose consensus around the idea that cholera was spread by human intercourse and that sanitary cordons were the best means of preventing its spread. But this position was gradually abandoned at the highest levels of the British administration. The government became increasingly opposed to the use of quarantines and stressed the desirability of an alternative course of action which concentrated on environmental improvements and sanitary education. Why did such a shift in policy occur? Historians agree that official doctrine on cholera from the late 1860s was closely tied to political and economic considerations such as pilgrimage and maritime commerce. However, they differ in their explanations of how these matters impinged upon the world of medicine. I have previously argued that the practice of land quarantine was generally – but by no means completely – abandoned because of concerns that it might provoke civil unrest, especially when it involved travel to and from places of pilgrimage. Secondly, I have argued that the government was opposed to maritime quarantine because it presented an impediment to commerce and communications, and because it created difficulties vis-à-vis its Muslim subjects. In order to defend both these positions, the government normally found it convenient to uphold medical theories opposed to contagion – in the case of cholera, at least. This 'anti-contagionist' doctrine was aggressively espoused by its Sanitary Commissioner, who located himself in an Anglo-Indian medical tradition which favoured environmental explanations of disease. Lastly, I observed that while the governments in London and Calcutta were both generally antagonistic to theories of contagion and quarantine, they had rather different political interests which sometimes led the British government to make concessions that the authorities in India disliked.[4]

Some aspects of this interpretation have been challenged by Sheldon Watts in an article of 2001. Firstly, he contests the idea that there was a distinctive Anglo-Indian medical tradition which claimed that cholera was a disease of locality. Secondly, and more importantly, he argues that it was the British government, rather than the Government of India, which was instrumental in forcing policy away from quarantine. In Watts's view the chief factor behind this decision was the British government's concern about maintaining the free flow of shipping through the newly opened Suez Canal.[5] The Government of India, in other words, was merely doing the bidding of its masters in London. This pressure brought about an abrupt change from what Watts sees as the 'official' view of cholera and its prevention before 1868 (i.e. pro-contagion and pro-quarantine) to one that was hostile to both. In his opinion, my emphasis upon the Government of India is misguided and a 'red herring meant to distract attention from the realities of power relationships between core and periphery'.[6]

The central figure in both interpretations is Dr. James MacNabb Cuningham (1829–1905), who held the post of Sanitary Commissioner with the Government of India from 1868 (at first in an officiating capacity) until 1884. During his long tenure, Cuningham exercised an important and often decisive influence on sanitary policy in India; one that became increasingly uncompromising in its opposition to the theory of contagion and the practice of quarantine. This much is agreed but Watts also alerts us to the fact that Cuningham's views on both matters appear to have changed around 1868. In the first report that he wrote on cholera (on the epidemic of 1867), while officiating Sanitary Commissioner, Cuningham took the view that the epidemic had been spread by human intercourse. At that time, he concluded there was no evidence to suggest any other cause. In view of this, he regarded land quarantines around military cantonments and towns in the path of returning pilgrims as wise measures, although he deprecated any general quarantine as impracticable and likely to generate unrest.[7]

Watts argues that Cuningham's report met with a 'frosty reception' in London, because measures such as quarantine entailed considerable expense.[8] He further asserts that:

> sometime in the summer or early autumn of 1868, London agents quietly talked to Cuningham, won him around to the [London] government point of view (quarantine was 'evil'), and saw to it that he was confirmed as full sanitary commissioner with the government of India.[9]

We then learn that Cuningham issued a directive to all new sanitary commissioners with provincial governments to examine and remove all 'local' causes of cholera, which Watts sees as proof that Cuningham had closed his mind to the possibility of contagion in any form. He then claims that Cuningham accumulated a mass of statistics which he manipulated to prove that cholera was not a contagious disease.[10]

In what follows I shall show that many elements of Watts's argument are unsubstantiated. While one cannot discount the possibility that Cuningham changed his mind about cholera to boost his career, there is no proof that he did so, or, more particularly, that he was pressurized into doing so by anyone in London. This is entirely a conjecture on Watts's part. Rather, a closer and more comprehensive review of the evidence shows that Cuningham changed his stance on cholera far less abruptly than Watts asserts, suggesting other factors were at work. I shall also show that after Cuningham did alter his opinion on cholera he was more uncompromising in his opposition to contagion and quarantine than either the Government of India or the government in London, and that this occasionally proved inconvenient for both. Lastly, this chapter presents further evidence to support my earlier contention that a substantial difference of opinion existed between the governments in London and Calcutta and that it was the latter which was by far the most hostile to quarantine.[11] Whatever the reason for Cuningham's change of heart, it is highly unlikely to have been due to pressure from London.

Unfounded assertions

Before examining additional evidence, I will begin by scrutinizing the assertions made by Watts. Firstly, it is necessary to consider his discussion of Cuningham's views while he was officiating Sanitary Commissioner and at the time that he wrote his report on the cholera epidemic of 1867. Watts is quite correct in his interpretation of this report. It is true that Cuningham accepted the theory of human intercourse as the most likely explanation of the 1867 epidemic and that he advocated the establishment of cordons to protect military cantonments and large cities. However, Watts does not mention that Cuningham was, even at this stage, opposed to the use of quarantine as a general measure, such as in preventing the movement of pilgrims. 'Such a measure could not be carried into effect without exciting the suspicions of the Natives', he wrote.[12] Nor does Watts mention that Cuningham already regarded the best means of preventing cholera as being the establishment of sanitary camps along pilgrimage routes and the cleansing of pilgrimage sites.[13] Although Cuningham believed that cholera was probably transmitted in the faeces of those suffering from the disease, he insisted that it could only thrive in insanitary conditions. Like many other British medical practitioners at the time, he used the analogy of a plant whose seeds could be propagated only in a favourable soil and climate.[14] This was not a narrowly contagionist position but one in which the spread of cholera was viewed as contingent upon other circumstances.

Watts points to the report of the cholera committee appointed by the Government of Madras (1868) as further evidence that the theory of human transmission was widely accepted by the late 1860s. The committee believed that pilgrims returning from Hardwar had been responsible for bringing the disease into the Madras Presidency and they recommended, *inter alia*, 'control' of the route of returning pilgrims and 'rigidly enforced conditions upon which fairs and festivals should be permitted to be held'. They also proposed a tax to pay for sanitary measures at pilgrimage towns.[15] Some previous investigations, such as that into the 1861 epidemic, had come to similar conclusions and were confirmed by many non-medical officials, such as army officers, civil surgeons and district collectors. Indeed, sanitary cordons were frequently resorted to in the wake of the Rebellion, the military response to which had been compromised by epidemics of cholera among British troops.[16] But Watts discusses only those documents (or parts thereof) which support his contention that there was a contagionist (pro-quarantine) consensus regarding the spread and prevention of cholera. Although he states that the Government of Madras recommended the committee's report to the Government of India,[17] he neglects to mention that some of the committee's main recommendations were subsequently regarded as impracticable. Indeed, the Madras government warned of the 'great difficulties attending the institution of a strict system of quarantine for bands of pilgrims'. For this reason, it was prepared to entertain sanitary cordons on a limited basis only, to protect towns and prevent outbreaks of disease spreading to other pilgrims. Like Cuningham, it also placed more emphasis on sanitary measures than on quarantine, particularly the conservancy of camping grounds.[18]

The response of other provincial governments to the Madras committee's report was equally circumspect. When reviewing the document, senior officials of the Government of Bengal were prepared to adopt the suggestion of a tax to pay for sanitary measures at pilgrimage centres such as Puri, but they emphasized that other recommendations were 'difficult if not impossible' to implement.[19] Among these were general quarantines and interdiction of pilgrims travelling to and from pilgrimage sites.[20] Whatever the theoretical desirability of preventing pilgrims from gathering in certain places, the feedback from the districts to government was that religious fairs could not be banned and that pilgrims ought not to be prevented from travelling. Persuasion could be used to dissuade such persons from moving when cholera had been reported, but never force.[21] Thus, by 1868, it was already recognized that sanitary intervention in pilgrimages would have to be designed so as not to offend the religious sensibilities of Indians.[22]

Despite the impression given by Watts that 'contagionist' and 'miasmatic' theories of cholera were mutually exclusive, most medical officials and administrators held views which contained elements of both. Sanitary conditions were generally thought to be linked to epidemics, if not always as a primary factor, then as an ancillary one. Such a view was entirely in keeping with Anglo-Indian opinion concerning cholera in previous decades.[23] Reports from local officials and civil surgeons in the 1860s confirm this view, as does the action taken by some local administrations to combat cholera. Most saw cholera epidemics as resulting from a combination of several factors: the movement of pilgrims, foul water, food scarcity, poor hygiene and accumulations of filth.[24] It was for this reason that the Deputy District Magistrate of Sholapur, in Bombay Presidency, proposed a tax to contribute towards the cost of sanitation in the town of Pandharpur. The Bombay government agreed and resolved that the irrigation branch of the Public Works Department would provide the town with a supply of clean water; that the sanitation of the town and its environs be made a matter of priority and that a pilgrim tax be levied at relevant times of the year.[25] Cuningham regarded the Pandharpur arrangements as a model for other pilgrim sites.[26] In Bengal, too, local sanitary measures were implemented specifically in order to deal with disease at pilgrimage sites, in some cases apparently to good effect.[27]

These local initiatives are significant because they indicate that there was a wide range of beliefs and practices relating to cholera in 1867–8, rather than a narrow, monolithic consensus stressing contagion and quarantine. The situation could hardly have been otherwise, for no one was in a position to impose any particular view or to engineer a consensus of medical opinion. Until 1868, the post of Sanitary Commissioner with the Government of India was occupied by a non-medical man, Lt. Col. G.B. Malleson. Like most army officers, he held opinions on the spread of cholera and its prevention which inclined towards the use of sanitary cordons – a long-standing military expedient in dealing with epidemics. In 1867 many, though by no means all, medical officers shared this opinion, one of whom was Cuningham, who worked as Malleson's secretary before officiating as Sanitary Commissioner. So, how and why did Cuningham move from an inclusive position (which embraced sanitation and limited use of quarantine) to an exclusive one which opposed contagion and quarantine in any form?

According to Watts, Cuningham changed his mind because he was pressurized into doing so by officials in London. But Watts adduces absolutely no evidence to support this assertion or his contention that Cuningham's report was badly received there. Nor does he tell us who disliked Cuningham's report or why. He merely speculates that 'it is not unlikely that' the expenditure sanctioned by Cuningham to deal with the 1867 epidemic 'was mentioned when persuading Cuningham to do an about face and dance to the government's tune.'[28] Again, no supporting evidence is provided. Moreover, Cuningham's own report makes it clear that the majority of expenditure had been incurred in promoting conservancy and other general sanitary works rather than in maintaining sanitary cordons.[29] Watts also fails to cite any sources which prove his assertion that the London government decided that it must develop a position on cholera that would disprove the relevance of quarantine control, its eyes allegedly fixed on the forthcoming opening of the Suez Canal. Instead he cites two reports which were commissioned, not by the India Office, or any other department of government in London, but by the Government of India – the importance of which he discounts. We then learn that 'Whitehall and the India Office decisively broke with the European consensus on cholera and set up a new agenda' in which cholera was to be 'compulsorily regarded as a disease of place' generated by insanitary conditions. As with Watts's previous contentions, the reader is left to guess when this decision was arrived at and by whom. The only source cited in support of this assertion is a document commenting on the insanitary state of Indian villages in 1883, some fifteen years after the alleged event![30]

In summary, Watts provides the reader with no evidence to show how, when and why (or, indeed, whether) the London government arrived at a position regarding cholera that was hostile to contagion or who the architects of this policy were. Although the opening of the Suez Canal is cited as the reason for this change, we are shown no proof that it was central to the government's thinking at this point. Having arrived at this unsubstantiated position, Watts then claims that the government in London 'leant' on Cuningham to change his mind. No evidence of any kind is provided to support this contention either, beyond the observation that Cuningham was appointed Sanitary Commissioner to the Government of India on a permanent basis 'sometime before 10 September 1868'.[31] The implication is that Cuningham was appointed because he had agreed to change his mind about both the transmission of cholera and the utility of quarantine. Leaving aside the fact that Cuningham was not actually appointed to succeed Malleson until 16 June 1869,[32] it is impossible to prove or disprove whether ambition played a part in Cuningham's change of heart. It would be naïve to suggest that it did not have some bearing on his opinions but whatever role ambition may have played, the tenor of Cuningham's reports and official communications over the next two years indicate that he changed his mind far more slowly than Watts would have us believe and that he did not do so as the result of any pressure exerted from officials, either in London or in India.

A change of mind

In charting Cuningham's course over the next two years, the obvious place to start is his second report as Sanitary Commissioner. The year 1868 was one in which cholera figured much less as a cause of death than in 1867, either among troops or civilians. But a few outbreaks were reported, as were the results of some ongoing investigations into the spread of cholera. In dealing with the often conflicting views expressed in these reports, Cuningham seems to have been fairly even-handed. He was favourably disposed to Dr. Bryden's statistical investigation into cholera outbreaks in India, which emphasized the meteorological causes of epidemics, and it may be that his growing scepticism towards the human transmission theory owed something to his much closer association with this fellow Edinburgh graduate.[33] In 1868 the post of Statistical Officer, which Bryden held, was attached to the office of the Sanitary Commissioner, which meant that the two men were often working in close proximity.[34] It was in that year, too, that Bryden placed on record the results of his statistical investigation of cholera in the Bengal Presidency, going back forty-two years. Cuningham reported that he had not yet made up his mind regarding Bryden's conclusion that cholera was spread by monsoonal air currents but praised his assiduity and the value of the data he had collected.[35] However, he was still some way from abandoning the human transmission theory. Cuningham did not dismiss the opinions of those, like Dr. Jardine, who believed that cholera had been imported into Jubbulpore by 'coolies', vagrants and travellers, although he cautioned that no positive proof had been sent to support his statements.[36] Thus, although Cuningham's tone was now more sceptical towards contagion, his report for the year 1868 shows no evidence of outright opposition to either contagion or quarantine.[37] On the contrary, Cuningham appears reluctant to rule anything out – even the use of quarantine on a limited scale. Indeed, in the same report, he actually recommended experiments with quarantine in jails:

> With special reference to Cholera, and in order that no measure may be wanting which is calculated to throw light on the manner in which it spreads, a few jails within the limits of the endemic area might be selected, and the effect of strict quarantine narrowly observed.[38]

While Cuningham may have hoped that these experiments would disprove the utility of quarantine, the fact that he was prepared to contemplate them suggests either that he had not fully formed an opinion or that he was hesitant about advancing it without further proof. His recommendations and the general tone of the report were very different from the dogmatic views he would express in the 1870s. Cuningham's official correspondence also suggests that he remained open-minded about cholera until at least the end of 1869, some months after he was confirmed as Sanitary Commissioner. In June of that year, when cholera was far more prevalent than in 1868, Cuningham wrote to the Government of India's Military Department offering advice to commanders on how to avoid it. His recommendations, made two days after he had been appointed successor to Malleson, stressed the removal of troops from infected localities but they also show that he was still prepared to contemplate the possibility of human transmission:

> In order to avoid the danger of communicating the disease to the place to which they are transferred, I would suggest that the troops should not move into the stations recommended, but they should be encamped in suitable topes in its vicinity . . . All communication should, indeed, be prohibited between the cantonment and the camp, and means of disinfection should be strongly carried out.[39]

The Government of Bengal also seems to have believed that Cuningham had an open mind and sent him various opinions regarding the causation and spread of cholera.[40]

It was at this point in time that Cuningham issued circulars to all commanding officers at military stations, as well as to all jails and civil surgeons, to which a pro-forma questionnaire was attached. The information elicited by these questions covered everything from the timing of cholera cases (which would have furnished evidence of importation) to sanitary and meteorological conditions, and the health and morale of the persons afflicted.[41] Watts construes this circular as an attempt to gather information which could be used to discredit the theory of contagion and the efficacy of quarantine. However, the construction of the forms, and the tenor of Cuningham's official communications and published reports, suggest that he had yet to form a definite opinion.

In any case, Cuningham's real change of heart came not in 1868, as Watts asserts, but at the end of 1869. From August to December 1869, Cuningham was not at his office in Calcutta but in the field, making a tour of cholera-afflicted districts and military stations. His observations and his conversations with medical practitioners, military men and jail superintendents appear finally to have convinced him that cholera was not spread by human transmission. Many towns and stations within afflicted districts were exempt from cholera while, in others, the evidence for importation was circumstantial at best. The epidemic thus appears to have lacked the clear pattern of spread observed in 1867, which strongly suggested its dissemination by pilgrims. Cuningham reported:

> From nearly every cantonment and from every regiment which was stationed in it, as well as from nearly every jail, the statement was made with a sameness that is almost monotonous, that no communication, either direct or indirect, could be traced between the person first attacked and any previous case of the disease.[42]

Moreover, Cuningham's experience in the field convinced him that: 'Even if it could be demonstrated beyond all doubt that cholera spreads by human intercourse, the difficulties of carrying out a really efficient system, of quarantine over one single district in this country, appear to be almost insuperable.'[43] He concurred with a recent statement made by the Sanitary Commissioner of the Central Provinces that quarantine was of little use in preventing cholera. In defence of his position, Cuningham cited those parts of his own report on the 1867 epidemic in which he had warned against the impracticability of general quarantine measures. This appears to have been the first time that Cuningham felt the need to refer to his earlier report and it suggests that he was conscious that his views were seen to be changing. That he had not done so before implies that he saw no major contradiction up to this point. Also significant is the fact that other sanitary officials were in advance of Cuningham in advising against quarantine. His own change of mind was therefore part of a general shift of opinion among medical men and other officials. Even then, his report for 1869 – signed off on 13 August 1870 – stressed the need for impartiality. Writing of the two major views on the spread of cholera – Bryden's air-borne theory and the human intercourse theory – he declared, 'Either of these views may be correct, but if the history of any epidemic is to be fairly considered, it is indispensable that both of them, for the time at least, be entirely set aside.'[44]

In the summer of 1870 Cuningham was evidently far from dogmatic about theoretical matters but he was more robustly pro-sanitarian and sceptical about quarantine than hitherto. Quarantine, he declared, 'could never be enforced with sufficient stringency to prove successful, and . . . its institution would lead to endless oppression and inconvenience'.[45] But the prospects for sanitary reform seemed brighter. The conclusions which Cuningham had reached on tour were confirmed by discussions with members of the British Army's Sanitary Commission (ASC) while on leave in England in early 1870. The ASC, which had close links with the reformer Florence Nightingale, had a strongly sanitarian ethos.[46] It was influential, certainly, but its jurisdiction did not extend beyond the British Army. It had no power over Cuningham or over how the Indian Army conducted its affairs. It is possible that Cuningham spoke to people at the India Office or others who encouraged him to abandon quarantine but there is no evidence of this. In any case, his mind seems to have been made up before he went on leave. The significance of the meeting with the ASC is that it suggested practical ways in which to demonstrate the relevance of sanitation. Provincial governments, such as the Government of Bengal, were initially sceptical about the ASC's proposal to create sanitary exemplars in cantonments, jails, villages, partly because they were unsure about the scope of the proposed scheme. But Cuningham reassured them that the proposals were modest, although he saw them as the first steps along a much longer road towards 'great sanitary reforms, especially in drainage and water supply'.[47] This more expansive vision had perhaps been encouraged by the formation, in 1868, of provincial sanitary commissions. Although these agencies were to prove less effective than Cuningham would have hoped, their creation may have encouraged those Anglo-Indians who saw it as their mission to sanitize, and therefore to 'civilize', India.

At this stage, however, it is far from clear that the Government of India was prepared to endorse Cuningham's vision of sanitary reform or to abandon the use of quarantine. The Inspector General of Hospitals of the Indian Medical Department considered the matter of quarantine as 'still *sub judice*'.[48] Although Cuningham insisted that land quarantine was impracticable, there were many military officers – especially in the army's chief garrison province, the Punjab – who remained attached to the practice and continued to use it. Responding to one such incident in 1873, Cuningham argued that 'the evils which attend the system are incalculable' and that there was no evidence that it had ever worked. In his support, he cited the opinions of Dr. A.C.C. De Renzy, Sanitary Commissioner of the Punjab, who, while differing from him of 'points of theory',[49] was 'as strongly convinced as I am that quarantine is practically useless, and that it ought to be prohibited'. He noted that, 'The stoppage of travellers, the herding together of large bodies of people in quarantine camps, the attempted isolation of infected villages, and the forcible removal of the sick to hospital' which had occurred in the Punjab the previous year had 'created very great and very natural dissatisfaction among the people' while having no impact on the spread of the disease.[50] However, some senior medical men disagreed with Cuningham and backed the army. The Inspector General of Hospitals replied that, while sanitary cordons could not shut cholera out of cantonments, they could interrupt communication with infected localities. The Sanitary Commissioner of Bombay Presidency also took the view that it was best not to close off any option,[51] although he agreed with Cuningham that insanitary conditions were responsible for most outbreaks of cholera.[52]

The issue of quarantine in the Punjab blew up again in 1876 when the Quarter Master General proposed to establish a sanitary cordon at Attock, along the banks of the Indus. Cuningham was resolutely opposed on the grounds that it was 'impracticable, injurious, and a derangement of commerce'. But as was usual in these cases, the Government of India decided to back the military authorities and permitted the quarantine to be established.[53] It was also prepared to ignore the civil government of the Punjab, which protested that

> the Sanitary Commissioner of the Punjab is . . . strongly opposed to quarantine as a preventive measure; and the Lieutenant-Governor concurs. Such being the case, it occurs to His Honor [sic] altogether inappropriate to override the opinions of the most scientific and experienced sanitary officials in favour of the views of the General Officer Commanding any division of the British Army in India, whose opinion on a matter of this technical sort must be held to possess very little weight.[54]

A.P. Howell, Secretary to the Home Department of the Government of India, was sympathetic and declared that this was 'a very reasonable remonstrance', noting that most scientific opinion, including that recently expressed by *The Lancet*, believed quarantine to be useless in checking the advance of cholera. E.C. Bayley, the Legal Member of the Viceroy's council, also disliked land quarantines but acknowledged that medical opinion was not unanimous and insisted that the council had already decided to support the military authorities.[55]

Thus, while official thinking was moving in line with Cuningham's views, the government still sanctioned quarantines when they were demanded by the military authorities. This pragmatism was at odds with the increasingly inflexible views of Cuningham and it is significant that Bayley remarked that, 'The "opinion of the best scientific authorities" is not all one way and cannot be quoted as conclusive'. This shows that the government's commitment to any particular position was provisional and, one can reasonably assume, made largely on grounds of expediency. It had no need to exert pressure on medical officers in order that they might arrive at opinions which were useful to the government; all it had to do was select whichever opinions justified its position. To Cuningham's intense frustration, these opinions were not always those of its Sanitary Commissioner.

Maritime quarantine

While Cuningham was on leave in early 1870, the Government of India passed the Indian Quarantine Act, which enabled provincial governments to establish quarantines and medical inspection in the ports under their jurisdiction. This statute seems to have been passed in response to demands from provincial governments which were anxious about yellow fever returning from the West Indies and Mauritius with indentured labourers. The Bengal government had already imposed such measures in ports such as Diamond Harbour near Calcutta and at Chittagong, albeit with dubious legality.[56] The passage of the Act indicates that the Government of India was prepared to countenance maritime quarantine but, as with its terrestrial equivalent, Cuningham was far less flexible than the government he served. He argued that to admit the utility of quarantine in India would strengthen the case of those who wished to impose it against Indian shipping. Up to this point, both Cuningham and the Government of India appear to have considered the problem of quarantine largely in relation to internal pilgrimages and not, as Watts suggests, principally in relation to maritime commerce. There is no mention whatsoever of maritime quarantine in the sanitary reports for 1867 and 1868 and it appears only tangentially in 1869, in relation to the recently passed Native Passenger Ships Act (1870). Indeed, when the matter of quarantine at Red Sea ports first came up in the wake of the Constantinople Conference, the Government of India was not overly concerned.[57] It complied with all requests from the Ottoman and Egyptian boards of health regarding regulations for pilgrim ship and bills of health for vessels leaving Indian ports. Nor was the government especially anxious about the quarantine proposed for pilgrims in the Red Sea, near Mokha.[58] At this point, the chief official concern arising from the Constantinople Conference related to the control of pilgrimages *within* India.

In early 1870, however, the Egyptian and Ottoman boards of health issued more stringent regulations against ships from ports potentially infected with cholera, fearing that the Suez Canal, which had opened in November 1869, would permit the rapid spread of the disease from pilgrimage sites in Arabia. These fears proved well founded. In 1871, cholera spread north from the Hejaz into Syria and southern Russia and across the Red Sea into the Sudan. Egypt was threatened from the north and the south, and imposed 10-day quarantines on all ships arriving at Suez from areas deemed to be infected. Much to the annoyance of the Government of India, these included its dependency, Aden, which was under the authority of the Government of Bombay. In the coming years, the Egyptian regulations became stricter (partly at French insistence), with a quarantine of around 30 days being imposed on all ships deemed to be in an unhygienic state or from ports considered likely to be infected.[59] Although the British consul in Egypt regarded the actions of the Egyptian Board of Health as justified because of the very real threat of cholera spreading there and the pressure exerted upon it by states along the Mediterranean, the Government of India was irritated by what it regarded as unwarranted interference with commerce. The major shipping companies – the Peninsular and Oriental Company and the British India Steam Navigation Company – also complained bitterly of the effects of the new regulations on their trade.[60]

It was therefore in 1870–1 that the issue of maritime quarantine became pressing; not, as Watts insists, in 1868. Having previously cooperated with the Ottoman and Egyptian administrations, the Government of India began to protest against quarantine with the backing of its Sanitary Commissioner. It could see the advantage of having someone with Cuningham's opinions in high office as they were generally compatible with the Government of India's interests (although not always those of the government in London). But, in 1870, it was Cuningham who took the initiative. It was he who pointed out the folly of passing the 1870 Quarantine Act, which had already allowed the governments of Burma and Madras to legalize quarantine measures in their ports. To endorse such actions while at the same time protesting against quarantine overseas smacked of double standards, he argued. But the Government of India was still in a position to stop the Bombay government from following suit. Bombay was by far the most important of India's ports for trade with the West, as well as being the main port of departure for pilgrims on the Haj. During the American Civil War (1861–5) it had grown immensely in significance as Britain began to obtain most of the raw cotton it needed for the clothing mills of Lancashire from western India. Cotton was one of those articles – along with wool – that had traditionally been regarded as susceptible of harbouring disease. Textile manufacturers in Britain and producing interests in India thus faced heavy losses from the disruption of navigation through the Red Sea and Suez Canal.

Once Cuningham had returned from leave, he advised the government to make no more concessions regarding quarantine. There is no suggestion that he was doing the London government's bidding but it would appear that the inconsistencies of the Government of India's position jarred with the theoretical position that he had formulated in 1869–70. Apart from its potential to disrupt trade, further restrictions upon the pilgrimage to Mecca were likely to annoy pilgrims and result in losses for Indian shipping companies, he warned. With the backing of its Sanitary Commissioner, the Government of India began to insist that there was no need for quarantine in Bombay or Aden. It considered its new Native Passenger Ships Act – which compelled pilgrim vessels to touch at Aden – and the arrangements already in force in that port to be adequate. The Bombay government continued to disagree. It professed concern about the spread of infectious diseases such as scarlet fever from Europe, arguing that growing traffic through the Suez Canal increased the risk of this occurring. It also demanded the appointment of a Port Surgeon at Aden who would have the authority to declare other ports in the Red Sea and along the coasts of Arabia and the Gulf infected and to place quarantine upon vessels leaving them.[61]

But the most likely reason why the Bombay government wanted quarantine was that it gave it the power to retaliate against Turkish and Egyptian quarantine measures which bore heavily on Bombay. In this sense, the concerns of the Bombay administration were closer to the government in London than to those of the Government of India. In May 1874, just two months before an international sanitary conference was due to be held in Vienna, the British Foreign Secretary inquired about the nature of sanitary laws in the Indian dominions (including Aden) following a request from the Turkish ambassador. As the conference approached, it was clear that Indian sanitary arrangements were coming under scrutiny and London was becoming concerned lest lax precautions in the Arabian Sea led to harsh measures against British shipping in the Red Sea and the Mediterranean.[62] The British government was more acutely aware of the problem than the Government of India because it was in constant touch with the embassies of foreign powers. It knew that some degree of compromise was necessary to secure British interests, which were not always identical to those of the Government of India. If the Indian government failed to take international concerns seriously, all British shipping in the Mediterranean was likely to be subjected to harsh retaliatory measures.

This proved to be the case. The Egyptian sanitary authorities and most of the foreign delegates to the Board of Health at Alexandria were growing impatient with what they regarded as prevarication on the part of the Indian government.[63] The Turkish consulate at Bombay also requested that they be given the right to check all bills of health issued at the port; a request which the Secretary to the Government of India thought 'utterly unprecedented'. It was 'virtually an imputation that our health officers are not to be trusted', he complained, and advised the government that the request ought to be resisted.[64] Cuningham also recommended that the government should resist the Egyptian order 'to the utmost'.[65] This was unwelcome news to the Government of Bombay which was more ready to comply with the demands of the Egyptian authorities than the Government of India. It did not want stringent regulations in the major ports under its control – particularly Bombay, Karachi and Aden – but to do just enough to prevent more damaging restrictions in the Red Sea and Suez. The Government of Bombay had already begun to tighten measures at Aden and the port's health officer and the harbour police placed vessels in provisional quarantine until they were inspected.[66] There was no basis for this practice in law but it had the tacit sanction of the authorities in Bombay. In 1873, when cholera was prevalent along the African shore of the Red Sea, the Egyptian Board of Health imposed quarantine against all vessels passing through the Red Sea, regardless of their port of origin. Aden responded to this by placing quarantine on all ships arriving from Egypt, which soon led, in turn, to Egypt removing restrictions against Aden.[67] These retaliatory measures seemed to be having the desired effect and, by 1874, the Bombay government wanted to place them on a permanent footing. It appointed a separate Port Surgeon to oversee sanitary arrangements at Aden and introduced a bill into the provincial legislature to establish a quarantine station under the provisions of the Act of 1870.[68]

The bill was not sanctioned by the Government of India but quarantine measures at Aden and other ports, including Bombay, continued on an *ad hoc* basis.[69] This situation continued until 1878, with the Government of India holding out against the implementation of the 1870 Quarantine Act despite the wishes of both London and Bombay. But in 1878 the British government was coming under increasing pressure from shipping companies such as the Peninsular and Oriental Company to prevent various alleged abuses of quarantine reported by the British consulates at Jeddah and Suez.[70] Representations were made to the Egyptian and Ottoman boards of health but it soon became clear that they were unlikely to secure the desired result – unless London could offer concessions. If quarantine procedures were tightened up in Aden and other Indian ports, the Ottoman and Egyptian authorities would have less excuse to interfere with British shipping. The Government of India's intransigence was all that was standing in the way of such a deal.

In September 1878, the British government had had enough. Lord Salisbury, the Secretary of State for India, ordered the Indian government to draw up quarantine rules applicable to all Indian ports, pointing out the importance of 'meeting the prejudices of other States as far as possible, so as to avoid the risk of restrictions being imposed on vessels passing through the Red Sea'. This marked the end of protracted debates between the home government, and the governments of India and Bombay, over whether or not to establish any kind of permanent sanitary regulation in Aden and Indian ports. As the Government of India was now forced to comply, all that remained to be decided was what form the rules should take and whether they would be acceptable to all the parties concerned. The Indian government laid down two basic principles for provincial governments to follow when drafting their rules: that a system of medical inspection should be introduced for vessels arriving with persons suffering from diseases endemic to India, and that quarantine should be reserved for occasions when there was a danger of diseases being imported, such as plague and yellow fever.[71] However, the draft rules sent to Calcutta by the provincial governments were inconsistent and, in February, the Secretary of State for India urged the Indian government to act, as the 'present state of affairs materially weakens the hands of Her Majesty's Government in protesting against bad quarantine arrangements at places belonging to foreign powers'.[72]

In response, Cuningham was charged with drafting clearer rules for the guidance of provincial administrations – something that went expressly against his wishes.[73] The draft rules effectively brought practices in India into line with arrangements in Britain.[74] It was recommended that medical inspection should entail minimal inconvenience to trade or passengers: vessels with just one or two cases of diseases such as smallpox or cholera were thus permitted to take up anchorage as normal and there was no need to detain healthy passengers pending inspection. All that was required was for the master of the ship to ensure that no passengers suspected of having disease were allowed to depart before the vessel was inspected. Passengers were to remain on the ship if two or more of them were suffering from disease and only then would the vessel be cleansed and fumigated. Even the quarantine regulations were liberal. They permitted vessels from infected ports, without cases on board, to proceed straight to the normal anchorage.[75] But the fact that India was forced to have such a system at all shows that no state, however powerful, could afford to ignore international opinion. Moreover, it demonstrates (*contra* Watts) that the London government was far more accommodating in respect of quarantine than either the Government of India or its Sanitary Commissioner.

Conclusion

While it has not been possible to address all the points made by Watts in his article on cholera and sanitary policy, such as those concerning Anglo-Indian medicine generally, it has been shown that his specific claims about the manipulation of medical opinion are entirely unsubstantiated. Cuningham was acutely aware of the political implications of what he said and wrote. That much has never been in doubt. It is also likely that he owed his long tenure as Sanitary Commissioner to the fact that his views on cholera tended to vindicate the policies of the Indian government, although by no means in all cases. But it is one thing to observe that Cuningham's opinions were used (selectively) to justify government policy and quite another to claim that Cuningham changed his mind about cholera because he was forced to do so, either by London or Calcutta. I have shown that these allegations are unsupported and that Cuningham's change of mind was far from abrupt. Firstly, it is clear that Cuningham's position in 1867 was not narrowly contagionist and that he believed that quarantine should play a subordinate role in tackling cholera – the emphasis being placed on sanitary improvements. This inclusive approach was broadly in line with that of most provincial administrators. Secondly, Cuningham's decisive break with contagionism came not in 1868, as Watts asserts, but in late 1869, following his tour of cholera-afflicted provinces. Cuningham had been growing more sceptical about the contagiousness of cholera and the practicality of quarantine over the previous two years, possibly as a result of his closer association with Bryden, but even after he had been confirmed as Sanitary Commissioner, in June 1869, he appears to have remained open-minded. He did not reject the human transmission theory outright and stressed that it was important to consider all views on the matter.

It was Cuningham's experience in the field, at the end of 1869, that seems to have convinced him to abandon the human transmission theory of cholera and to stress the importance of local sanitary reforms rather than quarantine. In making this decision, he was far from alone. Other medical officers and administrators were having doubts about quarantine on practical grounds and because of the uneven way in which cholera had spread during the epidemic of 1869. Although the 1867 epidemic had appeared to show clear evidence of human transmission, later outbreaks did not. At the very least, it seemed that some theory other than contagion was necessary to explain why cholera broke out in some places but not others. However, there were still some officials – especially military officers – who continued to see cholera as predominantly contagious and quarantine as desirable. Their views were sometimes upheld despite Cuningham's protests, showing that he was considerably less flexible than the government on such matters. There is therefore no evidence to suggest that his opinions on land quarantine were in any way manipulated by officials, whether in London or in Calcutta.

The same can be said of maritime quarantine, which was not prominent on the Government of India's agenda until 1870. Until that year, it was prepared to acquiesce in what was demanded of it by the Ottoman and Egyptian boards of health in the wake of the Constantinople Conference. It was not until after the opening of the Canal in late 1869 (not in 1868, as Watts claims) that quarantine in the Red Sea became a matter of great importance for the Government of India. Furthermore, there is no evidence that the Government of India was pressurized by London into becoming antagonistic towards quarantine. The situation was quite the reverse. London was generally more willing to make concessions regarding the use of quarantine than the Government of India. The latter was able to resist extension of the Quarantine Act to Bombay for nearly nine years despite mounting unease on the part of the Foreign Office and the Secretary of State for India. When the London government did finally intervene it was to ensure that quarantine was imposed uniformly in Indian ports, not to see it dismantled.

In presenting an interpretation that embraces the complexities of imperial governance I have not presented readers with a 'red herring' but with a version of events more compatible with the messy realities of imperial power. It is clear that both the British and Indian governments usually regarded quarantine as inconvenient and as detrimental to their commercial and political interests, but the relationship of medical theory to sanitary policy was far more complex and inconsistent than that presented in Watts's account. There is no evidence of any grand conspiracy of the kind that he alleges but rather of the selective, pragmatic and occasionally cynical use of medical expertise. For the most part, Cuningham's views were convenient for the Government of India, which made use of them to justify its hostility towards maritime quarantine. But they did not need to be as uncompromising as they were. Indeed, the position held by Cuningham was sometimes too inflexible for the government's liking. It was also increasingly at odds with the needs of the government in London which was becoming isolated internationally. That Cuningham remained steadfast in his opposition to quarantine and contagion throughout his tenure of office, despite the fact that he was sometimes ignored by his political masters and ridiculed by the medical profession in Britain,[76] suggests that he was a man of some conviction, however dogmatic he may have become.

Notes

1 Valeska Huber, *Channelling Mobilities: Migration and Globalisation in the Suez Canal Region and Beyond, 1869–1914*, Cambridge: Cambridge University Press, 2013; Birsen Bulmus, *Plague, Quarantines and Geopolitics in the Ottoman Empire*, Edinburgh: Edinburgh University Press, 2012; Valeska Huber, 'The Unification of the Globe by Disease? The International Sanitary Conferences on Cholera, 1851–1894', *The Historical Journal*, 49 (2006), 453–76; Norman Howard Jones, *The Scientific Background of the International Sanitary Conferences 1851–1938*, Geneva: WHO, 1975, 24–34.

2 Amir A. Afkhami, 'Defending the Guarded Domain: Epidemics and the Emergence of an International Sanitary Policy in Iran', *Comparative Studies of South Asia, Africa and the Middle East*, XIX (1999), 122–34.

3 See David Arnold, *Colonizing the Body: State Medicine and Epidemic Disease in Nineteenth Century India*, Berkeley: University of California Press, 1993, chap. 4.

4 Mark Harrison, *Public Health in British India: Anglo-Indian Preventive Medicine 1859–1914*, Cambridge: Cambridge University Press, 1994, esp. chaps. 4 and 5.

5 Sheldon Watts, 'From Rapid Change to Stasis: Official Responses to Cholera in British-Ruled India and Egypt: 1860 to c.1921', *Journal of World History*, 12 (2001), 335–7.

6 Ibid., 335.

7 *Fourth Annual Report of the Sanitary Commissioner with the Government of India 1867*, Calcutta: Office of Supt. of Govt. Printing, 1868, 129–36.
8 Watts, 'From Rapid Change', 349.
9 Ibid., 351.
10 Ibid., 352–3.
11 Harrison, *Public Health*, chap. 5; Mark Harrison, 'Quarantine, Pilgrimage, and Colonial Trade: India 1866–1900', *Indian Economic and Social History Review*, 29 (1992), 117–44.
12 *Fourth Report*, 131.
13 Ibid., 138.
14 Ibid., 135.
15 *Report of the Cholera Committee Ordered Under G.O. No. 216 of 27th February 1867, to Report Upon the Arrangements Which Should Be Made to Give Practical Effect in the Madras Presidency to the Recommendations and Suggestions of the International Sanitary Conference 1866*, Madras: Govt. Press, 1868.
16 Harrison, *Public Health*, 107.
17 Watts, 'From Rapid Change', 343–4.
18 R.S. Ellis to Sec. to Govt. of India, Home Dept., 27 April 1868, Proc. No. 12, July 1869, WBSA.
19 For a detailed study of sanitary measures in Puri, see Biswamoy Pati, 'Ordering "Disorder" in a Holy City: Colonial Health Interventions in Puri during the Nineteenth Century', in B. Pati and M. Harrison (eds.), *Heath, Medicine and Empire: Perspectives on Colonial India*, Hyderabad: Orient Longman, 2001, 270–98.
20 Marginal note written by the Officiating Junior Secretary to the Government of Bengal on document sent from 'The President and Members of the Cholera Committee of Madras', to the Chief Secretary to the Government of Madras, 4 December 1867, Proc. No. 12 Municipal Dept. (Sanitation), July 1869; A. MacKenzie to Under-Sec., Home Dept., Government of India, 8 July 1869, Proc. 14 Municipal Dept. (Sanitation), July 1869, West Bengal State Archives [hereafter, WBSA].
21 Additional Secretary to Govt. of Bengal to Magistrate Malda, 3 April 1868, denouncing suggestion by Sub-Asst. Surg. of Malda that the Magmurdum Churuck Mela ought to be prevented from taking place, 20 March 1868, Proc. Nos. 11–12, Municipal Dept. (Sanitation), 1868, WBSA.
22 For a detailed study of the politics surrounding the sanitary regulation of internal pilgrimages, see Amna Khalid, 'Disease and Pilgrimage in Northern India, 1867–1914', University of Oxford D.Phil Thesis, 2008.
23 See Mark Harrison, *Climates and Constitutions: Health, Race, Environment and British Imperialism in India 1600–1850*, New Delhi: Oxford University Press, 1999, 190–2.
24 E.g. Uday Chund Dutt, sub-Asst. Surg., to Officiating Magistrate, Puri, 1 December 1867, Proc. No. 54, April 1868, WBSA.
25 Deputy District Magistrate, Sholapur, to Collector and Magistrate, Poona, 30 March 1866, and Govt. of Bombay Resolution, Proc. No. 3, General, 1866, Maharashtra State Archives [hereafter, MSA].
26 *Fourth Report*, 130.

27 W. le F. Robinson, Officiating Commissioner of Rajshahye Division, Berhampore, to Sec. to Govt. of Bengal, 4 June 1868, Proc. No. 6, Municipal (Sanitation), August 1868, WBSA.

28 Watts, 'From Rapid Change', 349.

29 *Fourth Report*, 129–30.

30 Watts, 'From Rapid Change', 350, note 98.

31 Ibid., 351, note 103.

32 Notification – Home Department, Sanitary, Proc. No. 256, 16 June 1869, *Minutes of Proceedings of the Sanitary Commissioner with the Government of India*, 415.

33 Cuningham expressed his admiration for Bryden when writing his report on the 1867 epidemic, even though he did not then agree with him about how cholera was spread. See *Fourth Report*, letter from Cuningham to Sec. to Govt. of India, Military Dept., 11 September 1868, at front of report.

34 *Fifth Annual Report of the Sanitary Commissioner with the Government of India, 1868*, Calcutta: Office of Supt. of Govt. Printing, 1869, 61.

35 Ibid., 25.

36 Ibid., 24.

37 Watts, 'From Rapid Change', 324, note 8.

38 *Fifth Report*, 95.

39 Cuningham to Sec. to Govt. of India, Military Dept., 18 June 1869, Proc. No. 593, August/September 1869, *Minutes of Proceedings*, 595.

40 Officiating Junior Sec. to Govt. of Bengal to Cuningham, 24 August 1869, Proc. No. 223 August/September 1869, *Minutes of Proceedings*, 533–4.

41 Circular – Cholera Enquiry, 1869, Proc. 224 August/September 1869, ibid., 534–76.

42 *Sixth Report of the Sanitary Commissioner with the Government of India 1869*, Calcutta: Supt. of Govt. Printing, 1870, 53.

43 Cuningham to Under Sec. to Govt. of India, Home Dept., 4 November 1869, Amballa, Proc. No. 302, October/November 1869, *Minutes of Proceedings*, 301.

44 *Sixth Report*, 55.

45 Ibid., 69.

46 Jharna Gourlay, *Florence Nightingale and the Health of the Raj*, Aldershot: Ashgate, 2003; Harrison, *Public Health*, 66, 76–7, 109.

47 See correspondence in Proc. No. 142, July 1870, *Minutes of Proceedings*, 188, and No. 150, July 1870, 207.

48 Inspector-Genl. IMD to Sec. to Govt. of India, Military Dept., *Minutes of Proceedings*, 2 August 1870.

49 De Renzy was an ardent supporter of the water-borne theory of cholera, which led to a serious dispute with Cuningham and to the former's eventual relocation from the Punjab. See J.C. Hume, 'Colonialism and Sanitary Medicine: The Development of Preventive Health Policy in the Punjab, 1860–1900', *Modern Asian Studies*, 20 (1986), 703–24; Harrison, *Public Health*, chap.4.

50 Cuningham to Officiating Deputy Sec. to the Govt. of India, Military Dept., 28 April 1873; Cuningham to Sec. to Govt. of India, Home Dept., 5 May 1873, Proc. No. 511, 1872, MSA.

51 Inspector-Genl., IMD, to Sec. to Govt. of Bombay, Genl. Dept., 24 June 1873; James Lumsdaine to Chief Sec. to Govt. of Bombay, 17 June 1873, Proc. No. 511, 1872, MSA.

52 E.g. Lumsdaine to Chief Sec. to Govt. of Bombay, Genl. Dept., 18 December 1872, Proc. No. 7, 1872, MSA.

53 Col. H.K. Burne, Sec. to the Govt. of India, Military Dept., to QMG India, 3 August 1876, Proc. No. 64, Govt. of India, Home Dept., 1876, National Archives of India [hereafter, NAI].

54 Officiating Sec. to Govt. of Punjab to Officiating Sec. to Govt. of India, 18 August 1876, Govt. of India Home Dept., Proc. No. 67, 1876, NAI.

55 Memoranda from Howell and Bayley, 21 and 26 August 1876, respectively, Proc. No. 68, 1876, Govt. of India, Home Dept., NAI.

56 Officiating Sec. to Govt. of Bengal to Commissioner of Chittagong, 5 June 1867, General (Marine) Proc. No. 68; Officiating Master Attendant to Senior Officer at the Cruising Station, 5 June 1867, General (Marine) Proc. No. 71, June 1867; General (Marine) Proc. Nos. 73–5, June 1867, WBSA.

57 Memorandum, 'Establishment of a Quarantine Station Near Mokha', *General (Medical) Proc*, No. 77, February 1868, WBSA.

58 Home Dept. Resoln. 24 January 1868, Proc. No. 75; H.P.T. Barrow to Lord Stanley, Constantinople, 24 September 1867, General (Medical), Proc. No. 76, February 1868; E.C. Bayley to Sec. to Govt. of Bengal, 25 February 1867, General (Medical) Proc. No. 36, WBSA. For the sanitary aspects of the Haj generally, see Saurabh Mishra, *Pilgrimage, Politics and Pestilence: The Haj from the Indian Subcontinent 1860–1920*, New Delhi: Oxford University Press, 2011.

59 J. Netten Radcliffe, 'Memorandum on Quarantine in the Red Sea, and on the Sanitary Regulation of the Pilgrimage to Mecca', in *Ninth Annual Report of the Local Government Board 1879–80*, London: George E. Eyre and William Spottiswoode, 1881, 98–103.

60 Ibid., 103.

61 'Quarantine at Aden', Government of Bombay Nos. 1223–43, 27 April 1874, Home (Sanitary), No. 31 (A), June 1874, NAI.

62 Secretary of State for India to GOI, forwarding request from Secretary of State for Foreign Affairs, 21 May 1874, Home (Sanitary), No. 7 (A), July 1874, NAI.

63 Mr. H. Calvert, to Major-General Edward Stanton, 27 June 1874, Nos. 31–2 (A) Home (Sanitary) September 1874, NAI.

64 A.C. Lyell, memo., 7 September 1874, Nos. 31–2 (A) Home (Sanitary), Nos. 31–2 Home (Sanitary), September 1874, NAI.

65 J.M. Cuningham, memo., 4 September 1874, Nos. 31–2 (A) Home (Sanitary), September 1874, NAI.

66 Health Officer to Commissioner of Police, 12 January 1871, No. 430, Govt. of Bombay, Genl. Dept., Vol. 10, 1871, Maharashtra States Archives, Mumbai [hereafter, MSA].

67 Political Resident, Aden, to Sec. to Govt. of Bombay, 25 February, 1873, Govt. of Bombay, Genl. Dept., Vol. 70, MSA.

68 Government of Bombay to Government of India, 19 August 1874, Nos. 29–31 (A), Home (Sanitary), November 1874, NAI.

69 Government of India to Secretary of State, 6 December 1878, No. 16 (A) Home (Sanitary), December 1878, NAI.
70 T.V. Lister, Foreign Office, to the Hon. C. Vivian, HM Consulate, Alexandria, 17 May 1878, No. 6 (A) Home (Sanitary), December 1878, NAI.
71 Copy of Home Department Resolution, 19 September 1878, No. 7 (A) Foreign (General), May 1879, NAI.
72 Secretary of State to Government of India, 20 February 1879, No. 7 (A) Foreign (General), May 1879, NAI.
73 'C.B.', Memo., 11 March 1879; Government of India to Secretary of State, 16 June 1879, Nos. 17–38 (A) Home (Sanitary) June 1879, NAI.
74 See Ann Hardy, 'Cholera, Quarantine and the English Preventive System, 1850–1895', *Medical History*, 37 (1993), 250–69; Krista Maglen, 'The First Line of Defence: British Quarantine and the Port Sanitary Authorities in the Nineteenth Century', *Social History of Medicine*, 15 (2002), 413–29; John Booker, *Maritime Quarantine: The British Experience, c.1650–1900*, Aldershot: Ashgate, 2007, chap.16.
75 Appendices A and B, No. 7 (A) Foreign (General), May 1879, NAI.
76 Harrison, *Public Health*, 110–11.

3   Hakims and Haiza

Unani medicine and cholera in late Colonial India

Saurabh Mishra

Despite being mentioned in nearly all texts on the disease, mortality figures for cholera continue to shock us even today due to their magnitude. In India alone, the number of deaths is estimated to have reached the figure of nearly 40 million between 1817 and 1917.[1] Such massive mortality could not have failed to generate a climate of fear and anxiety; indeed, this sentiment was palpable across the globe, including those regions where fatalities occurred in relatively small numbers. As Christopher Hamlin puts it succinctly in his recent biography of the disease, 'much of cholera's story is a story of fear'.[2] This assertion is confirmed by other historians who describe how any real or supposed sign of a possible outbreak (e.g. the sighting of a 'cholera cloud') could cause great fear and anxiety across continents.[3] Despite the universal anxiety and fear, though, the disease arguably caused the greatest amount of distress in India where very few households were left completely untouched by it.[4] It is therefore surprising that, despite the large number of scholarly works on cholera,[5] there has been no attempt yet to produce a full-length social or cultural history of the disease in the subcontinent. Due to limitations of space, this chapter does not attempt to fill this rather large gap, but we will point toward the huge diversity in indigenous ideas regarding cholera by examining the writings of *hakims*.

One of the striking aspects of Unani tracts on cholera is their rather forthright admission of the ineffectiveness of most cures, with most *hakims* making a note of the fearsome and incurable quality of the disease. In fact one of them noted forebodingly that 'cholera is death's younger sibling' and again, a few sentences later, that 'the souls of the greatest physicians tremble with fear at the mere mention of cholera'.[6] Echoing similar sentiments, a reputed Unani journal noted that 'cholera is another name for death . . . if anyone is ever cured of the disease, this is owing to good fortune rather than medical expertise'.[7]

The helplessness of practitioners of all kinds is reflected in the fact that *vaidyas* sometimes fled the scene when their locality was visited by the epidemic.[8] Though such incidents were often interpreted by colonial officials as signs of 'native cowardice' or 'lack of character', Dhrub Kumar Singh notes that even colonial observers, on occasion, realized that the *vaidyas* fled due to 'the impossibility of affording any effectual medical aid from the suddenness of attack'.[9]

In such a scenario, where healers appeared powerless and all available treatments were ineffective, there was a greater willingness to try 'unconventional' remedies. Though such remedies were mostly peddled in the streets and bazars, or existed as folk remedies, some of them have found their way into written records as well. An anonymous author, in a tract titled *Mazarbat Akbari*, recommends the following cure: 'take a coloured piece of cloth, burn it to ashes, mix these ashes with urine, and get the patient to drink it.'[10] According to the author, this was a certain way of bringing back to life even those on the brink of death. Another author, from a village in Patiala, described how cholera faced little obstacle in carrying away most of the people from his village, until a *pansari* intervened and saved everyone's lives using a 'secret remedy'.[11] Apparently, the author had managed to cajole the *pansari* into revealing the ingredient of his pill which included, amongst other things, cloves, pepper and black salt.[12] These are only two examples out of several secret remedies, cures, charms, rituals and simples that were circulating throughout the subcontinent during the late nineteenth and early twentieth centuries.

The circulation of such cures led to a huge anxiety on the part of *hakims* and *vaidyas*, as they posed a challenge to their traditional authority. A lot of attention has been paid, until now, to the professionalization of Western biomedicine in Europe, and the challenges it faced from those who were defined as 'quacks';[13] a similar struggle was also going on between the latter and the practitioners of 'traditional' forms of medicine who had hitherto enjoyed great authority or recognition. Guy Attewell gives us examples of this while discussing Unani during the times of plague,[14] but similar examples can be found in the case of almost all other epidemic outbreaks as well. For example, when cholera broke out in Hyderabad, Mohammad Abbas Ansari Sayani – a self-styled doyen of Unani in the city – cautioned the public about various 'fake healers' making grand claims about their cures. Sayani claimed to have cured thousands of patients in the city and warned the public that a wrong prescription in the case of cholera – for example, prescribing pills that led to the retention of bodily waste instead of evacuation – could cause severe damage and even death.[15] Even Urdu newspapers warned of this danger, with the *Urdu Akhbar* publishing a long report on cholera aimed at creating awareness amongst the reading public.[16] The report started with a long diatribe against popular superstitions about the disease, noting that people often associated it with black magic or witchcraft, which led to the lynching or murder of those who are held responsible for it.[17] It cited the case of six people who had apparently been killed in this manner in Hyderabad during a recent outbreak.[18] The report was also sharply critical of the popular tendency to associate diseases with deities, ghosts and spirits.[19] While the *Urdu Akhbar* appears to have completely accepted the dichotomy between the scientific/rational and the religious/superstitious, and was consequently harsher on all kinds of 'quackery', even Unani tracts that were more respectful of the link between faith and healing were no less disapproving of such healers and their craft. It is clear, therefore, that epidemics brought to surface, in an amplified manner, the struggle for authority that was always lurking underneath. These struggles also alert us to the need for caution when using large, sweeping categories as 'indigenous practitioners' or 'indigenous medicine', as their use results in muting internal tensions between various kinds of 'native healers'.

Resisting biomedicine?

Greater caution in the use of such categories would also allow us to modify the simplistic picture of a straightforward rivalry between biomedicine and other forms of medicine. In fact much of the recent research has gone beyond the idea of an 'impact-response' framework which saw Western biomedicine as providing the stimulus for the growth of revivalist or reformist movements within 'traditional/indigenous medicine'. Guy Attewel notes, for instance, that 'the pressure for reform in unani tibb came from within an expanding and fractured unani profession. It did not result solely from a desire to imitate colonial institutional and professional models'.[1] 'The End of the Line? The Fracturing of Authoritative Tibbi Knowledge in Twentieth-Century India', *Asian Medicine,* vol. 1, no. 2 (2005), 397. This is not to underplay the impact that a state-backed system of medicine, with rapidly proliferating institutions, would have had on those who saw it as their main rival. However, there is a need to add nuance to some of these arguments.

Before we go into that discussion, though, it is important to point out that some of the tracts by *hakims* and others do indeed appear to directly confront European theories of cholera. In an impassioned argument that sought to refute the European charge that India was the original 'home of cholera', Babu Ganga Prasad Verma noted, in a text entitled *Dus Kanoon-I-Sehat*, that older Unani or Ayurvedic works made absolutely no reference to cholera, thus proving that it had been entirely absent from India in the past.[20] Noting that Europeans mistakenly saw insanitary conditions in the country as the chief cause for outbreaks, he argued that such conditions in fact created a slightly acidic tinge in the atmosphere, making it impossible for cholera to breed. According to him it was the cleaner environment of Europe that was more likely to (re)produce the disease.[21] While Verma's argument might appear untenable to scientists or medical men today, his rebuttal of the powerful European characterization of India is noteworthy for being rare. Generally speaking, the description of India as the 'home of cholera' has had such an influence that even historians writing today accept it uncritically.[22]

Most *hakims*, though not as sharply critical of European perceptions as Verma, showed an awareness of the international controversies surrounding the disease. In a *Tibbi* text that was written not long after the first outbreak of cholera epidemic at Mecca in 1865 – which led to an unprecedented degree of international focus on the disease – the author provided a brief narrative of the global spread of epidemics, referring also to some of the latest researches within Europe, including Snow's water-borne theory.[23] Another text titled *Shifa al-Insaan* made a note of the spread of the disease to Mecca in 1882. However, one of the first discussions on the global dimensions of the disease can be found in a Unani text written in Arabic and published in 1844, which dealt exclusively with epidemics.[24] Interestingly, the author translated his work into Persian a couple of decades later as, according to him, 'there was hardly anyone left [in the country] who could understand Arabic'.[25] In the text he identified cholera, as opposed to smallpox, as an exclusively European disease; according to him, smallpox was a disease of greater concern for people in the subcontinent whereas cholera was not a major issue at all.[26] The fact that the he still went on to discuss cholera in great detail is a significant indicator of the fact that Unani practitioners were not merely localized practitioners caught up in their own regional concerns, but showed a great awareness of global developments. This is not to set up an artificial hierarchy between those who were rooted within 'local traditions' and those who were trans-regional in their concerns, but merely to point out that while the local roots of Unani have been rightly emphasized by historians, there is also a need to take into account its global dimensions.[27]

Such a formulation would also allow us to challenge the idea that the basic tenets or ideas of Unani have remained constant/unchanged over time. In fact, when it comes to cholera, Unani texts show a distinct shift in terms of the predominant causative theories throughout the nineteenth and early-twentieth centuries. To what extent these shifts occurred because of an engagement with European theories of disease is one of the questions that we will seek to answer in the next section. Was there, for instance, an attempt to strike a distance with biomedical ideas in order to underline the independent identity of Unani? Or was there indeed a much greater overlap between these two theories than has been usually assumed?

Diet, morals and miasma

One of the distinguishing features of Unani discourses on cholera was the emphasis on diet as a causative agent. This included not just food items that were exposed to dirt and filth, but also other items that had the potential to disrupt the normal functioning of the body. Unripe fruits or vegetables were considered particularly dangerous, the logic being that they took a long time to digest, thereby festering in the stomach for days on end.[28] This theory continued to be popular for long – in fact one of the Unani texts that saw it as a dominant cause was published as late as 1936.[29] Underlining the importance given to died, one of the *hakims* went so far as to identify a separate strand of cholera that was linked exclusively with the consumption of food.[30]

The emphasis on certain kinds of food as causative agents was unique to Unani, though the growing concern with unhygienic or adulterated food was shared by large sections of the middle class in the nineteenth century.[31] Food, however, was seen not merely as the cause, but also as a cure. A number of *hakims* recommended, for example, the intake of 'cooling foods' such as ice made of milk (*doodh ka barf*), or rose water.[32] Further, easily digestible food was recommended not just for patients, but also for those living in close proximity with them. Also, quite a few of the pills prescribed by them were a mix of spices that were commonly used in households. This dual relationship with food was a long-standing feature of Tibbi medicine, but some of these ideas entered the Unani texts under the influence of new biomedical researches into nutrition, vitamins, fermentation and so forth. Certainly, at least in the case of Ayurveda, there was a greater recognition of the health-giving qualities of food items such as milk during the late colonial period as a result of the influence of new researches into nutrition.[33]

The other causative theory for cholera that stands out is the emphasis on the 'moral question'. To an extent this is part of the long-standing tradition within Islamic learning of linking epidemics and other calamities with the will of God.[34] This link was also made by several *hakims* in the case of cholera, with Safdar Hussain noting that the disease had been sent down by God as punishment as Muslims had become careless about the payment of *zakat*.[35] The moral question entered the discourse in other ways too – for example, some *hakims* underlined heightened sensuality as one of the reasons behind the growing incidence of the disease.[36] However, the explanation offered in this case was more physiological than moral – it was reasoned that excessive sexual activity led to weakness, leaving the body defenceless in the face of an attack of cholera.[37] The trope of excessive sensuality is one that recurs in Unani texts in the context of several other diseases as well, and is seen as one of those ills that defined the decadent modern age. Perhaps *hakims* who saw themselves as carrying forward the 'ancient legacy' of Unani consciously couched the idea of sensuality within strongly moral terms in order to separate themselves from 'quacks' and vendors who sold pills, elixirs and tonics to bolster sexual prowess.[38]

Theories regarding diet and sensuality were, however, secondary in importance to the theory of miasma, which appears to have found extensive mention in nearly all texts. Often called *Fasad-I-Ab-O-Hawa*,[39] *hakims* saw miasma or 'pollution' as the determining influence in the spread of cholera. The miasma, according to most of them, was caused by rotting vegetable or animal matter, by dead bodies left lying around during or after wars, or by marshes left filthy and unclean for too long.[40] However, though miasma was considered capable of quickly spreading across a large area, not everyone was seen as equally susceptible to it – a lot of stress was also laid upon the strength or resilience of the body. Dilating upon the idea of bodily resistance, Sayani narrated an incident where the son had died of cholera while his father, who came into contact with his son's bodily waste, survived. The same excreta, however, when placed outdoors, spread its infection to the entire neighbourhood, causing an epidemic.[41] The individual's susceptibility also depended on a number of factors related to their morals, lifestyle, diet and so forth. In fact one of the texts postulated a link between an individual's temper/temperament and his or her susceptibility, noting that Europeans had an acidic temperament (*talkh mijaaz*) and were therefore less likely to contract the disease.[42]

While the miasmatic theory appeared to be the most frequent explanation right from the 1840s onwards, we need to stress the fact that in most cases cholera's spread was explained using a wide range of factors. Apart from some of the causal explanations already mentioned, *hakims* also pointed towards meteorological conditions,[43] exceptional or anomalous weather (for example, sudden cold during the hot weather), exposure to extreme weather conditions,[44] wind direction,[45] large congregations of people at pilgrimage sites and insect-bites, amongst various other causes. Such was the fluidity of opinions that there was a lack of consensus even about the symptoms of cholera. Excessive vomiting and purging was considered the most reliable symptom, but this was contested by others who wrote of another variety of cholera called *band haiza* (literally, 'closed cholera') where the exact opposite could happen.[46] The susceptibility of certain age groups to the disease was also debated.[47] There was also, quite predictably, a great deal of uncertainty around the subject of cures. Many *hakims* recommended the use of fragrances to purify air, the administration of juice extracted from herbs, or of restorative fluids prepared with flower essences; some of them also advocated the consumption of human urine.[48] There was also some debate around the question of whether it was better to ensure a quick evacuation of poisonous bodily waste, or if it was necessary to retain bodily fluids.

The fluidity and multi-pronged nature of explanations was reflected in the work of individual practitioners as well. To cite just one example, Ghulam Nabi, who came into close contact with Anglo-Indian medicine in his official capacity as an assistant at a government hospital in Lahore, endorsed the official Indian stand on the disease, which was why his tract was published and actively disseminated by colonial authorities.[49] In his tract he talked about 'poisonous air', miasma, poorly sanitized areas, fermented food items and so forth – issues that were constantly raised by the Indian government as well.[50] He also acknowledged the primary role of internal pilgrimage sites in spreading the epidemic, noting that such places 'distributed cholera to the devotees like *prasad*'.[51] So well-informed was he about the Indian government's position that he also referred to the debates at the Vienna Sanitary Conference and the theory espoused by J.M. Cuningham, the Sanitary Commissioner of India.[52] However, the similarities with the official doctrine ceased when the text began to refer to Ibn Sina's stand on cholera and his theory of heavenly warnings of an imminent outbreak (shooting stars, comets, etc.). Quite interestingly, it also postulated a similarity in the cures for malaria and cholera, noting that 'malaria is the actual cause of cholera'.[53] Finally, going against the basic grain of the central 'official' discourse on cholera, he concluded in no uncertain terms that cholera was a contagious disease.

While *hakims* offer fluid explanations based on a combination of ideas, most of them foregrounded the idea of miasma. Over the course of the nineteenth century, though, other prominent explanations also began to make an appearance. This included the water-borne theory as well as the idea of a link between the disease and germs, or *jaraseem*, as germs were often called in these texts. In fact, at first glance there appears to be a parallel between the European trends and developments within Unani, especially as the latter began to show a greater recognition of the water-borne theory by the end of the nineteenth century. Some *hakims* like Sayani were so convinced about the accuracy of this new theory that they completely rejected older atmospheric ideas, noting that cholera had 'absolutely no connection with the quality of air'.[54] Others made a note of the spread of cholera through the railways and through sites of pilgrimage/fair.[55] However, despite this recognition, 'older ways' of looking at the disease persisted. In fact, even in the 1930s, when it became impossible to ignore/reject the germ theory for cholera, one could still find authors who were attempting to co-opt new developments within pre-existing ideas. Writing in 1938, Hakim Mohammad Ishmael Takabul noted that, if one looked closely, there was really very little that separated older miasmatic theories from recent bacteriological ones: any supposed difference between them could be attributed to the fact that, in the old days, when germs had not yet been discovered, they were referred to using shorthand terms such as miasma.[56]

This persistence of older ways was not unique to Unani, though; one can discern a similar pattern when one looks at Anglo-Indian medicine as well, as Mark Harrison and others have shown.[57] Yet, when it comes to Unani, there appears to be a greater willingness to generalize about its static nature. Contrary to such ideas it is possible to argue that, at least as far as cholera was concerned, Unani was characterized more by its dynamic and heterogeneous nature, with new dominant trends emerging every few decades. The question of what caused these changes or shifts is a difficult one to answer, though: did they occur due to the gradual spread of European theories, or simply because *hakims* gathered more empirical experience of the disease as it became far more widespread across the subcontinent? It certainly seems that the idea that *hakims* might be merely reacting to European or official Indian theories is a rather simplistic one.

Conclusion

To an extent the question of defining cholera is also related to the question of Unani's identity, which became a subject of great importance during the early twentieth century as it became linked with revivalist efforts and the nationalist upsurge. This could arguably explain the preference for miasmatic or atmospheric ideas, as they were more intimately connected to the humoural theory – often seen as the defining feature of Unani's understanding of disease and health. While this sounds plausible, it is difficult to sustain this argument on closer examination. After all, while it is possible to centralize institutions, ideas regarding disease are far more difficult to control. This was especially true during our period, as Unani texts began to be published not just from 'old centres of learning' such as Delhi and Lucknow, but also from small provincial towns such as Ara, tucked away in more remote corners of the country.[58] *Hakims* writing from such places showed an eclectic attitude towards cures, borrowing from various quarters without prejudice or partiality. Helen Lambert argues, in her study of contemporary rural north India, that patients and their families are remarkably flexible in their choice of healers, often accessing a range of them depending on availability, affordability and effectiveness.[59]

One could argue that a similar eclectic temperament also guided the cures prescribed by local *hakims* and other healers in the past. This is, of course, not to argue that the question of the professional identity of Unani was not an important question, or that the profession was untouched by larger political currents; it is merely to sound a note of caution that, while these questions were important both in the cities and provincial towns, not all actions or ideas of *hakims* all across the subcontinent can be understood within the framework of resistance, or impact-response. Finally, while I agree with Seema Alavi's work on Unani and cholera, where she highlights the areas of accommodation between *hakims* and Anglo-Indian practitioners during the early colonial period,[60] this chapter has shown that the picture might have changed by the late colonial period. Cholera began to attract a lot more attention from Unani experts during the late colonial period, which often led to a much more variegated picture where various local and global strands of various kinds jostled for space with each other. In highlighting this diverse picture, we hope to have pointed towards some interesting aspects that might attract more scholarly attention in future.

Notes

1 Thomas M. Leonard (ed.), *Encyclopedia of the Developing World*, Vol. 2, London: Routledge, 2006, 821.
2 'Preface', in *Cholera: The Biography*, Oxford: Oxford University Press, 2009, ii.

3 Projit Mukharji provides a graphic account of the anxieties that the alleged presence of a 'cholera cloud' provoked across the world, in 'The "Cholera Cloud" in the Nineteenth Century "British World": History of an Object-Without-an-Essence', *Bulletin of the History of Medicine*, 86 (2012), 303–32.

4 This is noted by some Unani practitioners as well. For example, Mohammad Abbas Ansari Sayani from Hyderabad noted that '*kum hi aise ghar honge jo is marz se bache honge*': Mohammad Abbas Ansari Sayani, *Risaala-I Haiza*, Hyderabad: not dated (hereafter n.d.), 6.

5 Prominent amongst the work published on the subject of cholera in South Asia are David Arnold's 'Cholera and Colonialism in British India', *Past and Present*, 113 (1986), 118–51; Mark Harrison, 'A Question of Locality: The Identity of Cholera in British India, 1860–1890', in D. Arnold (ed.), *Warm Climates and Western Medicine: Emergence of Tropical Medicine, 1500–1900*, Amsterdam: Rodopi B. V., 1996, 133–59; Ira Klein, 'Cholera: Theory and Treatment in Nineteenth-Century India', *Journal of Indian History*, 58 (1980), 35–51; Sheldon Watts, 'From Rapid Change to Stasis: Official Responses to Cholera in British-Ruled India and Egypt, 1860-c. 1921', *Journal of World History*, 12 (2001), 321–74; Jeremy D. Isaacs, 'D. D. Cunningham and the Aetiology of Cholera in British India, 1867–1897', *Medical History*, 42 (1998), 279–305; Dhrub Singh, 'Clouds of Cholera and Clouds Over Cholera', in Deepak Kumar (ed.), *Disease and Medicine in India: A Historical Overview*, New Delhi: Indian Historical Congress, 2001, amongst others.

6 The author noted that '*bahut bade doctor miya Haiza ki soorat dekhte hain to unki rooh kaanp uthti hai*': Hakim Saiyad Amaldar Hussain, *Tiriyak-I-Haiza*, Lucknow: Naval Kishore, 1883, 4.

7 Anonymous, *Intakhab al-Hikmat*, Lahore, May 1892, 8.

8 Dhrub Kumar Singh, 'Chlolera in Two Contrasting Pathies in Nineteenth Century India', 3. www.ihp.sinica.edu.tw/~medicine/ashm/award/Taniguchi%202016.pdf, accessed on 9 January 2016.

9 Singh, 'Clouds of Cholera and Clouds Over Cholera', 3.

10 Anonymous, *Mazarbat Akbari*, Lucknow: Naval Kishore, 1896, 66.

11 Many low-caste people were often ascribed with extraordinary powers to cure diseases. This can be seen in the case of Chamars as well, who were often asked to perform rituals to prevent cattle deaths due to epizootics. Chamar women also often acted as midwives and *dais*: see my 'Of Poisoners, Tanners and the British Raj: Redefining Chamar Identity in Colonial North India, 1850–90', *Indian Economic and Social History Review*, 48 (2011), 317–38.

12 Mohammad Rahmatullah, *Paisa Paisa Tibbi Chutkule*, Patiala: Rahmat-I-Ilahi, 1935 not paginated (herafter n. p.).

13 There is a huge amount of literature on professionalization of medicine in the European context. Some of the prominent ones include Roy Porter, *Quacks: Fakes and Charlatans in History*, London: NPI Media Group, 2003; Roy Porter, *Health for Sale: Quackery in England, 1660–1850*, Manchester: Manchester University Press, 1989; David Gentilcore, 'The "Golden Age of Quackery" or "Medical Enlightenment"? Licensed Charlatanism in Eighteenth-Century Italy', *Cultural & Social History*, 3 (2006), 250–63; Alison Klairmont Lingo, 'Empirics and Charlatans in

Early Modern France: The Genesis of the Classification of the "Other" in Medical Practice', *Journal of Social History*, 19 (Summer 1986), 583–603; John Burnham, *How the Idea of Profession Changed the Writing of Medical History*, London: Wellcome Institute for the History of Medicine, 1998; and M. Pelling, 'Medical Practice in Early Modern England: Trade or Profession?' in M. Pelling (ed.), *The Common Lot: Sickness, Medical Occupations and the Urban Poor in Early Modern England*, London: Orient Longman, 1998, 230–58.

14 Guy Attewell, 'Contesting Knowledges: Plague and the Dynamics of the Unani Profession', in *Refiguring Unani Tibb: Plural Healing in Late Colonial India*, Hyderabad: Orient Longman, 2007, 50–95. Projit Mukharji also makes a similar point in the context of Bengal. See his 'Lokman, Chholeman and Manik Pir: Multiple Frames for Institutionalising Islamic Medicine in Modern Bengal', *Social History of Medicine,* 24 (2011), 720–38.

15 *Risaala-I-Haiza*, Hyderabad: publisher not mentioned (not dated, perhaps late 1880s), 11.

16 The report was subsequently also published in the form of a short booklet, entitled *Haiza aur Iska Ilaz,* which was sold at an affordable price. The *Urdu Akhbar* was also published from Lahore.

17 *Haiza aur Iska Ilaaz*, Lucknow: Munshi Ram Agarwal, n.d., 1–2.

18 Ibid., 2.

19 Discussing this issue, the pamphlet noted pithily that 'man is the real enemy of man': *Haiza aur Iska Ilaaz*, 8.

20 *Dus Kanoon-I-Sehat*, Lucknow: J. P. Verma and Brothers Press1884, 148-9.

21 *Dus Kanoon-I-Sehat*, 149. This argument about acidity is interesting, as some colonial researchers also argue that the cholera bacillus was unable to survive in an acidic medium. One wonders whether Varma borrowed the idea from colonial scientific publications. See, D. D. Cunningham, *Scientific Memoirs by Medical Officers of the Army of India: On Milk as a Medium for Choleraic Comma-Bacilli*, Calcutta: Government Printing, 1890.

22 Christopher Hamlin points towards the Asianizing of cholera in his biography of cholera: *Cholera: The Biography*, 39. Projit Mukharji notes that, despite Hamlin's work, India continues to be seen as the 'home of cholera': 'The "Cholera Cloud" in the Nineteenth Century', 314.

23 Anon, *Nuskha-I Amal-I Tibb*, Hyderabad: Masih Us-Zama 1873, 133.

24 Asghar Hussain, *Shifa al-Waba*, Agra: Matba Education Press, 1867 (originally published in 1844).

25 Ibid., 2.

26 Ibid., 3.

27 For a fascinating argument in favour of global histories of medicine, see Mark Harrison, 'A Global Perspective: Reframing the History of Health, Medicine, and Disease', *Bulletin of the History of Medicine*, 89 (winter 2015), 639–89.

28 Sayani, *Risaalah-I Haiza*, 29.

29 Hakim Mohammad Wahid, *Risaala-I-Haiza*, New Delhi: Maqbool Barki Press, 1936.

30 The author called it *Haiza-I- Ghazai*, Wahid, *Risaalah-I Haiza*, 6.

31 On the subject of middle-class anxieties around the subject of food, see the chapter entitled 'Food adulteration, public health, and middle-class anxieties' from my book *Beastly Encounters of the Raj: Livelihoods, Livestock and Veterinary Health in North India, 1790–1920*, Manchester: Manchester University Press, 2015, 102–22; see also Srirupa Prasad, 'Crisis, Identity, and Social Distinction: Cultural Politics of Food, Taste, and Consumption in Late Colonial Bengal', *Journal of Historical Sociology*, 19 (September 2006), 245–65.

32 In fact these cures were often also recommended by those who did not see themselves as Unani practitioners. See, for example, Mukund Ram, *Dushman-I-Amraz*, Badayun: Nizami Press n.d., 62.

33 See, for instance, Acharya Shri Chatursen Shashtri, *Arogya Shashtra*, New Delhi: Sanjeevni Institute, 1932, 238; Ganpati Verma Singh, *Dugdh Gun Vidhan*, Bikaner: publisher not mentioned, 1934, 19–26; Tarachandra Doshi, *Dugdhopchar aur Dugdh ka Khana*, Sirohi: Publisher not mentioned, 1918.

34 Attewell notes in the context of plague that 'in Islamic learning there was a body of authentic hadith (traditions) that relate to plague specifically . . . In addition, there was an authoritative tradition which was founded on hadith but then developed into its own genre relating Tibb to Islamic learning, Tibb al-Nabi (medicine of the Prophet)': *Refiguring Unani Tibb*, 53.

35 *Risaala-I-Haiza*, Patna, n.d., 3. In fact Hussain does not present this as his own view, but the view of noted *maulanas*.

36 Saiyad Ghulam Yahya, *Risaala-I-Haiza Wabai*, Ara: Nisha Arba 1873, 8.

37 Interestingly, the same text also dissuaded people from doing too much physical exercise. According to the author, this opened up the pores of the body, allowing the poisonous atmosphere (*fiza*) to enter the body: Yahya, *Risaala-I-Haiza Wabai*, 8.

38 For an interesting account of the medical market in these kinds of substances, see Joseph Alter, *Moral Materialism: Sex and Masculinity in Modern India*, New Delhi: Penguin Books, 2011. Seema Alavi notes how Unani *hakims* almost banished the idea of sensuality from their texts, even when offering advice on the question of procreation: 'Unani Medicine in the Nineteenth-Century Public Sphere: Urdu Texts and the Oudh Akhbar', *The Indian Economic and Social History Review*, 42 (2005), 109.

39 The term is used by Hakim Mohammad Abdul Wahid, but the same idea is to be used in a number of Unani texts. See Wahid, *Risaalah-I-Haiza*, Delhi: Maqbool Barki Press, 1936, 4.

40 Saiyad Ghulam Yahya is one of those who explicitly mention wars as the main cause for dead and decaying bodies, but the role of decaying animal matter in forming miasma is acknowledged by all *hakims* who believe in the theory of miasma.

41 *Risaalah-I-Haiza*, 49.

42 Babu Pyare Lal, *Jauhar-I-Hikmat*, Aligarh: Institute Press 1895, 342.

43 Saiyad Ghulam Yahya, *Risaala-I-Haiza Wabai*, Ara, 1874. Asghar Hussain also mentions it in *shifa-ul-Waba*, where he calls it 'sitaron ki gardish': 6.

44 Ghulam Yahya names *hararat, burudat, rutubat and paivast* as the four chief causes: *Risaalah-I Haiza Wabai*, 8.

45 The Southerly wind was thought to be the bearer of disease, while the Easterly was held to be good for health. Mohammad Akbar, *Aksir-ul-Kulub* (publisher and date not mentioned).

46 Abdul Wahid, *Risaalah-I-Haiza*, New Delhi: Makbul Barki Press, 1936, 12. The various other varieties of the disease mentioned by him and other authors include *dry cholera, ambulatory cholera, malignant cholera, muttalakh haiza,* and *Haiza-I-Ain*.

47 Authors like Babu Pyare Lal, amongst others, argued that younger men were more susceptible to the disease.

48 See for instance Anonymous, *Risaala Matlub wa Atalbeen*, Kanpur: publisher not mentioned 1897 (third edition).

49 More than a thousand copies of the text were distributed on more than one occasion. Ghulam Nabi, *Risaala-e-Haiza*, Lahore: Victoria Press 1884 (third edition).

50 The exact term used by many texts is *zahrila madda*, which can be more accurately translated as 'poisonous matter' polluting the air.

51 *Prasad* is an offering of food made to deities. Nabi, *Risaala-I-Haiza*, 15.

52 *Risaala-I-Haiza*, 20.

53 It must be clarified here that he did not use the term 'malaria' as referring to 'bad air' but to the specific disease caused by mosquito-bites. In *Risaala-I-Haiza*, 25.

54 '*Iska hawa se koi taalluk nahin hai*', 29.

55 Nabi, *Risaala-I-Haiza*, 13.

56 *Tibbi Kadeem Aur Tibbi Zadeeb*, Hyderabad, 1938, 63.

57 See 'A Question of Locality: The Identity of Cholera in British India, 1860–1890'; see also his 'Quarantine, Pilgrimage, and Colonial Trade: India 1866–1900', *Indian Economic and Social History Review*, 29 (June 1992), 117–44. I have also discussed, elsewhere, the changing definitions of cholera espoused by the Indian government in the context of the international spread of the disease: 'Cholera, Commerce and the Ka'aba: Epidemics and the Haj from India', *Pilgrimage, Politics, and Pestilence: The Haj from the Indian Subcontinent*, New Delhi: Oxford University Press, 2011, 53–80.

58 We are referring here, of course, to the text written by Saiyad Ghulam Yahya, entitled *Risaalah-I Haiza Wabai*. Not much can be gleaned from his texts about the man himself, but Yahya was clearly a prolific writer on medical themes such as uroscopy and cholera; he also wrote other general treatises prescribing remedies for a wide variety of ailments.

59 Helen Lambert, 'Popular Therapeutics and Medical Preferences in Rural North India', *The Lancet*, 38 (1996), 348, 1706–9.

60 Alavi also makes the fascinating argument that these early interactions, and the consequent reactions against cholera, might have provided a sort of template for the public health response against cholera in Britain in the 1830s: *Islam and Healing: Loss and Recovery of an Indo-Muslim Medical Tradition, 1600–1900*, Basingstoke: Palgrave Macmillan, 2008.

4 Of cholera, colonialism and pilgrimage sites

Rethinking popular responses to state sanitation, c.1867–1900

Amna Khalid

In June 2013 *Foreign Policy*, a news magazine, published the following rather alarming news item regarding the forthcoming Hajj pilgrimage in Saudi Arabia:

> Today, the Middle East is threatened with a new plague, . . . the Middle East respiratory syndrome . . . This novel coronavirus was discovered in Jordan in March 2012, and as of June 26, there have been 77 laboratory-confirmed infections, 62 of which have been in Saudi Arabia. . . [T]he disease is raising anxiety throughout the region . . . This fall, millions of devout Muslims will descend upon . . . Saudi Arabia's holy sites in one of the largest annual migrations in human history . . . And having a large group of people together in a single, fairly confined space threatens to turn the holiest site in Islam into a massive petri dish . . . The disease is still mysterious. Little is understood about how it is transmitted and even less regarding its origins. But we do know that MERS is deadly, with a mortality rate of about 55 per cent.[1]

The connection between pilgrimage and disease is certainly not new. In the nineteenth century cholera, the transmission of which was a matter of intense medical debate for the better part of the century, was closely associated with pilgrimage. The pandemic of 1865–66 spread to Europe via an outbreak at the Hajj in Mecca in 1865 and Muslims pilgrims from India were believed to have brought the disease with them.[2] The third International Sanitary Conference, organized in the wake of this pandemic, took a contagionist stance and concluded that pilgrimage was 'the most powerful of all the causes which conduce to the development and propagation of epidemics of cholera'.[3] But it was not the pilgrimage to Mecca that the conference was referring to; rather 'places where congregations of Hindoo pilgrims take place' within India, which was rendered 'the home of [Asiatic] cholera'.[4]

Hardwar and Allahabad, two pilgrimage sites along the banks of the Ganges in north India, were specifically named as starting points for cholera epidemics 'almost every year'.[5] Pilgrimage fairs, particularly the Kumbh melas – special pilgrimage fairs that convened every twelve years and attracted exceptionally large crowds – thus came to be seen as especially dangerous in terms of their potential to spread disease. Much like the way in which *Foreign Policy* refers to how the gathering of large groups of pilgrims threatens to turn Mecca into a 'petri dish' for the mysterious MERS, in the colonial imagination pilgrimage fairs at Hardwar and Allahabad loomed large as hotbeds for cholera in the nineteenth century and the average Hindu pilgrim came to be seen as the root cause of epidemic outbreaks. The colonial archive constructs the pilgrim as filthy, superstitious, inherently irrational and resistant to sanitation measures that the state introduced.[6] The state almost always blamed the pilgrims' rejection of the basic principles of sanitation and their unsanitary habits and customs for cholera outbreaks. Interestingly much of the scholarship on public health in British India also notes Indians' rejection of state-introduced public health measures, though it is framed in ideological terms: as resistance to state interventions to contest colonial rule rather than an 'irrational' reaction to the logic of sanitary science. The secondary literature accommodates accounts of Indians who favoured state-introduced sanitary measures by claiming that it was only a small minority of elite, educated Indians who subscribed to Western medicine and sanitary science while the majority did not.[7] However, I contend that a close reading of popular explanations shows that far from resisting the tenets of sanitary science people were demanding that the state provide better sanitation, the very thing the state was blaming them for rejecting. In fact, they saw the colonial state's sanitary neglect as the source of cholera epidemics. Yet in colonial discourse the pilgrim continues to feature as essentially dirty, embodying disease and posing a serious threat to public health. The question that I am addressing in this chapter is why did the construct of the irrational and dirty pilgrim become such an enduring one in colonial discourse?

In the first section of this chapter I examine the public health measures put into place at pilgrimage sites, namely, Hardwar and Allahabad, during the latter half of the nineteenth century. This section focuses on cholera outbreaks during five large fairs (1867, 1879, 1882, 1890 and 1892) and draws mainly on the vernacular press[8] as a means to gauge popular responses to state intervention. These five fairs represent key moments that capture the ways in which people explained the epidemic outbreaks and encompass the main thrust of people's complaints. They also show that while initially some were sceptical of the new measures and indeed, offered explanations invoking the divine for cholera visitations, the majority of popular explanations focused on the flawed and inadequate sanitary arrangements. They held the state's wilful neglect responsible for creating the conditions that facilitated the spread of disease.

The second section then considers the ways in which colonial officials accounted for the same cholera epidemics and shows how their explanations squarely laid the blame on the unsanitary habits and customs of the pilgrims.

Section three considers why, despite evidence to the contrary, colonial medical discourse continued to view the pilgrim as representing danger and disease. I argue that this image of the pilgrim in fact served key purposes at three levels: the political, the administrative and the ideological. At the political level, it rationalized state surveillance of pilgrimage sites for political ends in the name of public health. At the administrative level, it masked and deflected attention from the colonial administration's own shortcomings and inefficiencies. And at an ideological level it served to reify the difference between the colonizers and Indians, thereby legitimizing the colonial project.

Prior to delving into the ways in which the pilgrims and colonial officials explained cholera outbreaks, I would like to note briefly that places such as Hardwar and Allahabad became sites of contestation between the population more generally and the colonial state, as well as among colonial officials themselves. At one level these sites represented a flashpoint between two distinct world views: that of a modernizing state, determined to control the spread of infectious disease for economic and political reasons that looked upon pilgrimages as a sanitary problem; and a subject population that viewed these places as essentially sacred. At another level, these places also became sites of contestation between colonial officials. For most of the nineteenth century there was considerable debate about how cholera was transmitted. The sanitarianists/anti-contagionists subscribed to the miasmatic theory of cholera transmission, which considered disease to be specific to locality, i.e. the result of the atmospheric and sanitary conditions of a place; whereas contagionists believed human agency played a central role in spreading the disease. While the Government of India (GOI) did take an anti-contagionist stance, there were a number of provincial administrators who dissented.[9] This then formed the basis of considerable debate among the contagionists and sanitarianists about which measures were appropriate for pilgrimage sites – and often the measures taken were a combination of what the two schools of thought prescribed. However, despite these differences the two schools of thought converged in their view of the average pilgrim. Both medical discourses relied on and reinforced the image of the pilgrim as backward and essentially filthy. Section three of this chapter will discuss this feature in more detail.

Popular explanations for cholera outbreaks: government intervention as cause of sickness

In 1867, just a year after the International Sanitary Conference had issued its indictment of pilgrimage sites, a Kumbh mela was due to take place at Hardwar. Given that the Kumbh took place only every twelve years and was considered to be especially auspicious, these gatherings were far larger than annual fairs. Since the sanitary and medical administration of India was organized along provincial lines, it fell to the government of the North-Western Provinces (NWP) to oversee pilgrimage fairs at Hardwar and Allahabad, both sites falling under its jurisdiction. But this year the anticipation of an exceptionally large gathering compounded the enormity of the task. Anticipating a large gathering, and feeling the pressure of foreign states keenly observing the outbreak of epidemics in India, the GOI and the government of NWP were meticulous about planning the fair site, paying particular attention to sanitary, medical and supervisory matters. On the chief bathing day of the fair, around 3 million people were present.[10]

To begin with, the location was surveyed. The valley close to Hardwar was categorized as 'intensely malarious'.[11] This further underscored the need for precautions against potential cholera outbreaks. The local government mapped out the entire site, cleared the undergrowth to render it more salubrious and imposed a grid-like order on it. It clearly demarcated hospitals, latrines and police stations, and predetermined the exact width of roads and passages between pilgrim camps to allow for free passage of air to deodorize the site.[12]

Perhaps the most important organizational question was how to dispose of excrement. Given the extremely crowded nature of the site at such times, effective conservancy (i.e. disposal of human waste) was a challenge. Most of the accounts of previous melas penned by British travellers and officials refer to the 'intolerable stench' emanating from human waste piled up and lying exposed to the sun and wind.[13] The sanitarian's gaze was almost exclusively on excrement and dirt.

Consequently, extensive conservancy measures were introduced. Almost 30 per cent of the entire expenditure of the mela was on conservancy arrangements.[14]

Special stone kilns were built to burn filth and excrement collected at the site. A system of trench latrines was also introduced whereby people were encouraged to relieve themselves only in the trenches. These ditches were then covered with dry earth. This system, at least initially, seemed to work as can be gleaned by the Commissioner of Meerut's statement that 'not a single Anglo-Saxon, a race far more sensitive to foul smells than Natives, perceived it [any smell]'.[15] However, these latrines were not popular with everyone, for the Commissioner of Meerut also made the following note: 'I have heard from a "native" gentleman, that rather than go to public latrines, many people, women particularly abstained from relieving themselves during the two or three days the fair lasted.'[16]

But the big blow came with torrential rains just a day prior to the chief bathing day. Rainwater saturated the ground and trench latrines became cesspools; the fair site began to reek of excrement. The day after the chief bathing event, cholera broke out among the dispersing pilgrims. Neighbouring districts, divisions and provinces were telegraphed immediately to be vigilant of returning pilgrims and to institute measures to prevent the spread of the epidemic among the general population, prisoners and European troops. Commissioners of Delhi, Hissar, Umballa, Jullundar and Lahore divisions were instructed to arrange for medical inspection of pilgrims that passed through their jurisdiction and to quarantine those showing signs of the disease. The quarantine period ranged from 48 hours up to 5 days. Moreover, to protect large centres of population, the pilgrims were diverted and put on alternate routes bypassing cities. For instance, pilgrims approaching Lahore were told not to proceed by train but to go via the Grand Trunk Road to protect the military cantonment lying close to the train line. The Multan line was redirected through Umritsar to protect Lahore.[17] The health of troops was of prime importance for the colonial state and every effort was made to protect military cantonments.[18]

Nonetheless cholera spread in the wake of returning pilgrims erupting into a full-blown epidemic in north India. What concerns us here is the manner in which pilgrims, and the population more generally, explained the outbreak. There were indeed those who viewed it as divine retribution, the manifestation of Kali's (the goddess of protection) wrath for having allowed the colonial state to enter this holy space and implement disease prevention measures thus doubting her powers of protection.[19] However, the vast majority of explanations did not make any recourse to the supernatural. Rather, they were rational critiques of the sanitary arrangements put into place by the authorities. Indigenous *hakeems* and physicians attributed the outbreak to the smoke emanating from the furnaces the government set up at the fair site to burn filth and waste.[20] They also blamed the nature of the conservancy system, claiming that the trenching of filth, and the humid, moist stench that emanated from the trenches after the rain had caused the outbreak.[21] Furthermore the latrines were criticized for having been too close to pilgrims' sleeping camps which meant that with the onset of the rains the contents of the latrines overflowed into the soil on which the sleeping quarters were laid out.[22] The following excerpt from an article that appeared in a vernacular newspaper best reflects popular sentiment:

> This year one or two such measures were introduced into the Government arrangements as *were calculated to cause sickness* . . . the conservancy arrangements were so bad, and filth was thrown in such places as were not deep enough, and on which so little earth was thrown that the rain falling on it caused a bad smell, and thus induced cholera.[23]
>
> (Emphasis mine)

It is interesting to note that such explanations were not dissimilar to the miasmatic theory of disease that held considerable cache with colonial sanitary authorities of the time – yet as we shall see in the following section the sanitary administration was reluctant to see this outbreak as the consequence of their arrangements and instead blamed the habits of 'uncivilised natives'.

Along with condemning the sanitary measures, people objected to the ways in which pilgrims were diverted and rerouted on their return journeys; the government was blamed for creating conditions that increased the cholera death toll. *Rohilcund Ukhbar*, a vernacular paper noted that

> such a check was placed upon pilgrims and people generally, returning from the fair, that they were not allowed to enter cities or villages, and could not make the necessary arrangements to provide for their daily food on the roadside . . . water was not procurable for them; and *this great check from Government created such alarm among them as was sufficient to produce sickness.*[24]
>
> (Emphasis mine)

Similar criticisms were to reverberate twelve years later upon the breaking up of the Kumbh mela when pilgrims were diverted from their original return routes to protect big centres of population. Preparations were made well in advance for the 1879 Kumbh. The numbers expected were considerable; according to the official report of the mela, on the main bathing day, April 12, 600,000 people were present in Hardwar.

On April 8, sporadic cases of cholera at the site began to be reported. Simultaneously, it was reported that there was severe cholera among the hill people, pilgrims from Kumaon and Garhwal. These people had camped at Chandi, a hilly and sandy area on the eastern bank of the Ganges. The administration felt that an epidemic was looming and decided not only to cut communication between those at Chandi and those across the river, but also to disperse the crowds at Chandi. The police were instructed to break up the gathering and clear the site but they encountered considerable resistance from the crowd.[25] Hill pilgrims were forced to return by an alternate route in order to protect major cities on the way.[26] The new route was incredibly arduous and no provisions were made along the way for the pilgrims. Many died en route: of the 6,902 people that went from Kumaon to Hardwar for the mela, about 24 per cent died and almost 4 per cent were unaccounted for, quite likely dead as well.[27] According to the Senior Assistant Commissioner of Kumaon, '[i]n ordinary years the route by which these people were ordered to travel is very short of water. This year, owing to prolonged drought, there was great scarcity of water.'[28] Moreover, food was hard to procure as there were few shops along the road, 'and in all probability most of the banias (shop owners) went off when they heard of the out-break of cholera.'[29] The vernacular press immediately seized upon this and blamed the actions of the government. The press claimed that the death toll was high not because of cholera deaths but because of those who died en route unable to get basic amenities. *Almora Akhbar*, one of the major vernacular papers of NWP, reported:

> The road from Hardwar to Almora was covered with corpses for several days . . . As soon as cholera appeared at Hardwar, they were compelled to . . . return to their homes, but they were not permitted to pass through towns and villages, and had to travel through forests, where they could get neither food nor water, and died of thirst and hunger.[30]

A compounder at a dispensary along the road confirmed this noting, 'hundreds of people died from thirst'.[31] Even the Senior Assistant Commissioner acknowledged this, though not publicly, when he said, 'I have not the least hesitation in saying that a great deal of the mortality . . . was caused by the people having to traverse long distances under a burning sun, without water, and with, in many instances, insufficient food.'[32]

The next major religious fair was the Kumbh mela scheduled for January 1882 at Allahabad. A total of 3 million people attended.[33] Despite the precautions taken, sanitary conditions at the fair quickly deteriorated, and night-soil trenches soon became watery and muddy. According to Dr. Planck, the Sanitary Commissioner of NWP, the unsanitary state of the ground was 'widespread and general, to an extent surpassing anything of previous experience in all my years of Sanitary Commissionership'.[34] He noted, the 'drainage-ways [were] choked with sweepings, chiefly large leaves in which food had been purchased – moistened with much refuse water used for cooking or washing, with great suspicion of urine admixture.'[35] The accumulation of filth was apparently so rapid that the supply of sweepers was rendered utterly inadequate to clear the site. Until 15 January, there was no report of any cases; however, on that day a few cholera cases came to light and on 18 January, cholera was found to be rife among the *sadhus* [Hindu ascetics] at the fair. Soon thereafter, cholera seemed to spread along the return routes of pilgrims.

When it came to making sense of the outbreak once again people pointed the finger at the sanitary administration. They did not oppose the arrangements per se, but rather the ineffectiveness of the measures put in place. *Hindi Pradip* blamed the outbreak on the deficient sanitary provisions.[36] *Sahas*, another vernacular paper, wondered why, when large crowds were anticipated, had the administration not hired sufficient sweepers and conservancy carts.[37]

The 1890 cholera outbreak at the Magh mela at Allahabad was also framed in terms of the incompetence of sanitary authorities. The trench latrines came under fire again. The Ganges meandered and changed course every year altering the space available for the fair and that particular year the river swelled to submerge most of the fair site leaving little space to accommodate the pilgrims. Trenches were dug for the disposal of night soil, but given the spatial constraints, they were located unusually close to the pilgrim camps. The proximity was accentuated by fact that the crowd gathered for the fair was larger than usual – on the main bathing day, January 20, there were between 300,000 and 400,000 people. Just two days after the chief bathing day, cholera broke out at the fair.[38] The vernacular press was quick to blame the defective sanitary measures. *Hindustan* noted:

> The Municipal Commissioners in charge of the management of the fair are really to blame, and are responsible for all the deaths

that have occurred. They have made latrines near the fair, and the filth is buried close by: the filth rots in the underground water which is close to the surface at the place and poisons the air. The latrines should have been made at a greater distance, and the filth should have been immediately removed from the latrines by the municipal conservancy carts.[39]

In light of its experience of cholera, the administration redoubled its organizational efforts for the next Kumbh mela at Hardwar scheduled for April 1891. Preparations started as early as December the previous year and sanitary measures were sketched out with great care: the site was thoroughly cleaned, undergrowth cleared and bridges constructed well in advance to ease the flow of pilgrims and to prevent overcrowding. Temporary latrines and hospitals were set up, extra sweepers were called in from neighbouring municipalities and the site was divided into eight sanitary sections where each section was under the charge of a separate sanitary patrol composed of constables, chaukidars and vaccinators. Particular attention was paid to conservancy arrangements, especially after the criticisms levied against the arrangements at the Kumbhs of 1867 and 1879. In 1891, almost 30 per cent of the total expenditure on the mela was reserved for conservancy, whereas at the previous Kumbh of 1879, conservancy expenditure was barely 10 per cent of the total budget. According to the Sanitary Commissioner of NWP, the crowds were considerable and on the four nights leading up to the chief bathing day of April 12, 'the town . . . was simply one mass of human beings stretched along roof, verandah and every open space, and crowding all the available accommodation in dwellings.'[40] A cholera outbreak was anticipated, but much to the surprise of the administration, there was no serious outbreak. This is the only Kumbh mela at Hardwar, in the period under study, when cholera did not erupt. It was a moment of considerable relief for the provincial government and the Sanitary Commissioner was quick to credit the arrangements. In his annual report he wrote:

> The 'unparalleled result' of an almost total immunity from cholera was only obtained . . . by rigid personal attention to sanitary details, to the careful and early removal and isolation of suspicious or actual cases of disease, and to the clearance and disinfection of supposed areas of contamination and infection.[41]

The degree of self-congratulation is almost palpable in the reports of the colonial officials responsible for arrangements at the fair. The following quote from the Superintendent of Dehra Dun's report to his superior is one such example:

> The wonderful cleanliness of the fair was the general subject of remark; not a sign of filth was lying about, and not a bad odour was anywhere perceptible. The people, who had no doubt dreaded the sanitary regulations terribly, soon got accustomed to them, and began to take pride in carrying them out. One continually heard the remark from passing pilgrims 'what and excellent *bandobast* the Sirkar has made.'[42]

There was renewed faith in the effectiveness of sanitary measures; the authorities believed they had found the key to cholera prevention. The Sanitary Commissioner for NWP noted that finally it had been proved that 'cholera is a preventable disease' and that no 'practical illustration of this truth has ever been placed on record than the immunity from cholera following the late great fair . . . of 1891.'[43] Indeed the local press also acknowledged the efforts of the administration and congratulated colonial officials. *Hindustan* for instance was very keen to publicly praise the arrangements noting, 'Mr. Patterson and other officials associated with him in the management of the fair are entitled to the gratitude of the public.'[44]

Freedom from cholera at the mela of 1891 may indeed have partly resulted from the close attention paid to sanitation at the site. All filth and refuse were removed from the inhabited quarters and if there was any doubt about whether an area was unclean, it was disinfected with a solution of perchloride of mercury.[45] But perhaps a major contributing factor was the meagre attendance. Many people, from Saharanpur in particular, did not attend the mela, most probably for fear of an outbreak at the site.[46] In fact the authorities of neighbouring districts were expressly instructed to dissuade residents from going to the Kumbh as cholera was almost certain to break out at Hardwar.[47] Another reason for the relatively fewer numbers may have been the more auspicious event of the Mahavaruni mela, scheduled for the following year. Many pilgrims quite possibly deferred their visit until the Mahavaruni mela. Interestingly the NWP Sanitary Commissioner does not mention this in his report. In fact, he made a point of stressing that the body of pilgrims gathered was considerable – this made his achievement of preventing an outbreak at the mela seem grander. Since the arrangements had been made with a larger crowd in mind than those that eventually came, it was probably not a great challenge for the sanitary authorities to maintain sanitary standards. The sanitary authorities basked in their success.

But this moment of success was short-lived – the management of the Mahavaruni mela of 1892 proved challenging indeed. The last Mahavaruni mela was in 1865 and according to an officer present at that mela, 'there was no one who had seen such a crowd collected anywhere before, and that the multitude was far greater than that of any Kumbh year.'[48] Expecting a gathering at least as large as at a Kumbh mela, the Magistrate of Saharanpur started preparations early. He oversaw the construction of an extensive system of bridges to facilitate pilgrim traffic and attended to conservancy arrangements carefully, acquiring 150 permanent iron latrine seats and erecting temporary latrines. An army of hired sweepers cleared the undergrowth and set up camps for pilgrims.

Despite these seemingly elaborate arrangements cholera reared its head during the fair. The Sanitary Commissioner and the medical officer on duty decided that the disease was bound to spread and that the gathering ought to be dispersed at the earliest. They took immediate action and instructed all railway companies to suspend train services to Hardwar. The next step was to force pilgrims out of Hardwar. This met with considerable opposition; people perceived this measure to be a direct contravention of the government's promise of religious tolerance.[49] Pilgrims, who were chased from different areas of the fair site, 'came back to the same place by another road'.[50] About 50,000 people openly defied the orders and refused to turn back shouting '*nahaenge, nahaenge*' [Will bathe, will bathe] and 'moved down the riverside getting a dip where they could'. Others squatted by the river and shouted, 'You must throw us out otherwise we will not go.'[51] They refused to budge claiming, 'It is better to die here; we won't go home (*behtar hai marna yahin; ham nahin jate ghar*).'[52] Lodging houses were crammed to the brim. As the police emptied them, many of the pilgrims, 'instead of going to the railway station or leaving the town by road managed to make their escape into other streets and were taken into other lodging houses.'[53] It took two days to clear the site; finally, a day before the chief bathing day the authorities managed to send back most of the pilgrims. About 17,000 were sent on special trains requisitioned for this express purpose. Despite the strict instructions to stay clear of the sacred pool, a large number of pilgrims lingered in neighbouring towns hoping to get access to the river. Finally, by that evening all pilgrims were evacuated. Just when the authorities thought the crowd had been successfully dispersed, it transpired that late that night approximately 10,000 of them returned to a neighbouring town under the cover of darkness. What's more, this crowd included several cholera victims. The next day, the authorities herded them out again.

Special cordons were set up to block all the roads leading to Hardwar for the following few days as another fair, the Somwati Amwas, was scheduled to take place two days later.[54]

Finally, the crowds were disbanded but the incidence of cholera among returning pilgrims was considerable. Once again, the pilgrims and the population at large blamed government measures for the epidemic. The vernacular press was awash with criticisms of the dispersal of the gathering.[55] *Rahbar* noted, 'The outbreak of cholera [at Hardwar] was a matter of doubt, but the panic created by the dispersion was a fact that led to the epidemic.'[56]

Moreover, there was a tendency to blame the conditions on return trains for cholera's appearance in pilgrims that were sent back. The carriages were extremely overcrowded. They were referred to as 'Black Holes' into which people were crammed. It was alleged that had people not been forced into these rail wagons, many lives could have been saved.[57] The dispersal of the 1892 fair is significant for it brought to light yet another popular explanation for the outbreak of disease: the railways were blamed for spreading the epidemic. They were not censured for spreading the disease farther and faster on account of their speed, rather sanitary and other arrangements at stations and on board were targeted. An article in *Bharat Jiwan* outlining these problems is worth quoting at length:

Religious gatherings have been liable to outbreaks of cholera since the extension of railways. When there were no railroads, pilgrims travelled on foot or in carriages at their ease, with due regard to their health. They freely attended to the calls of nature, obtained wholesome food and had good rest at night. But they are exposed to great ill-treatment, especially on occasions of large fairs, on railways. Enormous crowds of men have to lie on the ground at railway stations, where they have no shelter from the inclemencies of the weather, receive bad food, and are unable to get sound sleep at night. They experience great difficulties in obtaining tickets and access to the platform. Carriages are overcrowded to suffocation, as if passengers were not considered as men by the railway officials, but merely cattle. When carriages are not available, passengers are required to travel in dirty wagons which have no ventilation and are reeking with malodours and vermin. Again, they are unable to obtain potable water, to satisfy the calls of nature, or to have any rest during their journey. It is no wonder that pilgrims who travel hundreds of miles in this way get sick. Hence it will be perceived that the outbreak of cholera at religious gatherings is chiefly due to the hardships and privations which pilgrims have to endure in railway travelling.[58]

After an outbreak of cholera at the Somwati fair at Hardwar in 1901, another vernacular paper of considerable circulation criticized the manner in which diseased passengers were shoved together with healthy ones in the same wagon and warned that 'if there is no improvement in railway administration, India will always continue to be a prey to one epidemic disease or another'.[59]

The condition of rail carriages, particularly those used for pilgrim traffic, was subject to extensive criticism. Most pilgrims travelled third class, and sanitary standards were so appalling that the Magistrate of Saharanpur wrote a special report on the treatment of third-class rail passengers journeying to Hardwar. In his report, he noted that often closed goods wagons with iron roofs and no lighting or vents were used to transport pilgrims; the temperature inside them rose rapidly in summer. Moreover third-class carriages had no latrines.[60] For large fairs the number of pilgrims crammed into a wagon far exceeded the maximum number allowed, causing much inconvenience.[61] It altered the pilgrimage experience by affecting the quality of the journey.[62] A medical official in Panjab commenting on the state of train carriages of pilgrims returning from the Hardwar mela of 1879 observed, 'The cruel way in which natives are crowded into railway trains in the hot weather is a most fertile source of disease.'[63]

Thus, popular explanations of cholera outbreaks during pilgrimages tended to blame government-introduced measures. Pilgrims and the general population pointed the finger at the way in which the pilgrimage experience had changed as a result of state intervention: both through sanitation measures implemented at the sites as well as the conditions for transportation of pilgrims via rail. However, the condemnation of public health measures should not simply be understood as outright resistance towards everything colonial – rather a closer reading shows that far from opposing the sanitary logic of the administration, the complaints in fact focused on precisely the inadequacy of the sanitation measures introduced. They held the government responsible for not doing enough. At other times, such as when gatherings were dispersed on account of cholera, state measures were seen as having gone too far in terms of their heavy-handedness. Not only did people see this as directly contravening the state's own policy of non-interference in religious matters, but they also held the methods of dispersing the gatherings responsible for precipitating the outbreaks. Popular explanations time and again stressed that cholera outbreaks were the result of a lack of willingness on the part of the colonial administration to introduce serious sanitation and public health measures at pilgrimage sites.

Official explanations for the outbreaks: 'native antipathy to conservancy'

Official explanations for the outbreaks of cholera at pilgrimage fairs were diametrically opposed to popular ones. Accounting for the cholera outbreak at the Kumbh mela of 1867 J.M. Cuningham, the Sanitary Commissioner with the GOI, repeatedly emphasized the actions and rituals of the pilgrims at the site, holding them responsible for the epidemics. The blame was squarely put on local atmospheric conditions and the 'insanitary habits' and the religious rites of Hindus: bathing in and drinking the Ganges water.[64] Furthermore, Cuningham discredited popular objections by stating that it came as no surprise to him that the 'natives' blamed the sanitary measures for the outbreak, for they were 'ignorant and terror-stricken'.[65] In the same vein the Commissioner of Meerut, who was directly responsible for the organization of the mela, completely disregarded the opinion of *hakeems* that smoke from furnaces burning waste was responsible for the outbreak. In addition, he completely denied that trench latrines reeked of excrement saying, 'I think this hypothesis is due to the Native antipathy to conservancy.'[66]

Similarly, the NWP Sanitary Commissioner held people's rejection of the new latrines (different from trench latrines) responsible for the outbreak at the Allahabad pilgrimage fair in 1882. He was appalled by pilgrims answering calls of nature in all manner of places other than the designated latrines. Despairing of these 'habits' of pilgrims, the Sanitary Commissioner wrote, 'this great evil never was and never could be properly dealt with.'[67] Yet another sanitary official at the fair noted,

> Latrines may be put up: but native habits . . . are determinedly against using them, except under compulsion. In this locality we failed altogether in this respect. And it was only by turning ourselves into head scavengers, and employing every available official from the Tehsildars downwards for the same purposes, that with great exertions we managed to clear up the area after its contamination by the fair goers.[68]

The introduction of latrines was indeed not an intervention that the majority of pilgrims were enthused about. The majority preferred to use nearby woods instead.[69] As the Commissioner of Allahabad noted in his report on the Magh mela of 1882, 'Notwithstanding the latrines provided and punishments awarded for not using them, it was impossible to prevent thousands – who preferred it – resorting to the fields; and it was hopeless to expect any other result when such multitudes had to be dealt with.'[70] The 'difficulty of restraining them [the pilgrims] from insanitary practices' and how these 'habits' formed the basis of cholera outbreaks are constant refrains in the reports and proceedings of the Sanitary Department.[71] In the colonial imagination pilgrims were an especially unclean lot and their resistance to latrines confirmed the state's perception of them as 'irrational', 'backward' and hostile to sanitary logic.

However, a closer analysis of the sources provides a very interesting insight into pilgrims' aversion to latrines – one that shows that in fact this may have been a 'rational' choice. The key lies in examining the nature of these latrines, something that hardly any of the reports comment on. Built as confined enclosures the rationale behind them was to designate a space where the excreta and the resulting odours could be contained. However, they were designed for mass use and did not have separate compartments and thus afforded little privacy. In 1883 as an experiment some of latrines were fitted with separate compartments and not surprisingly the authorities found more people making use of them for 'the privacy thus gained was appreciated'.[72] Given that this was only a one-off small experiment and other latrines continued to be built on the previous model, it is small wonder that many people, especially those from higher castes and women, chose the nearby forests over latrines.

Colonial officials viewed the habits, customs as well as religious rites of Indians generally, and pilgrims particularly, as medically 'dangerous'. Traditions such as joint-family life and purdah – important aspects of Indian culture – were seen as aiding overcrowding and sickness.[73] A practice particular to pilgrimage that colonial officials saw as unsanitary and aiding the spread of cholera was the taking back of *Ganga Jal* (holy water from the Ganges) to share with their friends and relatives at home.[74] This water would often be used for purposes such as blessing the infirm/sick and purifying water wells. Even the food people brought along was considered suspect and a vehicle for disseminating disease.[75] Indeed the entire practice of pilgrimage was seen as posing a threat to public health. The following statement made by the Sanitary Commissioner for Madras epitomizes this,

The intensity of cholera, and the prolongation of its epidemic visitations, are, I am convinced, largely due to the habits of people in gadding about to diverse places where festivals are held, and by their unnatural modes of living during such seasons of festivity.[76]

This image of the unsanitary pilgrim stuck. Even in the twentieth century during a cholera outbreak at the Hardwar Kumbh, the Sanitary Commissioner of NWP framed it as the 'problem' of the 'exceptionally filthy habits' of the pilgrims.[77] In official discourse pilgrims certainly represented the worst of the Indians and even among them certain communities were considered worse than others. For instance, those coming from the hills to Hardwar were regarded as especially backward and insanitary. During the epidemic at the 1879 Kumbh, the Civil Surgeon at Saharanpur reported that the disease broke out first and foremost among the *paharis* (hill people) because of their 'dirty habits'.[78] Similarly when cholera reared its head at the Magh mela of 1891 it was noted that the disease was 'chiefly among hill-men, whose unclean habits are well known'.[79] In that instance since the disease did not become epidemic, it was seen as testifying to 'the excellence of the sanitary and other arrangements', whereas disease among the hill people was attributed entirely to their inability to observe basic hygiene.[80] The Jhariyas from the Central Provinces also came under attack. They attended the Magh mela of 1883 and the administration kept a close eye on them as they were seen as a group 'whose native habits so often cause sickness'.[81] Among the *sadhus*, certain sects, such as the Bairagis, were also believed to pose a special danger to public health and safety. According to the Sanitary Commissioner of NWP 'Bairagis are nearly always the worst offenders against cleanliness and truculent in their manner . . . In cholera times their habits are dangerous to the whole community.'[82]

Thus, in the official imagination pilgrims and travelling *sadhus* were suspect. Colonial medical discourses furthered this impression by casting pilgrims and *sadhus* as the embodiment of public health risk by virtue of what was termed their 'dirty habits' and 'unnatural modes of living'. Yet the discussion in the first section of this chapter has shown that far from being averse to sanitation measures, pilgrims were in fact asking the state to provide more and better sanitation. This then raises the question: why did the archetype of the dirty pilgrim continue to persist in and inform colonial discourse? The next section offers an analysis of the significance of this pilgrim archetype.

'Dirty', 'dangerous' and 'diseased': the significance of the pilgrim archetype in colonial discourse

While pilgrimages had been identified as one of the key avenues for cholera dissemination early in the nineteenth century,[83] it was the cholera epidemic of 1865 that reached Europe via Muslim pilgrims that cemented the association between pilgrimage and disease. The Sanitary Conference of 1866 reified the negative image of pilgrims within India by casting them as the chief propagators of Asiatic cholera.[84] Moreover, both sanitarians and contagionists constructed the typical pilgrim in a negative way. While the two schools of thought differed in the ways they explained the spread of disease, they both perceived the pilgrim as a potential public health risk. Sanitarians viewed pilgrims as an unhygienic, filthy group that were responsible for creating the conditions that gave rise to cholera outbreaks. They believed that pilgrims soiled the fair site by defecating which in turn bred the miasma they saw as causing cholera. The contagionists, in turn, saw pilgrims as a dirty lot that spread cholera in their wake. The mere fact of being pilgrims implied a fear of contamination. Writing in the 1890s, Charles Banks, Civil Medical Officer of Puri, noted that pilgrims and cholera were almost inseparable, the ebb and flow of disease correlating to the surge and decline of pilgrims.[85] The archetypal pilgrim according to both schools of thought was primarily uneducated – for 'rational' thinking did not allow for such customs and beliefs. Hence both contagionists and the sanitarians held the pilgrim as the epitome of the unhygienic and uneducated 'other'.[86] Both medical discourses warranted close surveillance of pilgrims and travelling *sadhus* and were used by the state as justification to track their movements and activities.

The archetype of the filthy and irrational pilgrim helped serve political, administrative as well as ideological ends. The colonial state viewed pilgrimage sites, pilgrims, priests and *sadhus* as politically suspicious and dangerous. After the 1857 rebellion the state became extremely wary of large religious gatherings as they had the potential of turning seditious and rebellious. *Pandas* in particular were highly suspect after it came to the fore that during the 1857 revolt, the *pandas* (priests) at Allahabad joined the rebellion and were active in perpetuating unrest in Allahabad.[87] In Bihar too the initial plot for the rebellion in 1857 was hatched at a fair, namely, the Sonepur mela, where already in 1845 Hindu and Muslim notables had covertly met to plan an anti-British movement.[88] Moreover, the 'frightening maze of narrow streets and blind alleys' of cities and pilgrimage sites in particular evaded state surveillance, adding to the administration's suspicion of possible 'internal conspiracy, rebellion, or sabotage'.[89] As it stood, itinerant groups, such as pilgrims and travelling *sadhus*, provoked state anxiety, for they crossed geographic boundaries and were difficult to monitor and control. Perceived to be a potential threat to social and political stability, such groups were stigmatized and at times criminalized by the colonial state.[90] But the state was also bound by Queen Victoria's proclamation of 1858 that guaranteed the colonial state's detachment from the religious matters of the subject population, thereby limiting state surveillance of pilgrimage sites. The construction of pilgrims and *sadhus* as dirty and squalid then opened the door for subjecting them to the colonial gaze. The connection between pilgrimage and disease further stigmatized pilgrims and travelling *sadhus* and justified close surveillance of them in the guise of public health. So, in this context medical discourse and its construction of pilgrims (and travelling *sadhus*) as medically dangerous by virtue of their 'antipathy' to hygiene served not only to justify policing them from a public health perspective but also allowed the state to keep an eye on political developments at pilgrimage sites.

But the archetype of the 'irrational', 'filthy' pilgrim was not only useful in justifying surveillance for political reasons. In fact, it also served administrative ends for it was necessary to mask the inadequacy of the sanitary policy and practice. The sanitary administration faced substantial financial constraints. These monetary limitations were the result of Lord Mayo's policies during his time as governor general (1868–72). He devolved the responsibility of public health from the central to the provincial governments in order to address the budgetary deficit created under the previous governor general's governance. Provincial governments struggled to raise sufficient funds to cover the cost of extensive and effective sanitation and in turn passed on the responsibility of generating funds from local taxation to the municipalities.[91] Since the elective principle was deemed a pre-requisite for raising money through local taxation to cover better sanitation, representation was granted to Indians on municipal commissions and boards.[92] However, municipalities were in no position to raise the requisite monies for extensive sanitary projects. Even the United Provinces Pilgrim Committee, which was instituted to report on the sanitary conditions of pilgrimage sites, noted in its final report in 1913 that 'adequate sanitation' required the introduction of piped water supply, construction of drainage and sewage systems, building of hospitals and the maintenance of better-qualified and better-paid staff; and that such 'comprehensive schemes of sanitation' were 'far beyond their [i.e. municipalities'] resources'. The Committee recommended that the central and provincial governments pay for at least the initial outlays for such projects.[93] But the central and provincial governments refused to make financial provisions for these schemes and instead blamed the stunted growth of the sanitary infrastructure on the indifference of the elected members of municipal boards (who were Indian) towards Western ideas of sanitation. Official discourse is replete with statements of the 'native antipathy' to hygiene and municipal boards stalling sanitary reform.[94] Pointing the finger at the attitudes of Indians towards sanitation served as a tool in the hands of colonial officials to explain the lack of a sanitary infrastructure and absolved them of any responsibility. The archetype of the 'dirty' and 'backward' pilgrim then provided a scapegoat for official explanations for epidemic outbreaks at pilgrimage sites and in this way detracted from the deficient public health measures of the administration.

In addition to serving political and administrative ends the image of the disease-spreading dirty pilgrim also served an important ideological purpose – by branding the customs and habits of pilgrims as inherently unsanitary, especially their religious rites and practices such as drinking *Ganga Jal*, the colonial state was also casting Hinduism in a negative light. As David Arnold has argued that state intervention at pilgrimage sites in the name of controlling cholera 'was also an attack on Hinduism, one which appeared all the more authoritative for its invocation of medical science'.[95] Furthermore, essentializing Indians generally (pilgrims in particular) as tradition-bound and resistant to sanitary improvements worked to portray the administration in a sympathetic light – as wanting to help the people but faced with the insurmountable challenge of the unchanging beliefs and incorrigible ways of Indians. In many ways the construction of pilgrims as a major public health risk and challenge also legitimized and justified the imperial project. Despite evidence to the contrary the archetype of the unsanitary pilgrim endured in colonial discourse, for it became a necessity for the state to defend itself against charges of sanitary neglect and at the same time provided a means of rationalizing colonial presence in India.

Conclusion

Pilgrimage and cholera came to be closely associated in nineteenth-century India. An analysis of popular and official explanations for epidemic outbreaks at pilgrimage sites reveals a fundamental disconnect: while pilgrims and *pandas* blamed the inadequacy of sanitary arrangements, state explanations pointed the finger at the inherent 'antipathy' of 'natives' towards sanitary principles. The discussion in this chapter shows that firstly, while there were a few instances of the new sanitary measures being opposed, these were mainly confined to the earlier fairs; secondly, even in the case of some of these rejections, such as of latrines, a closer reading reveals that their refusal was not based on an outright rejection of the principles of sanitary science; and thirdly, that contrary to the assertion in official discourse of Indians as incapable of understanding the logic of sanitary science, popular opinion (and not just that of the educated elite) was using the very logic of sanitation to blame the administration for epidemic outbreaks, and asking the state for more of the very sanitary measures the administration insisted the pilgrims were resisting.

I have argued that the reason why, despite evidence to the contrary, the archetype of the dirty and irrational pilgrim endured in colonial discourse was that it helped legitimize state presence in a religious domain and facilitated the political surveillance of pilgrims and *pandas* in the name of public health. Furthermore, this construct of the pilgrim provided the perfect scapegoat that detracted from the colonial sanitary administration's inadequacies and failings and lent legitimacy to the colonial project.

Notes

1 Laurie Garrett and Maxine Builder, 'The Middle East Plague Goes Global', *Foreign Policy*, 28 (June 2013).
2 Saurabh Mishra, *Pilgrimage, Politics and Pestilence: The Haj from the Indian Subcontinent 1860–1920*, New Delhi: Oxford University Press, 2011.
3 A.H. Leith, *Abstract of the Proceedings of the International Conference of 1866*, Bombay, 1867, 14.
4 Ibid., 10.
5 Ibid., 20–1.
6 In the interest of brevity and readability I am using the term 'pilgrim' to signify the way in which colonial discourse constructs both pilgrims and *sadhus* and *pandas* (priests) who travelled to pilgrimage sites. The archetype of the dirty and irrational pilgrim reflects how pilgrims as well as priests figured in the imagination of the colonial state.
7 See for instance David Arnold, 'Smallpox and Colonial Medicine in Nineteenth-Century India', in David Arnold (ed.), *Imperial Medicine and Indigenous Societies*, Manchester: Manchester University Press, 1988, 45–65; David Arnold, 'Cholera and Colonialism in British India', *Past and Present*, 113 (1986), 118–51; Mark Harrison, *Public Health in British India: Anglo-Indian Preventive Medicine 1859–1914*, Cambridge: Cambridge University Press, 1994, 107.

8 I am drawing on the official translations of vernacular newspapers that were authorized by the colonial state mainly as a means to take the pulse of political developments on the ground. While the literate population in India was not large, vernacular newspapers had a wide 'readership' as often newspapers were read aloud in groups allowing the not-literate sections of the population to partake. Indeed, the fact that the state set up a department to survey, monitor and translate selections from these newspapers in itself points to their value as a reliable means to gauge popular sentiment.

9 For an overview of the critique of the official stance on cholera see the debate between the Sanitary Commissioner for the GOI and the Sanitary Commissioner for Panjab. Harrison, *Public Health*, 100–5.

10 *Annual Report of the Sanitary Commissioner with the Government of India 1867*, Calcutta: Government Press, 1868, 8 [hereafter *Report of Sanitary Commissioner GOI*].

11 *Report of Sanitary Commissioner GOI 1867*, 3.

12 Ibid., 5–7.

13 NWP General Proceedings A, August 1867, Proceedings 122–3, India Office Records [hereafter IOR]: P/438/30.

14 *Report of Sanitary Commissioner GOI 1867*, 130.

15 NWP General Proceedings A, August 1867, Proceedings 122–3, IOR: P/438/30.

16 Quoted in Katherine Prior, 'The British Administration of Hinduism in North India, 1780–1900', Cambridge University Ph.D. thesis, 1990, 187.

17 *Report of Sanitary Commissioner GOI 1867*, 137.

18 David Arnold and Radhika Ramasubban have argued that the institution of public health in India in fact emerged out of concern for the health of the army. See David Arnold, *Colonizing the Body: State Medicine and Epidemic Disease in Nineteenth-Century India*, Berkeley: University of California Press, 1993; Radhika Ramasubban, 'Public Health and Medical Research', Swedish Agency for Research Cooperation with Developing Countries Working Paper, 1982.

19 *Report of Sanitary Commissioner GOI 1867*, 18.

20 Report on the Hardwar Fair by F. Williams, Commissioner of Meerut: NWP General Proceedings A, August 1867, Proceedings 122–4, IOR: P/438/30.

21 NWP General Proceedings A, August 1867, Proceeding 127, IOR: P/438/30. Note that this critique drew on colonial discourse of smell signifying disease and used it to challenge the measures introduced by the administration.

22 *Report of Sanitary Commissioner GOI 1867*, 18.

23 *Rohilcund Ukhbar*, 7 Dec. 1867, *Selections from the Vernacular Newspapers for the Punjab, NWP, Oudh and Central Provinces* [hereafter *SVN*], 1868, IOR: L/R/5/45.

24 *Rohilcund Ukhbar*, 7 Dec. 1867, *SVN* 1868, IOR: L/R/5/45.

25 *Report of Sanitary Commissioner NWP 1878*, 43–4.

26 NWP Sanitary Proceedings A, September 1879, Proceeding 6, IOR: P/1280.

27 Ibid.

28 Ibid.

29 Ibid.

30 *Almora Akhbar* 1 May 1879, *SVN* 1879, IOR: L/R/5/56.
31 NWP Sanitary Proceedings A, September 1879, Proceeding 8, IOR: P/1280.
32 NWP Sanitary Proceedings A, September 1879, Proceeding 9, IOR: P/1280.
33 *Annual Report of the Sanitary Commissioner with the Government of NWP 1881*, Allahabad: Government Press, 1882, 44 [hereafter: *Report of Sanitary Commissioner NWP*].
34 'Cholera at the Allahabad Fair in 1882, and Its Dissemination Through the Surrounding Districts by Pilgrims,' in *Proceedings of the Allahabad Medical Society*, 1, 5 (October 1882), 140.
35 *Report of Sanitary Commissioner NWP 1881*, 50.
36 *Hindi Pradip*, Jan 1882, *SVN* 1882, IOR: L/R/5/59.
37 *Sahas*, 28 Jan 1882, *SVN* 1882, IOR: L/R/5/59.
38 NWP Miscellaneous Proceedings A, May 1890, Proceeding 1, IOR: P/3597.
39 *Hindustan*, 8 February 1890, *SVN* 1890; *Prayag Samachar*, 10 Feb 1890, also attributed the outbreak to 'burial of all filth underground at the fair', *SVN* 1890, IOR: L/R/5/67.
40 *Report of Sanitary Commissioner NWP 1891*, 18A.
41 Ibid., 22A.
42 Ibid., 27A.
43 Ibid., 22A.
44 *Hindustan*, 17 April 1891, *SVN* 1891, IOR: L/R/5/68.
45 *Report of Sanitary Commissioner NWP 1891*, 22A.
46 NWP Miscellaneous Proceedings A, January1892, Proceeding 14, IOR: P/4061.
47 NWP Miscellaneous Proceedings A, January1892, Proceeding 17, IOR: P/4061.
48 NWP Miscellaneous Proceedings A, January1893, Proceeding 2a, IOR: P/4296.
49 *Gosewak* 22 December 1892, *SVN* 1892, IOR: L/R/5/69.
50 NWP General Proceedings A, March 1893, Proceeding 77, IOR: P/4294.
51 Ibid.
52 Ibid.
53 NWP Miscellaneous Proceedings A, January1893, Proceeding 2a, IOR: P/4296.
54 Ibid.
55 See *Subodh Sindhu*, 19 April 1892, *Bharat Jiwan*, 23 May 1892, *SVN* 1892, IOR: L/R/5/69.
56 *Rahbar*, 1 July 1892, *SVN* 1892, IOR: L/R/5/69.
57 *Rahbar*, 24 April 1892, *SVN* 1892, IOR: L/R/69.
58 *Bharat Jiwan*, 5 September 1892, *SVN* 1892, IOR: L/R/5/69.
59 *Oudh Samachar*, 7 August 1901, *SVN* 1901, IOR: L/R/5/78.
60 This was a grievance that was voiced very often in the vernacular press, see for instance *Hindustan*, 27 April 1893, *SVN* 1893, IOR: L/R/5/70.
61 NWP Miscellaneous Proceedings A, May 1893, Proceeding 69, IOR: P/4296.
62 Ian J. Kerr, 'Reworking a Popular Religious Practice: The Effects of Railways on Pilgrimage in 19th and 20th Century South Asia', in Ian J. Kerr

(ed.), *Railways in Modern India*, New Delhi: Oxford University Press, 2001, 316.

63 *Annual Report of the Sanitary Commissioner with the Government of Panjab 1879*, Lahore: Government Press, 35. In 1912 the GOI suggested appointing special committees in the provinces to consider ways to improve the sanitary state of pilgrimage sites. The resulting reports of the Committees for United Provinces (1913), Bihar and Orissa (1913), Madras (1915) and Bombay (1916) all dedicated significant space to documenting the deficient nature of sanitary arrangements made by railway companies catering to pilgrim traffic. Both the committees for UP and Bihar and Orissa noted that they were 'inundated' with complaints about how pilgrims travelling by rail were treated. *Report of the Pilgrim Committee, United Provinces, 1913*, Simla: Government Central Branch Press, 1916, 40; *Report of the Pilgrim Committee, Bihar & Orissa, 1913*, Simla: Government Central Branch Press, 1915, 31.

64 *Report of Sanitary Commissioner GOI 1867*, 20–3.

65 Ibid., 18.

66 NWP General Proceedings A, August 1867, Proceedings 122–3, IOR: P/438/30.

67 *Report of Sanitary Commissioner NWP 1881*, 49.

68 NWP General Proceedings A, October 1882, Proceeding 68, IOR: P/1812.

69 *Report on the Sanitary Arrangements at the Gurhmooktessur Fair of 1868*, Allahabad: Government Press, 1869.

70 NWP General Proceedings A, October 1882, Proceeding 65, IOR: P/1812.

71 See for instance NWP Miscellaneous Proceedings A, May 1890, Proceeding 12, IOR: P/3597.

72 NWP General Proceedings A, August1883, Proceeding 19, IOR: P/1996.

73 J.A. Turner and B.K. Goldsmith, *Sanitation in India*, Bombay: Times of India, 1922, 938–9.

74 NWP Sanitary & Medical Proceedings A, June 1894, Proceeding 40, IOR: P/4506.

75 NWP General Proceedings A, August 1867, Proceeding 124, IOR: P/438/30.

76 William Robert Cornish, *Report on Cholera in Southern India for the Year 1869*, Madras: Morgan, 1870, 149–50.

77 *Annual Report of the Sanitary Commissioner with the Government of United Provinces 1915*, Allahabad: Government Press, 1916, 22.

78 NWP General Proceedings A, February 1880, Proceedings 66–7, IOR: P/1458.

79 NWP Miscellaneous Proceedings A, June 1891, Proceeding 3, IOR: P/3829.

80 Ibid.

81 NWP General Proceedings A, July 1883, Proceeding 4, IOR: P/1996.

82 NWP Miscellaneous Proceedings A, July 1902, Proceeding 8, IOR: P/6295. Other communities were also stigmatized as 'dirty'. In the context of pilgrimage in Orissa, low-caste Bengali women were seen as carriers of disease; their presence in large numbers at pilgrimage sites was considered the cause for cholera outbreaks during fairs. Charles Banks, *Observations on Epidemics of Cholera in India with Special Reference to Their Immediate Connection with Pilgrimages*, Cuttack, 1896.

83 Arnold, *Colonizing the Body*, 185.
84 Leith, *Abstract of Proceedings of International Conference*, 14.
85 Banks, *Observations on Epidemics of Cholera*.
86 Pamela Gilbert notes some other groups of Indians were also seen as threats to public health in the official mind. Coolie labour gangs were seen as transmitters of disease as they were migratory labour. But she notes that they 'were more problematic scapegoats [compared to pilgrims] since they were following the labour market created by British industry and agriculture'. Pamela Gilbert, *Mapping the Victorian Social Body*, Albany, NY: SUNY Press, 2004, 167.
87 Kama Maclean, 'Making the Colonial State Work for You: The Modern Beginnings of the Ancient *Kumbh Mela* in Allahabad', *The Journal of Asian Studies*, 62, 3 (2003), 882–3.
88 Anand Yang, *The Limited Raj: Agrarian Relations in Colonial India, Saran District, 1793–1920*, Berkeley: University of California Press, 1989, 18. Even in the twentieth century pilgrimage sites were used as platforms and recruiting grounds by various political movements; Nandini Gooptu points out that the 1928–29 Kumbh mela at Allahabad was a prominent site for the propagation and proclamation of Adi Hinduism, an anti-caste movement. N. Gooptu, 'Caste and Labour: Untouchable Social Movements in Urban Uttar Pradesh in the Early Twentieth Century', in Peter Robb (ed.), *Dalit Movements and the Meaning of Labour in India*, Oxford: Oxford University Press, 1993, 289; for the Kumbh mela as a site for nationalist propaganda see Kama Maclean, *Pilgrimage and Power: The Kumbh Mela in Allahabad, 1765–1954*, Oxford: Oxford University Press 2008, 145–90.
89 Veena Talwar Oldenburg, *The Making of Colonial Lucknow, 1856–1877*, Princeton: Princeton University Press 1984, xv.
90 Nomadic tribes, such as the Banjaras, were criminalized. See Ian J. Kerr, 'On the Move: Circulating Labor in Pre-Colonial, Colonial and Post-Colonial India', in Ran P. Behal and Marcel Van Der Linden (eds.), *Coolies, Capital and Colonialism: Studies in Indian Labour History*, Cambridge: Cambridge University Press, 2007, 100.
91 Harrison, *Public Health*, 105.
92 Ibid., 166.
93 *UP Pilgrim Committee Report*, 64.
94 See for instance Letter from Commissioner Jhansi Division to the Secretary of Government, UP, dated 8 May 1926, in Notes and Orders Regarding the Pilgrim Committee's Recommendations about Conservancy. Uttar Pradesh State Archives, File 416E, Box 326.
95 Arnold, *Colonizing the Body*, 188.

5 Western science, indigenous medicine and the princely states

The case of Ayurvedic reorganization in Travancore, 1870–1940

Burton Cleetus

This chapter seeks to address the process of indigenous therapeutic reorganization in the princely state of Travancore under colonial dominance. Questions concerning the attitude of princely states towards social modernization, in comparison to those of the British presidencies, have evinced profound interest among scholars working on the different state systems in India.[1] One basic premise from which such enquiries emerged was the realization that the princely states used tradition as a powerful means towards consolidating their legitimacy as well as offering a cultural resistance to the colonial state. Thus what was witnessed within most parts of princely India was the active intervention and engagement by the princely states towards consolidating and repositioning art, architecture, music, dance and medicine, which were deemed essential parts of the collective cultural past of the Indian subcontinent, to which the nineteenth-century princes laid claim. Barbara Ramusack remarks that 'the princely patronage of religious specialist and institutions, visual and performing arts, luxury crafts, secular scholarship, and sports will reveal how princes fostered cultural nationalism while fulfilling their princely dharma'.[2] Such attempts at installing tradition also went alongside a vigorous attempt at administrative modernization and the introduction of Western medical, educational and technological institutions. The twin agenda of modernization through the introduction of Western institutions while building a network of elaborate cultural symbols and forms was seen as a way of consolidating legitimacy in an age in which status, rights and political power were fluid, and perceived to be under threat from the overarching reach of the colonial state.[3] Princely India therefore witnessed a new configuration of ideas and institutions, deemed cultural and traditional, which coexisted alongside Western networks of bureaucratic state-centred institutions.

By the latter half of the nineteenth century, princely India witnessed active intervention from the ruling dispensation to structure administrative machinery and to modernize institutions of the state. An active revival, restructuring and institutionalization of art forms and therapeutic practices considered essential to a broader Hindu religious and nationalist identity was undertaken. The institutionalization and reorganization of the state and the elaboration of rituals also enabled locally bounded princely states to extend and lay claim to a new identity, which was both nationally and religiously bounded. While the elaboration and the institutionalization of cultural forms in art, dance and music generated a new genre of tradition, it was in the domain of traditional medicine that a crisis emerged, which the state both in colonial and postcolonial contexts found it difficult to overcome.

Studies on state policies both within British India and in the princely states brought to light the wide gap between state objectives and their actual realization at the level of policy implementation. Though the state connected disparate practices, 'classical' and 'local' practices were transformed through negotiation and restructuring at multiple levels. As the modern state system is based on a constellation of ideas and practices that connected the state to its subjects and vice versa, during the late nineteenth and twentieth century, its principal collaborators among the social elites were repositioning themselves in relation to the changing values of modernization. The state thus introduced and familiarized new cultural motifs that emerged from the desires of the social elites. State sanction for such motifs also ensured that they received official recognition as well as a wider reach, for such images could be replicated throughout the institutional structures of the state. The state revived and reinstalled certain rituals and rites, and the elaboration and extension of such rituals allowed the state to extend its power and influence over its subjects. Hence, state attempts at modernization were channelled by the desires of elites in a changing social system. However, the capacity of the state to control and reorganize practices through institutional structures raises questions about the character of the state and the manner in which it was able to regulate and control the knowledge forms, institutions and therefore the lives of its subjects. The state therefore remained as a central regulatory authority and pivotal structure through which the dissemination of knowledge forms was made possible. Medicine was a significant cultural motif as both the social elites and those desirous of a higher position within the social order embraced text-bound classical traditions as a means to ascend the social hierarchy.[4] Yet institutionalization and extension of the text-bound medical knowledge posed serious questions about the introduction and extension of science by the Travancore state, which considered itself to be 'progressive', modernist and receptive to Western science and technology.

By the closing decades of the nineteenth century, Travancore, a region within the southwestern part of the Indian subcontinent, emerged as an important space in which social modernization progressed significantly. In the domain of medicine, this became evident, paradoxically, in the mandatory imposition of classical Sanskrit texts like *Charaka Samhita, Sushruta Samhita, Ashtangahridhayam* and their later commentaries from which Ayurveda had to be practised. Even when the classical texts emerged as the envisaged fulcrum for the dissemination of indigenous medical knowledge, the difference between state-supported 'classical' medicine and 'local' practices was constrained by the limitations imposed by the state.

Institutionalization and state-organized dissemination of Ayurvedic knowledge was constrained by alternative understandings of the body familiarized by Western medicine. Though the integration of anatomical and physiological knowledge familiarized by Western medicine into the indigenous medical tradition was desired, there remained difficult questions about its compatibility with the theoretical understanding of the body in classical Ayurvedic medicine, especially the role of the five elements or *panchamahabhootam*, the three energies (*doshas*) and the seven elements (*datus*). The constitution of the body, its etiology and physiology were incompatible with Western medical understandings of the body and its ailments. Even when the proponents of the state and reformers in medicine confidently asserted the possibility of integration between Western medicine and Ayurveda, being guided by a belief in the universality of science, the integration of different epistemic structures failed to materialize.

One the major concerns about institutionalization was that it made medicine distant from the cultural beliefs in which it had been formerly located. The human body, its ailments and cures, were part of a larger cosmology.[5] The institutionalization of medicine was also driven by the aim of secularizing Ayurveda, constituting it as a system of medicine that was devoid of cultural beliefs. The reformulation processes that happened in India under colonial dominance were seen as a form of resistance by those engaged in the reform of medical practice. K.N. Panikkar writes that reformers in medicine were not blinded by tradition but critically engaged with both Western medicine and the classical texts in creating a new paradigm for Ayurveda.[6] Deepak Kumar also argues that, even in resistance, there was an implicit acceptance of the standards set by the colonizer.[7] Both Kumar and Panikkar recognize the significance of Western medicine as a hegemonic epistemic practice and argue that modernization of Ayurveda essentially meant the reorganization of the practice in accordance with the changing contexts of modernity. One needs to look at integration beyond the frameworks of resistance and accommodation, which had predominated the thinking of Ayurveda. As Kavita Philip remarks, attempts to locate social change through the framework of protest and resistance have often undermined the nuances of transformation.[8] What is significant is the manner in which colonial standards came to be accepted and integrated into the domain of medicine. Though Travancore was a regional entity, modernization of Ayurveda reflected the state's attempt to become part of a nationalist identity that located itself within a larger Hindu cosmology, in which social status, identity and political power were classically defined.

Recent scholarship on the history of Western science has questioned attempts to locate the global and the local as unrelated and distinct entities. Kapil Raj argues that the global was shaped by close interaction with the local and non-European knowledge forms and practices were integral to the emergence of Western science.[9] Mark Harrison argues that the colonies also opened up important spaces for investigation and experimentation in Western science and medicine.[10] Projit Bihari Mukharji argues that hybridization of Western and Indian medicine resulted in multiple modernities, in which different versions of Western medicine and indigenous medicine emerged in various contexts.[11] Mukharji and Hardiman's work on medical marginality further challenges the division between Western medicine, text-bound Ayurveda and localized forms of medicine.[12]

One important question emerging from this scholarship is the relationship between state-centred institutionalized medical practices and local healthcare traditions. While the need to integrate Western medical practices remained central to the concerns of the policy makers and those of the state with regard to Ayurveda, the standards that defined Western science also became the basic framework through which Ayurveda was understood. This prioritized homogeneity and hierarchy, and the need to produce knowledge through rational and materially grounded enquiries. One of the central elements of this programme was the need to define therapeutic practices using classical texts such as the *Charaka Samhita*, *Sushruta Samhita*, *Ashatangahridhayam* and their later commentaries.

Colonialism in its Indian context established benchmarks for the ways in which the state, nation, bureaucracy, systems of enumeration, maintenance of records, revenue collection, education, census and the past came to be figured. Writing on European states and society in the post-Enlightenment era, Foucault argues that medicine acquired an important position in the 'administrative system and the machinery of power';[13] similarly, though indigenous medical knowledge was one among the many forms of knowledge disseminated from the state to its subjects, the role of healthcare, as a means of saving and disciplining sick bodies, emerged as an important arena in which the state could exercise social control and governance, and thus articulate its sovereignty.[14] In an age in which princely states were considered by the British to be remnants of the old feudal order, they sought to distance themselves from such stereotypical representations. One way of doing so was to make fundamental changes in the administrative structures of the state, on the model prevailing in the British Indian provinces, so that they were seen as front runners of change and modernity. The princely states also considered the sustenance and modernization of indigenous cultural traditions as forms through which sovereignty was extended within their geographical domain. Accordingly, by the latter half of the twentieth century, states like Baroda, Mysore, Travancore and Punjab came to be considered as models due to their increasing affinity with Western knowledge and their huge investments in infrastructure, education and healthcare.[15]

The emergence of Travancore as a model state under colonial constraints reflected the intensity with which this princely state adhered to standards of administrative reorganization expected of modern state systems. Yet the changes introduced in the princely states, though seemingly alike, differed fundamentally in certain measures, in comparison with those of the British presidencies. This was because of its use of classical symbols in consolidating sovereignty, as well as a means of resistance against the domineering influence of British colonialism. Philip argues that this was a counter-hegemonic strategy, designed to carve out and maintain the social self, so that it would not be lost to the principles of colonialism.[16] The history of the reorganization process is therefore replete with contestations, integration and the further reformulation of a hybridized identity for indigenous medicine. While it is generally recognized that from the mid-nineteenth century onwards, across the subcontinent, there were conscious efforts by the state, individuals, organizations and groups towards repositioning Ayurveda in accordance with the epistemic paradigms familiarized by Western medicine, Kavita Sivaramakrishnan argues that such endeavours were primarily a reflection of the aspirations of the new social classes within the changing social order brought about by modernity.[17] Desire for social aspirations did play a significant role in shaping knowledge forms and repositioning identities. However, the extent to which modern institutional structures redefined the practice remains questionable. Apologists for institutionalization argued that while there was integration of Western medical paradigms into the domain of Ayurveda, in terms of familiarizing new understandings of the body, bringing about advanced pharmaceutical methods of production and standardization, or disseminating it through an organized curriculum, Ayurveda remained essentially the same in terms of diagnosis and etiology; and that the production of drugs continued to be based on the classical texts and their commentaries.[18]

However, those opposed to the changes argued that these institutional changes fundamentally altered the basic character of Ayurveda and created a hybridized identity that deviated in a large measure from its essential character. The underlying logic of those who argued in favour of the *shuddha* (pure) and *mishra* (integrated) Ayurveda was that contemporary Ayurvedic medicine was a failure as local physicians had deviated from the texts. Thus, those who argued in favour of pure or integrated Ayurveda based their premise on a realization of failure in the present; classical Ayurveda, however, was regarded as scientific, and it was thought that this tradition should be reinstated as a scientific enterprise. The debate between the *shudda* and *mishra* in Ayurveda failed to engage with the idea of the 'authentic' and 'integrated' and how the notion of the authentic was brought about by concerns that were generated within the contexts of colonial modernity. Thus, as Paul Brass notes, 'while revivalist leaders had great respect for the truly competent traditional physicians, for their abilities to heal, and for the traditional guru-disciple system of teaching, the primary orientation of the supporters of Ayurveda was towards the revival, restoration, and further development of ancient science rather than to the maintenance of contemporary traditional practices.'[19] Secondly, the project of integration was often beset with problems as attempts to institutionalize the practice in accordance with the standards and principles of Western science and medicine was negotiated through complex relationships that often undermined the state's efforts to institutionalize.

The princely state in modern parlance was seen to reflect the 'collective will' of the people against the domineering influence of Western medicine and colonialism. However, in its relationship with British colonialism, proponents of the state realized that the colonial presence could not be easily discarded; rather, the newly emerging cultural contexts of the late nineteenth and twentieth centuries were based on a nuanced relationship that was defined both through similarities as well as differences with the West. While similarity was depicted through an affinity towards administrative modernization by incorporating Western knowledge forms and practices within its domain, difference was highlighted by maintaining a culture based on Sanskrit symbols and forms.[20] Though such imagery was created without controversy in the domain of arts, the possibility of creating an indigenous therapeutic domain was replete with problems.

As the state emerged as the prime agency for preserving and sustaining tradition, it had to reposition the cultural symbols necessary to actualize desires for social mobility. This was in tune with the interests of the emerging social elite, whose redefined economic status within nineteenth- and early twentieth-century Travancore demanded an elevated social position. Such desires for social mobilization shaped the way in which cultural identities came to be reconstituted in princely India. Though open to Western ideas of change and modernity, the proponents of the state channelled and shaped tradition as possible frameworks through which state and society could be reorganized and represented. Thus, the reframing of tradition emerged in response to demands made by the dominant section of society, to which the Travancore state responded positively as it believed that state sovereignty rested on the support of emerging social elites. Hence, it was a two-way process – while the support extended by the social elites was essential for the indigenous state system in an age of emerging nationalism, state initiatives in the repositioning of cultural symbols as tradition aimed to satisfy the desires and expectations of its preferred subjects. As Charles Leslie observes, the reorganization of indigenous medicine was fundamentally aimed at adopting institutional forms, concepts and medications from Western medicine.[21] This re-creation, codification, reorganization and the consequent dissemination of a classical Hindu tradition and culture, primarily through the language of Sanskrit, was based on the premise that a revived classical culture represented indigenous society in terms of its culture, truth and identity.[22]

This new version of tradition was, nevertheless, far removed from the socio-cultural life of most Indians. In Travancore such desires for social mobility were represented through an engagement with various art forms such as music, dance, fine arts and medicine among many others, and also in the reformulation of Malayalam as a language, by defining through an engagement with the Sanskrit textual tradition. Lloyd Rudolph and Susanne Rudolph argue that the key objectives of the Indian princely rulers were to preserve and protect social formations that existed prior to the state, such as the customs, castes, sects, status orders and guilds.[23] Contrary to what Rudolph and Rudolph argue, the princely states, though not keen on altering social norms and practices in the context of social modernization and administrative reforms, accepted that the reorganized and repositioned tradition was, to a larger measure, distinct from the social arrangements of an older era. Underlined by the changing contours of state and society, pre-state caste structures, occupational patterns and priorities underwent fundamental change. In this new context, the state realized the necessity of repositioning itself in accordance with the norms of modern state structures, familiarized by the colonial presence.

By the mid-nineteenth century, Travancore state abolished the *Ootupura* system, a practice of providing free meals to the Brahmans, and the utensils were transferred to the Ayurveda College for the preparation of drugs.[24] This reflects the larger picture of the changing state preferences in the new context and the changing status of tradition. Hence, the key objective was not merely to preserve the status of pre-state ideas and institutions but to reposition society and state in accordance with the needs of the emerging socio-political contexts generated under colonial conditions. The state had to present itself as a distinct entity with roots in the past, as well as being receptive to change: a dual identity that could be bridged through a reworking of tradition. Partha Chatterjee argues that colonized societies had to incorporate material aspects of the European world in their projects of reorganization, while maintaining a distinct spiritual essence, in order to prevent the erosion of their national identity.[25]

Tradition therefore became a powerful mode of resistance; it encompassed different shades of power that could be wielded against colonialism. Rejuvenated traditions could redefine power relations between indigenous states and colonial authorities. In the context of indigenous state reorganization in Travancore, what occurred was not a preservation of tradition but the constitution of an alternative practice as tradition, organized above the cultural practices of the contemporary society.[26] The new medical practice that was constituted from this emerged as different and distinct from those practised within indigenous society. The question remains, as Andrew Brennan asks: once matter is displaced from its cultural context does it still have meaning?[27]

Scholars analyzing the changing status of health and healthcare in the colonial context often sought to locate the process of reorganization in a nationalist framework, as a form of resistance against the domineering influence of Western medicine.[28] Though it was a sense of marginalization, defined through national boundaries, which forced proponents of indigenous medicine to embark on a process of therapeutic modernization, the privileging of the idea of the nation in healthcare practices under colonial conditions had lasting impact on the future of Indians. Such metanarratives of the nation led to the homogenization of tendencies and neglect of the multiple relationships that existed within the Indian therapeutic domain. What was overlooked was the question of caste, as a unit of social division, in shaping cultural patterns and therapeutic practices in a society in which dissemination of knowledge was shaped by the constraints of Sanskrit language, within which the textual tradition was codified. However, there were attempts by members of the lower castes to argue that a Sanskrit-based textual tradition had been widespread in pre-colonial society, irrespective of caste differentiation.[29]

The indigenous healthcare practices of Travancore, during the period under study, included many that were intermingled with the belief systems of contemporary society, including specialized methods of treatment like *Vishavaidyam* (treatment for poison), *Marmavaidyam* (massage), *Manthram* (exorcism), *Jyothisham* (astrology) and so forth, which were accompanied by specialized forms of treatment methods like *Ottamoolichikilsa* (a single medicine which was supposed to have magical powers and which could be used as a panacea for all ills), *Yukti Chikilsa* (treatment through logic), *Kaipunyam* (divine powers possessed by the vaidyan) and others, underlining the predominance of the physician in locating the disease, in contrast to the sort of predominance that the classical tradition came to acquire in defining what constitutes 'the indigenous' in the late nineteenth century. A synoptic view of contemporary healthcare practices is presented in the census of India, 1901, which states that:

> the astrologer, the exorcist and the physician were 'all in attendance' at the sick bed of a person. The astrologer divined the causes and prescribed propitiatory remedies; the exorcist performed a ceremony to drive out the demons and spirits and finally the physician or vaidyan treated the patient.[30]

It is in this domain of the indigenous that the state sought to reorganize health practices. Captivated by a belief in the classical tradition, members of the princely state of Travancore state like kilamanoor, Attingal and Kodungaloor like Ananthapurathu Moothakoil

Thampuran, harippad Rajaraja varma Moothakoil Thampuram and others stepped in to disseminate sanskrit based textual tradition to the wider society. In this, caste differences were often overlooked to an extent, as attempts were made to engage with an emerging social elite amongst the Ezhavas and other subordinate castes who were hitherto considered as untouchables.[31] Such initiatives had an over-bearing influence on the circulation of forms of knowledge. Castes other than Brahmans like the Ambalavasis and Nairs, and even lower castes like the Ezhavas who learnt classical knowledge in medicine, in turn, disseminated the same to the members of their own community. The transition to a text-based tradition among caste groups who occupied subordinate positions within the social hierarchy was also possible due to the desire amongst the lower-caste groups to climb the social ladder through the strength of tradition. Secondly, almost all social groups within the state practised medicine locally, which made it relatively easy for castes to attain upward mobility. Given the significance of the indigenous state system that aimed to encompass different sections of its population within its ambit, it sought to ensure that textual knowledge in medicine had a wider circulation, which within the larger domain of social relations of the nineteenth century, without the intervention of the state system, was difficult to realize. Thus, the state as a new centre of power functioned as an intermediary between those who possessed textual knowledge about healthcare and the majority members of the non-caste groups in transgressing knowledge and practices in the nineteenth-century colonial context.

Centralized dissemination of knowledge forms in medicine, and its institutionalization under the aegis of the state, based largely on the Ashtangahridaya text, had multiple objectives. Prime among them was the need to constitute an authentic version of healthcare, and therefore tradition, which the Travancore state claimed to represent. Those practitioners who did not adhere to a centralized and unified system of medical practice based on the Sanskrit textual tradition were considered to be quacks as their presence was deemed to question the basic structure of a unified edifice marked by an assertion of indigenous cultural forms. As C.A. Bayly argues,

> Oriental scholarship was not a homogenous mode of gaining power over India. It was rather an arena of debate in which the more powerful – the British and the Indian elites – attempted to appropriate themes and symbols which suited the political needs and chimed with features of their intellectual culture.[32]

Similarly, in colonial Travancore, while the reconstituted Ayurveda had on the one hand sought to distance itself from the multiple health-care practices of indigenous society, the proponents of this medical practice had to seek legitimacy by defining it through Western medical categories.

Organized dissemination: the emergence of the patasala

The establishment of the Ayurveda Patasala was a major step towards the realization of the state's objective to cross the epistemological boundaries that separated Ayurvedic medical knowledge and Western medicine. As the demand for the new Ayurvedic practice increased, and as the palaces could no longer accommodate the increasing number of students, the system of Ayurvedic schools was transplanted from the palaces to the Ayurveda *Patasala* or schools. This move also reflected the perceived need to disseminate indigenous medicine as an institutional and scientific knowledge through an organized curriculum. A new notion of governance also emphasized that 'it is the bounden duty of the state to create an atmosphere favourable to the maintenance of at least a minimum standard of professional efficiency among the practitioners of (our) Indian systems'.[33] The establishment of the Ayurveda Patasala at Trivandrum in 1889 and the introduction of the grant-in-aid in 1896 were important stages towards the realization of this end.[34]

However, by the late nineteenth century, Ayurvedic learning moved out of the palaces and came to be disseminated through the patasala established by the state in Trivandrum and also by individual initiatives in other regions of the state. Proficiency in Sanskrit was considered a basic criterion for admission to these schools, in the hope that once students were familiarized with all the classical Sanskrit texts, an authentic and scientific version of Ayurveda could be constituted.[35] This was primarily because it was believed that all knowledge of indigenous society was embedded within a tradition that was defined through classical Sanskrit texts. The underlying belief was that the patasala would function both as a means of dissemination of knowledge as well as the space through which institutionalization of indigenous medicine could be actualized. Similarly, the objective of the Ayurveda Patasala was to create a new generation of practitioners who would not merely able to possess the 'authentic form' of Ayurvedic medical practice, but would, in turn, propagate it within society. Though the basic objective of the patasala system was to enable a return to the classical past, it was soon realized that the pressing need of such institutionalization processes should also be to define the classical in accordance with notions of health, science and medicine popularized by Western medicine. Nonetheless, Ayurvedic instruction imparted through the patasala, based exclusively on Sanskrit, failed in defining indigenous bodily understandings akin to those of Western medical categories. Based on this realization, a communication was sent to the mangers of the Ayurveda schools in 1904 instructing that:

> students should be taught western medical system also so that they would be able to have a conceptual knowledge about both the western forms of understandings of the human body and its pathology, as well as what is enunciated by the ancient Ayurvedic texts. They should be given training in surgery and midwifery . . . As per the new syllabus modern anatomy and its laboratory practical training has to be imparted to the students, and for this, the services of an Allopathic doctor has to be made available in all Ayurvedic schools.[36]

Though the prospects for collaboration between both systems of knowledge remained uncertain, it was expected that by the introduction of Western science and medicine, the patasala would, in the long run, produce a synthesis between the two streams of medical practice. Over time, however, it was realized that the classical tradition disseminated through the Ayurveda Patasala had failed in its objectives of formulating a scientific domain for 'the indigenous' by incorporating standards of Western medicine into the classical. It was soon felt that a radical change in the form and content of the overall teaching and practice of Ayurveda was needed. The proponents of change were harping on the idea of science as a mode of rational enquiry to be incorporated into the textual tradition. Demanding urgent change, the committee for the reconstitution of the Ayurveda Patasala argued that:

> Ayurveda is based upon the properties of the irreducible living protoplasmic cells. Many of our ancestors had spent their lifetime in the study of this science. The valuable truth discovered by them had been by our negligence drowned in the sea of oblivion. The little that remains had to withstand the ravages of a series of predatory invader systems of foreign medicine. The survival of this system after the death struggle is in itself a sufficient proof of its soundness and efficacy. Research work in this department will surely increase the stock of knowledge and add to the material prosperity.[37]

The demand for research and reorganization of Ayurveda was therefore based on an understanding of the reverse flow of history, wherein the present was seen as a failed representation of the past. Such an understanding was familiarized by James Mill in his multi-volume *History of British India*,[38] and remained in colonial discourse leading to the establishment of a powerful branch of ancient Indian learning known as Indology. Indian social reform movements and nationalist assertions were premised on this assertion of the reverse flow of history and aimed to correct the past by repositioning the contemporary in accordance with the notions of science and modernity familiarized by Western science and medicine.

There was a growing conviction among the reformers of the indigenous therapeutic domain that the inculcation of Western medicine and science into the curriculum would enable students to understand the scientific notions ingrained in the Ayurvedic texts better. Yet, in the academic practice of knowledge dissemination through the Ayurveda Patasala, the principles of Western science and medicine remained distinct from those of Ayurvedic textual knowledge, even though attempts were made towards the integration of both. There were also doubts about the success of the patasala experiment, as the dominant belief was that as far as its basic objective of defining Ayurvedic medical categories in biomedical terms was concerned, it was heading towards failure. It was this that prompted the Director of the Ayurveda Patasala in Trivandrum to make a polemical attack on the existing system of Ayurvedic instruction. In a letter addressed to the Principal of Ayurveda he pointed out that:

> The students who were given admission to the patasala were those who have had no benefit of a liberal education. Their stock of knowledge derived solely from *Sanskrit Kavyas* consisted of a few exaggerated notions of an imaginary world like the proverbial lotus-eaters. They accordingly live in a dreamy life in the patasala, where their fond fancies are carefully nurtured till they come out of it to look in the world full in the face. They shrink, they fail in the unequal combat, and the failure is naturally attributed to the system of medicine of which they are exponents.[39]

The underlying belief was that the integration of the methodologies of Western science and medicine, in terms of their understanding of human anatomy and physiology, as well as the clinical observation of drugs and their compounds, would in the long run lead to the demonstration of indigenous medicine as science. However, the problems attached to the functioning of indigenous medicine under the influence of Western science and its societal principles resurfaced. Neither did the integration of indigenous medicine lead to a synthesis between 'systems', Western and Eastern, nor did they function in harmony, accepting or rejecting hypotheses and theories. The major step towards the realization of this objective was formulated in 1917, when a committee was established by the government of Travancore for the reorganization of the Ayurveda Patasala. One of the major demands of the committee was to restrict admission to students who had at least completed the school final course.[40] Thus entry into the new mode of Ayurveda came to be limited only to those students who had prior knowledge of Western science, with which they were supposed to understand the basic structures of Ayurveda. The students were henceforth expected to visualize Ayurveda through the metanarratives offered by Western medicine. Although the object of enquiry remained the same, the subjective perception that guided the ways in which the 'indigenous' was looked at was undergoing a fundamental transformation. David Arnold writes that Western science in India was repositioned in accordance with the beliefs and preferences of the indigenous societies.[41] Yet, the beliefs and practices were constantly evolving in accordance with the ways in which Western science was understood and positioned.

Similarly, many terms and categories that were prominent in the domain of the indigenous, in this new context, became redundant. The committee for reconstitution of the Ayurveda Patasala remarked that

> in the new context the term 'native vaidyasala', became an 'uncouth' expression, which did not connote the 'scientific aspect' of the Ayurvedic system of medicine and therefore propose[d] that the highly suggestive expression of 'Ayurveda Vaidyasala' in Malayalam and 'Ayurvedic institutions' in English be adopted in lieu of existing names.

In addition, the name of the Ayurveda Patasala became

> old and uninviting and he therefore suggested that the name of the institution be changed to 'Ayurveda College' and the designation of the Director of Ayurveda be changed into the 'Principal of Ayurveda College'. It was also desired that all further correspondence concerned with the Ayurveda College and department be made in English.[42]

As classical knowledge forms in medicine were to predominate over local healing techniques, attempts were made to translate a large number of Sanskrit texts into Malayalam, the native language of the people of the state.[43] Texts like *Ashtangahridhyam, Astangasamgraham, Suthrasthanam* and *Madhavanidhanam* were translated and various versions of such texts came to be available in the market.

In response to the report on Ayurvedic modernization, a committee was set up to reformulate the syllabus of the Ayurveda Patasala, which included prominent vaidyans trained in the *Ashtangahridaya* texts, assisted by a biomedical physician.[44] The fundamental initiatives in this regard were to rearrange curricula in such a way that 'whatever is weak in the indigenous system would be supplemented and strengthened by western system of medicine'.[45] A five-year degree course was formulated based on the expectation that:

> In the course of the 5 years of study the student is expected to gain all necessary knowledge in all sciences that would stand him in good stead and practice of Ayurveda. A detailed study of the Physical environment and their influences, the elemental construction of matter (analytical and synthetic chemistry) the biological evolution of man, specialization of organs and the differentiation of types would enable an intelligent student to understand the real meaning of the essential principles of Ayurveda based upon the natural properties of the irreducible, elemental protoplasmic cells of living bodies.[46]

There was, however, opposition to the proposed move towards institutionalization of the practice, basing itself entirely on the classical textual tradition. Opponents argued that both systems of knowledge, Western and indigenous, were in fact distinct entities with incompatible paradigms, hence the proposed attempts at integration would be futile. Similarly, there were protests against the government's move to restrict practice only to those who had received their education from formal institutions of Ayurvedic dissemination. Such voices of concern found expression even in a letter written by the Dewan of Travancore to the Chief Secretary, who contested the decision of the government to restrict contemporary therapeutic practitioners in the award of the grant. Elaborating on the problems attached to the new regulation he writes that such a sweeping restriction is not practically workable under the existing conditions of the state. He further writes that:

> the population that are not resorting to formally qualified doctors or native Vaidyans form only a very trifling proportion to the vast

number that are daily seeking relief from native Vaidyans learned in the *Ashtangahridayam* or *Chintamani* system but who holds no certificate or diplomas. This latter class of physicians is rendering inestimable services to the public in quite an ostentatious manner and at very little expense on the part of the patients . . . Each village however unimportant whether in the interior or in the towns, has its own physicians with whose service the villagers are ordinary content. Driving people to the necessity of going to a diploma holder for treatment even in petty cases such as a cold or indigestion is putting them to unnecessary trouble and expense against their will especially when the strength of medical men in the state possessing recognized qualifications is quite inadequate to the demand of medical aid. The restriction that is imposed on private Ayurvedic medical practice cannot but work hardship on the public especially the poor and the inhabitants of the country parts, not to speak of the disappointment and humiliation that will be caused to many able and deserving native physicians, who now carry on their worthy profession without holding any certificate or diplomas.[47]

Similarly, the inspector of Ayurveda expressed his dissent and stated that the arrangements and the 'initiatives taken by the government for the improvement of the indigenous medical system was not in the right direction'.[48] Protests against the standardization of the practice were expressed by communities and regions in support of practitioners who were earlier catering to the health needs of the locality. Joint petitions signed and submitted by the people from across the state demanded that indigenous practitioners who had commanded the trust and confidence of the people of the locality may be supported by state grant, and not those who had a degree from the Ayurveda schools.[49]

Botanical gardens were established for the upkeep of medicinal plants so as to enable the students to be familiar with them. These were to be made part of the process of organizing indigenous medicine through a curriculum and forms of learning.[50] The report also suggested the establishment of a committee for the revision of the curriculum, which included prominent *Ashtangahridaya* vaidyans along with a Western medical physician.[51]

The concentric system

Proponents of reform were well aware of the multiplicity of medical practices within the contemporary society of Malabar. Standardization and institutionalization under the aegis of the state was possible only by limiting the total number of drugs, and forms of enquiries on health and healthcare, within the larger domain of indigenous health. M.C. Koman, who conducted an extensive survey of the healthcare practices in the province of Madras, identified more than 8,000 forms in which fever was perceived and understood.[52] The director of Ayurveda writes that 'given the multiplicity of healing techniques, the total number of prescriptions that a vaidyan had to remember for the successful treatment of all diseases of the human system ranged from 8,000–10,000'. Institutionalization of Ayurveda was possible only by limiting the total number of therapeutic enquiries and drugs from the large number of healthcare practices of indigenous society.[53] The process of limiting the drugs and practices at the very outset visualized drugs as independent of the cultural world and belief systems that accompanied healing techniques. Named as the concentric system, the director of Ayurveda explained that the system was formulated with 'a view to build up the syllabus on a scientific basis laying considerable importance on the fundamental principles which are for the most part neglected by vaidyans who take to the practice of Ayurveda'.[54] The Director went on to elaborate that he had

made a special study of the published and unpublished available works on Ayurveda and without deviating from the general principle enunciated, assorted all medicinal plants into various groups noting with care the properties of each group according to science as far as it could help and based especially on my own experience of treatment for many years. Drugs are prepared according to these medicine groups, which form the base as it is called. These drugs prepared out of various groups can be compounded according to certain definite laws and principles, which have also been established after careful investigation. The basic preparations are supplied to the Ayurveda hospitals from the Ayurveda pharmacy and the Vaidyan in charge of the Ayurveda hospital prescribes medicines by combining two, three or four according to the conditions of the patient. Thus it is that the Vaidyan is enabled to give medicines to all patients who go to him for medical aid. According to the old and time honoured method each patient must have his own medicine prepared according to a standard prescription which will be practically impossible in a hospital where the attendance ranges from 200 to 300 per day. If the old system is followed and medicines are sent to the hospital according to that system, the medicines will have to be kept in a stock till suitable patients go for consultation. Moreover many medicines could not be kept long as they get spoilt soon. Thus there will be considerable difficulty in treating patients besides great wastage and loss . . . This is a novel system based on the science of Ayurveda and it has been found by experience that it admirably suits modern condition of life.[55]

This was at a time when in most parts of rural Travancore the patients themselves prepared drugs, in accordance to the instructions laid down by the physician. However, the introduction of pharmaceutical production techniques in the domain of indigenous healthcare, under the aegis of the state, not only sucked indigenous drugs out of their cultural domain but transformed the relationship between the physician and the patient in finding common arenas of collaboration, in terms of disease etiology and the preparation of drugs. In the new context, drugs came to be sold as over-the-counter products in contrast to the sort of relationship that was prevalent within the indigenous therapeutic domain. Such transformations were to be pushed forward through state aid and came to be known as grants-in-aid given by the state to the indigenous medical practitioners.

As a counter-strategy, people collected signatures and protested before the inspector of Ayurveda vaidyasala against the imposition of Sanskrit-based textual knowledge acquired from the government-sponsored Ayurveda Patasalas as a necessary condition for the award of the grant-in-aid.[56] They also tried to convince the administration of the mystic power yielded by the physicians who did not have formal training from government recognised Ayurveda schools and colleges.

Grants-in-aid and the disciplinary mechanisms of the state

Ayurveda as an organized academic discipline had to be not merely sustained by borrowed biomedical standards of institutionalization but had to be supported by the state, if it were to be sustained in the long run. With this objective in mind, the grant-in-aid system was introduced in order to ensure that a certain amount of money was given to Ayurvedic practitioners as state aid. Grants from the state were important for various reasons. Firstly, the grant supported practitioners in a society in which healthcare was not sustained primarily by a desire for economic advancement. Indigenous therapeutic practices were generally non-monetary in nature and it became difficult for practitioners to sustain themselves without the support of the state. Financial assistance was extended by the Travancore state to traditional practitioners as sustenance in an age of therapeutic transformation, driven by Western medicine. Grants were also made in recognition of the services of indigenous practitioners from the state as a symbol of maintaining authenticity in an age of emerging cultural nationalism. Heightened nationalism resulted in a situation in which those who did not cater to the dominant text-based tradition were regarded as aberrant, for they clearly did not display a homogenous national identity. Though the articulation of nationalism in medicine led to the revival of a tradition that claimed to be all-encompassing, in its actual practice it reinforced the idea of exclusion. While the revival and institutionalization of indigenous medicine was a nationalist response to the influence of Western medicine, the grants forced local practitioners to adhere to the norms and standards set by the state and in the long run were able to convince society to accept the Sanskrit-based tradition as sole standard of authenticity.

In 1889, detailed guidelines were issued by the government to indigenous practitioners who wished to be considered for a grant-in-aid. The minimum qualification for an award was a certificate of having passed the highest test in *Ashtangahridayam* from the medical school in Trivandrum.[57] Though it seems that the grant was, primarily, a form of sustenance for indigenous medical practitioners, it compelled them to adhere to the norms of the state. Periodic inspection notes prepared on the status of Ayurveda vaidyasalas, towards the award of aid, reflect state priorities in the award of these grants. Practitioners were directed to raise a botanical garden at the vicinity of their vaidyasala and to use medicinal plants in their practice. However, the terms and conditions defined in the award of the grant undermined relationships which hitherto existed in indigenous society. The report for the award of the grant in aid stated that all practitioners were to maintain a vaidyasala or clinic with spacious rooms, properly ventilated and in most instances in accordance with the building plan described by Perkins, who was the inspector for Ayurveda Vaidyasalas in Travancore. Practitioners were also supposed to have ready-made medicines in stock, preserved in bottles ready for public consumption. They were also supposed to maintain records of the patients treated, and at the same time, to ensure that public health concerns were addressed with diseases like cholera, malaria, plague and other contagious diseases. British personnel in the administrative structures of Travancore had a prominent role in the transformation of localized indigenous medical methods into an organized clinically bounded practice.

As Ayurvedic dissemination was undertaken through the Ayurveda Patasala, and as those who had at least a basic training in the schools were considered for the grant, those who joined the new stream of Ayurvedic practice were not necessarily from the traditional community of practitioners, and many lacked knowledge about medicinal plants and their therapeutic uses. The necessity of familiarizing the students of the Ayurveda Patasala with these plants and their medicinal uses was recognized, and a botanical garden was raised within the premises of the Ayurveda Patasala at Trivandrum. In an age of therapeutic modernization medicinal herbs thus came to be removed from their socio-cultural environment and relocated in a new 'rational' framework. Similarly, as medical practice shifted from home-based remedies to clinically bounded practice, all vaidyasalas were to have a botanical garden adjacent to them. Medicines were to be made readily available and preserved in bottles with labels pasted on them. All records of the patients treated were to be maintained with details of the diseases treated.[58]

As the state was well aware of the impact of infectious diseases on its efficiency, it relied on Western medicine for public health initiatives that aimed to combat them. Indigenous practitioners were enrolled in an attempt to supplement practitioners of Western medicine in addressing these concerns. Those indigenous practitioners who addressed contagious diseases were deemed by the state to be advanced in their understanding of health issues and were sometimes considered for grants-in-aid. But these were not always successful. Muthuswami Pillai, for example, requested state assistance on the strength of his claim that he had found a medicine for cholera and had cured patients with it.[59] The state, however, did not entertain such claims on the grounds that indigenous medicines were unable to cure contagious diseases.[60] By the 1930s, as a nationalist upsurge overtook state preferences in medicine, the state sought to gain insights from similar attempts to revive traditional medicine in the larger Indian cities, such as Calcutta, Madras, Bombay and other prominent centres of therapeutic modernization. Gopala Pillai, a student of the Ayurveda Patasala, was sent to Calcutta for training under Gananath Sen, the prominent figure in Ayurvedic reform in India. Thus, from the corridors of the palace in the mid-nineteenth century, Ayurveda emerged as an academic domain that incorporated many different practices within the subcontinent.

Conclusion

The institutionalization of Ayurveda under the aegis of the princely state in Travancore offers an interesting site in which to examine the restructuring and reordering of non-European knowledge forms and practices through the administrative structures of the state. This process raises the questions of what it means to be an institution and how states come to accept, integrate or exclude forms of knowledge and practice. In principle, the state becomes the final arbiter and regulator of practices as it reserves the right to legally validate a practice. In practice, however, institutional structures remained limited and non-institutionalized medical practitioners continued to thrive in a medical market in which multiple stakeholders coexisted. As Charles Leslie points out, the standardization 'movement was an ideological failure judged by its goals of restoring the scientific authority of ancient medical texts and of creating an autonomous medical system based upon traditional concepts and therapeutic practices'.[61] Similarly, as Guy Attewell argues in his study on the reorganization of Unani Tibb, the very notion of a ' "unani system of medicine", as it had been unreflectively termed, is a product of the colonial era – of the will to systematize, demarcate, represent knowledge and practice as a coherent whole'.[62] In reality, practices have always been more diverse.

The extent to which indigenous medical cosmologies could be overcome and undermined by the institutional efforts of the state remains to be examined, as efforts to institutionalize medical knowledge continued to be challenged – cosmological ideas and older notions of the body continued to coexist alongside newer ones derived from the Western model. While the princely state stepped in to reorder traditional cultural forms in accordance with the sensibilities of the late nineteenth and twentieth centuries, as formed by British colonialism in India, the reordering of a medical domain raised fundamental questions about the relationship between traditional knowledge forms and Western science and their use in public health. Travancore state, as a repository of an alternative power, was bounded by culture as a significant element of consolidating sovereignty. Commitment to the creation of an organized structure for Ayurveda and its sustenance through state-centred institutions meant that it had a strong commitment to traditional symbols and forms. The state's effort at reinstating a text-bound Ayurveda tradition installed a new version of Ayurveda that subjected disparate local practices to marginalization, compelling them to survive without state support. While one cannot draw a sharp distinction between the elite and the local within the Ayurvedic tradition, the state's interventions tended to undermine the fluid relationships which existed between practitioners of different traditions within Travancore. Institutionalization of Ayurveda, rather than undermining the relationship between the local and the classical in medicine, highlighted the close relationship between the two – one which the Travancore state tried to undermine.

Notes

1 Barbara Ramusack, *The Indian Princes and Their States*, Cambridge: Cambridge University Press, 2005; Robin Jeffrey, *People, Princes and Paramount Power: Society and Politics in the Princely States*, Oxford: Oxford University Press, 1978.

2 Ramusack, *Indian Princes*, 132.

3 Aya Ikeyama, *Princely India Re-Imagined: A Historical Anthropology of Mysore from 1799 to the Present*, Abingdon: Routledge, 2012.

4 Burton Cleetus, 'Subaltern Medicine and Social Mobility: The Experience of the Ezhava in Kerala', *Indian Anthropologist*, 37, 1, (January–June 2007), 147–72.

5 Harish Naraindas, 'Preparing for the Pox: A Theory of Small Pox in Bengal and Britain', *Asian Journal of Social Science*, 31/2 (2003), 304–39.

6 K. N. Panikkar, 'Indigenous Medicine and Cultural Hegemony: A Study of the Revitalization Movement in Keralam', *Studies in History*, 8/2 (1992), 283–308.

7 Deepak Kumar (ed.), *Disease and Medicine in India: A Historical Overview*, New Delhi: Manohar, 2004, xviii.

8 Kavita Philip. *Civilizing Natures: Race, Resources and modernity in Colonial South India*. New Brunswick. N.J, Rutgers University Press, 2004.

9 Kapil Raj, *Relocating Modern Science: Circulation and the Construction of Knowledge in South Asia and Europe, 1650–1900*, London: Palgrave Macmillan, 2007; Harold Cook, *Matters of Exchange: Commerce, Medicine and Science in the Dutch Golden Age*, New Haven: Yale University Press, 2007; Biswamoy Pati and Mark Harrison (eds.), *Health, Medicine and Empire: Perspectives on Colonial India*, Hyderbad: Orient Longman, 2001.

10 Biswamoy Pati and Mark Harrison (eds.), *The Social History of Health and Medicine in Colonial India*, Abingdon: Routledge, 2009, 173–94.

11 Projit B. Mukharji, *Nationalising the Body: The Medical Market, Print, and Daktari Medicine*, New York: Anthem Press, 2009.

12 Projit Mukharji and David Hardiman (eds.), *Medical Marginality in South Asia: Situating Subaltern Therapeutics*, Abingdon: Routledge, 2012.

13 Michel Foucault, *Birth of the Clinic: An Archaeology of Medical Perception*, New York: Pantheon Books, 1973, 5.

14 Ishita Pande, *Medicine, Race and Liberalism in British Bengal: Symptoms of Empire*, London: Routledge, 2010, 1–17.

15 Robin Jeffrey, *The Decline of Nayar Dominance: Society and Politics in Travancore, 1847–1908*, New Delhi: Vikas, 1976.

16 Kavita Philip, *Civilising Natures: Race, Resources and Modernity in Colonial South India*, Hyderabad: Orient Longman, 2003, 17.

17 Kavita Sivaramakrishnan, *Old Portions, New Bottles: Recasting Indigenous Medicine in Colonial Punjab, 1850–1945*, New Delhi: Orient Longman, 2006.

18 Gita Krishnankutty, *A Life of Healing: A Biography of P. S. Varier*, New Delhi: Viking, Penguin, 2001.

19 Paul Brass, 'The Politics of Ayurvedic Education', in H. Rudolph Sussanne and I. Rudolph Lloyd (eds.), *Education and Politics in India*, Studies in Organization, Society and Polity. New Delhi: Oxford University Press, 1972, 344.

20 Ikeyema, *Princely India Re-Imagined*.

21 Charles Leslie, 'The Professionalising Ideology of Medical Revivalism', in Milton Singer (ed.), *Entrepreneurship and Modernisation of Occupational Cultures in South Asia*, Programme in Comparative Studies in South Asia, Durham, NC: Duke University Press: Monograph and Occasional Papers Series, No. 12, 1973, 217.

22 Ramusack, *The Indian Princes and Their States*, 132.

23 Lloyd I Rudolph and Susanne H Rudolph. *The Modernity of tradition: Political Development in India*. University of Chicago Press. Chicago and London. 1967, p. 251.

24 Reorganisation of te Ayurveda Patasala. File No. II-17 of 1918. Vol-I General. B. No 172.

25 Partha Chatterjee, 'Colonialism, Nationalism and Contested Women: The Contest in India', *American Ethnologist*, 16/4 (2005), 622–33.

26 Eric Hobsbawm and Terrance O. Ranger (eds.), *The Invention of Tradition*, Cambridge: Cambridge University Press, 1983, 1–14.

27 Andrew Brennan, 'Asian Traditions of Knowledge: The Disputed Questions of Science, Nature Ecology', *Studies in History and Philosophy of Biological and Biomedical Sciences*, (2002), 567–81.

28 Panikkar, 'Indigenous Medicine and Cultural Hegemony'; Kumar, *Disease and Medicine in India*, 285.

29 Richard Grove, 'Indigenous Knowledge and the Significance of South-West India for Portuguese and Dutch Constructions of Tropical Nature', *Modern Asian Studies*, 30/1 (1996), 121–43.

30 *Census of India*, 1901, Vol. XX, Cochin, Part, I Report, Government Press, Ernakulam, 24.

31 Who is Who in SNDP.

32 C.A. Bayly, *Empire and Information: Intelligence Gathering and Social Communication in India, 1780–1870*, Cambridge: Cambridge University Press, 1996, 252.

33 *Report of the Committee on the Indigenous Systems of Medicine*, 2 Volumes, Madras: Madras Government Publications, 1923, 20, Kerala State Archives (hereafter KSA).

34 *AyurvedaGrant in Aid Rules*, Bundle No. 223, File No. C. 15349, 1896, KSA.

35 Ibid.

36 *Letter from the Office of the Director of Ayurveda, Personal Assistant for Honorary Secretary, to the Managers of Ayurveda High Schools Who Receive Grants-in-Aid*, 1904, 7, KSA.

37 *Reorganization of the Ayurveda Patasala: A Scheme for the Expansion of the Ayurvedic Patasala into an Ayurvedic College*, Bundle No. 172, General, File No. II-17 of 1918, Vol. I, 7–8, KSA

38 James Mill. *The History of British India*. James Madden. London, 1848.

39 *Reorganization of the Ayurveda Patasala: A Scheme for the Expansion of the Ayurvedic Patasala into an Ayurvedic College*, General, Bundle No. 172, File No. II-17 of 1918, Vol. I. 4. KSA

40 Ibid., 6.

41 David Arnold, *Science,Technology and Medicine in Colonial India*, New Cambridge History of India, Cambridge: Cambridge University Press, 2000.

42 *Rules for Grant-in-Aid to Vaidyasalas: Powers of the Director*, Bundle No. 164, File No. II /5 of 1917, 2, KSA.

43 *Reorganization of the Ayurveda Patasala: A Scheme for the Expansion of the Ayurvedic Patasala into an Ayurvedic College*, Bundle No. 172, General, File No. II-17 of 1918, Vol. I, 2, KSA.
44 Parameswaran Moothathu, Cunnhamangalam Kochu Krishna Panikkar, Cheeroony Koil Tampuran and Vaisakkara Moosu, and others were included in the committee for the revision of the Ayurveda curriculum; they were assisted by K. Kesava Pillai, an allopathic medical practitioner of 1096 M.E (1920 A.D). Similarly, practitioners like Pandit Gopala Charlu of Madras, Gananath Sen, Kaviraj Nagendra Sen of Calcutta and others who were considered to be the leading figures of Ayurveda were persons who were deemed to be successful in negotiating with the Western system of medicine in their attempt at reorganizing the indigenous medicine on 'scientific lines', ibid., 12.
45 *Danwantri*, March 1917, 35.
46 *Reorganization of the Ayurveda Patasala: A Scheme for the Expansion of the Ayurvedic Patasala into an Ayurvedic College*, Bundle No. 172, General, File No. II-17 of 1918, Vol. I, KSA
47 *Regarding the Imposition on Certain Restriction on Private Medical Practice: Budget for the Ayurveda Department for the Year 1106 M.E.*, Bundle No. 156, File No. 7/31, LGB, 1931, Ayurveda Department, KSA.
48 Ibid., 5–6.
49 *Petition for the Establishment of a Vishavaidyasala at Nedumangad*, Bundle No. 138, File No. II-2 of 1915, KSA.
50 Ibid., 9.
51 Ibid., 12.
52 Ayurvedic Patasala: Opening of Ayurvedic Botanical Garden, Proceedings of His Highness the Maharajah of Travancore. From Rao Bahadur MC Koman, Honorary Physician, General Hospital, and Officer, In charge of investigation into indigenous drugs. To the Honorable Surgeon General, Government of Madras, I.G.O. No. E. 1282, Dated the 18th April, 1918, KSA.
53 *Regarding the Appointment of the Inspector of* Ayurveda, Bundle No. 201, General, File No. 1581, KSA.
54 Ibid.
55 Ibid., 1–2.
56 *Ayurveda Grant in Aid Rules*.
57 Ibid.
58 *Award of Grant to the Ayurveda Hospital at Nagercoil Conducted by Vaidyan B. Nilakandan*, Ayurveda Department, Bundle No. 148, File No. 106 A/30, 9, KSA.
59 Ibid.
60 Medicine for cholera found by Muthuswami Pillai. No. 2948. 1890.
61 Charles Leslie, 'The Ambiguities of Medical Revivalism in Modern India', in Charles Leslie (ed.), *Asian Medical Systems: A Comparative Study*, New Delhi: Motilal: Banarsidass, 1998, 357.
62 Guy Attewell, *Refiguring Unani Tibb: Plural Healing in Late Colonial India*, New Delhi: Orient Longman, 2007, 3.

6   Christian missionary women's hospitals in Mysore state, c.1880–1930

Barbara N. Ramusack

In India we can observe a difference between the response to medical missionaries in regions ruled by Indian Princes and the areas ruled directly by the British . . . In part, the princely ruler of Rajasthan appreciated the medical missionaries as they wanted trained western doctors without having to provide for any great outlay, and mission doctors came at a bargain price . . . The Hindu princes were not much concerned about their being Christians, for they had a longstanding tradition of patronizing a whole range of religious bodies and sects, and they saw the missionaries as just one more such group worthy of support.[1]

In his study of medical missionaries who worked with the tribal Bhils in Rajputana David Hardiman has highlighted how the princes of India patronized purveyors of social or cultural services regardless of their personal religious/confessional commitments. Besides tribal groups, medical missionaries focused on Indian women. Research on women medical missionaries in India such as the pioneering work of Antoinette Burton, Ruth Compton Brower and Rosemary Fitzgerald has focused on British women medical missionaries who laboured in British provinces in north, central and western India.[2] In south India research has concentrated on the American Arcot Mission that established the renowned medical complex at Vellore in Tamilnadu.

Through an analysis of five hospitals that missionary women established in the princely state of Mysore, my essay illuminates the diversity in structure, personnel, funding and programmes among their hospitals. It delineates how one princely state supported missionaries willing to work in locations and medical specialties that Mysore did not offer. Moreover, the British were willing to provide funding for specific projects. These five institutions established at the cusp of the twentieth century reflect significant changes from existing scholarship on missionary institutions during the nineteenth century. The foreign medical women who staffed these hospitals in Mysore exhibited greater professionalization, earlier reliance on Indian medical women and possibly more political and fundraising acumen than the pioneer medical women of the late nineteenth century. The willingness of the Wadiyar rulers of Mysore, known for their Hindu orthodoxy and progressive economic and social initiatives, to extend economic support to Christian missionaries for whom evangelization was the ultimate goal further illustrates Hardiman's argument. That four of the five missionary institutions that I analyze survived the transition to independence as private medical institutions of high repute affirms their continuing value for their patients and the state of Karnataka.

St. Martha's Hospital that the French Sisters of the Convent of the Good Shepherd founded in Bangalore, the Mary Calvert Holdsworth Memorial Hospital in Mysore city and the Redfern Memorial Hospital in Hassan city in the Shimoga district of the Wesleyan Methodists and the Zenana Hospitals in Bangalore and Channapatna of the Church of England Zenana Missionary Society (CEZMS) reveal the varied clienteles of medical mission work, why Indians might have been attracted to these hospitals, the sometimes tense relationship between the male missionary hierarchy and female medical missionaries as well as the differential financial relationships between mission hospitals and the Mysore state. Besides establishing how a princely state would rely on missionary hospitals for medical aid in geographical areas where state employees did not wish to serve and for services that the state did not provide, I argue that the trajectories of these institutions reflect changes that were occurring. By the early 1910s it was increasingly difficult to attract educated British women doctors to decades of missionary work in contrast to the late nineteenth century when British (and American) women doctors served for their adult lives in India. Consequently Indianization of medical staff began earlier in these hospitals than in some colonial institutions. Moreover, both British missionary and Indian women physicians were earning higher levels of professional qualifications than many of the pioneer medical women had achieved in the nineteenth century.

St. Martha's – the Catholic anomaly

French Catholic nuns and not English Protestants were the first missionaries to provide medical care in Mysore. As women they were a relatively recent participant among Roman Catholic missionaries who had been active in Mysore from the late seventeenth century. Begun in 1641 at Caen as a branch of the Order of Our Lady of Charity that had autonomous establishments, the Good Shepherd sisters had a cloistered branch and a group that sought to reform girls and women of 'dissolute' habits, implying sex work. In 1835 St. Mary Euphrasia formed the independent Congregation of the Good Shepherd Sisters and expanded their work to the United States, Africa and Asia. Travelling by bullock cart from Pondicherry, the seat of the French bishop overseeing the Catholic diocese of south India, the first Good Shepherd sisters, 18–26 years old, arrived in Bangalore on 15 August 1854. Although they initially opened homes for orphans and for 'rescued' women, they soon established the Good Shepherd School for Girls, still an elite institution in the heart of Bangalore on Residency Road.

In the early 1880s Mother Mary of the Visitation Leusch (1838–1893), the first superior or superioress as Mysore officials would address her of the Convent of Good Shepherd, proposed that the Good Shepherd nuns should establish a hospital primarily for Europeans and Eurasians in the Cantonment of Bangalore.[3] Evidence about her motivation is limited. A Centenary Souvenir and my conversations with hospital administrators in 1996 cite the impact of a severe drought, the subsequent famine in 1876 and 1877 and plague and cholera epidemics in 1878 in Mysore state. During these years the Good Shepherd nuns did 'simple' nursing in their convent and two nearby government camps.[4]

Initially Mother Visitation faced opposition from the Superior General of her order and British officials. Although she lacked medical training and support from France, she overcame this resistance. In June 1883 Mother Visitation advised Seshadri Iyer, the diwan (chief minister) of the Mysore Durbar (state government), that after entreaties from the Pettah, the area in Bangalore under the control of the Durbar, she decided to situate the hospital to serve Indians there.[5] A few weeks later A. Sreenivasa Charlu, the vice president of the Bangalore Municipal Commission, advised her that the diwan authorized a grant of 5,000 rupees towards a building. The Pettah municipal government promised a monthly grant of 200 rupees for the operation of the hospital 'so long as it is efficiently managed and the caste wards are kept up'.[6]

Mother Visitation proposed to purchase the land, to partially support building expenses, to be responsible for the administration, to provide nurses ['Sisters of Charity, whose devotedness and skillfulness are worldwide known'[7]] who would 'conform' with suggestions of the doctors and to respect 'the customs and prejudices of caste and religion' of patients.[8] Four months later she asked J.B. Lyall, the British

Resident in Mysore, to grant land in the Pettah, 5,000 rupees towards the building and a monthly grant of 200 rupees for maintenance that his predecessor had promised for the C&M hospital.[9] He refused advising that the Mysore government should provide such a hospital managed by their medical officers.[10] Not to be deterred, she next appealed to the public.

On 22 March 1884 Mother Visitation asked for subscriptions of any size to enable the sisters to care for 'sufferers of every rank and denomination'. She enticed subscribers with the benefit of daily prayers by poor invalids.[11] By July 1884 A.H. Macintire, the president of the Bangalore Municipal Commission, advised the Lady Superior that she could take possession of 21 acres for the hospital in the Pettah.[12] Maharaja Chamarajendraraja Wadiyar was recorded as the donor.

Although Dr. J. Henderson, the surgeon in charge of the Government Dispensary in the Pettah, wanted the Municipal Board to manage St. Martha's,[13] Mother Visitation argued that her convent should administer the hospital but without control over the physicians (male) who would be employees of the Mysore Durbar. She asserted that 'if comparison were drawn between institutions governed by the latter [religious corporations], and those administered by secular bodies, the Lady Superior thinks that religious communities may stand the comparison'.[14] Mother Visitation prevailed. After St. Martha's Hospital opened in 1886, the Mysore government abolished its dispensary and hospital in the Pettah and transferred its medical personnel to St. Martha's on 14 August 1887. However, in 1892 this arrangement was terminated.[15] Then in 1901 St. Martha's became an independent house of the Good Shepherd Order based in Augers, France.[16]

St. Martha's was a most unusual mission hospital in India. At first Roman Catholic nuns were the administrators and supervisors of nursing care but most physicians were male and paid employees. Although some Catholic orders of nuns such as the Sisters of Charity have a long history of nursing work, canon law forbade Roman Catholic nuns to pursue medical education to become physicians until the late 1920s. Here again, St. Martha's was different. Its staff included Sister Mary Martha (d. 1935) and Sister Aloysius Fernandes (d. 1950s) who were nuns with degrees from Bombay and Madras Medical Colleges, respectively.[17] Second, St. Martha's was a general hospital that had an equal number of beds for men and women. It did not open a separate maternity ward until the 1950s. It differed from most mission hospitals which British and American women physicians established where the focus was on women patients, especially their maternal health.

Over the years the Mother Superiors of Good Shepherd continued to solicit financial support from the Mysore Durbar. After thanking her for some artichokes that were a treat in the nuns' refectory (but which she could not eat because of her 'old complaint'), in 1913 Sister Emphani asked the wife of Dr. McGann, the former Senior and Durbar Surgeon, for advice from her husband on how to approach the Mysore Durbar for funds to build a 'comfortable and airy house' to ensure the good health of sisters who work in the hospital.[18] Without any comment Dr. McGann forwarded her letter to the Durbar. The Second Councillor of the Mysore government argued that St. Martha's 'has been generously treated by government already', and the request was denied.[19] In 1913 St. Martha was receiving 200 rupees each month from the Mysore state and the Bangalore City Municipal Council. The Mysore Durbar now was supporting other missionary medical institutions.

Wesleyan Methodist Mission Hospitals

By 1913 four more mission hospitals had joined St. Martha's. The devastation wrought by a plague epidemic that reached Mysore city in 1898 demonstrated to the Wesleyan missionaries, Reverend H.H. and Mary Calvert Holdsworth, the need for a hospital. After ill health forced them to return to England, Reverend George W. Sawday campaigned for a hospital. He quickly enlisted the approbation of Mary Calvert Holdsworth, known for her visits to offer emotional support and sanitary advice to Indian families during the disastrous plague.[20] Dying in England in 1903, Mary Holdsworth embodied the transition in missionary medicine from pre-professional health visiting to institutional missionary medicine that surged in the early twentieth century. On 14 September 1905 Sawday petitioned the Mysore Durbar for a grant of 34,000 rupees, one-third of the cost of the building being erected in the 'most densely crowded area of the [Mysore] city' that is 'most in need of medical help'. Based on the medical complex at Vellore he estimated monthly expenses would be 1,000 rupees. He then asked for a monthly grant of 400 rupees, the amount that another institution in Bangalore (meaning St. Martha's) received.[21] The Senior Surgeon, Dr. J. Smyth, I.M.S., supported this request because

> [The hospital] will not only be an ornament to the city, but be of the utmost service to its population. These missionaries have ways of getting at people of which we Government officers know little or nothing.[22]

Here and elsewhere Mysore state officials acknowledged the attraction of mission hospitals for their subjects.

Smyth added that such a hospital at a cost to the Mysore government of an initial grant of 34,000 rupees and 400 rupees monthly would be 'practically' a free gift to Mysore city and to the district of Mysore.[23] The Wesleyan institution would be supported by its home organization and private contributions from Britain and India. The Mysore State Council decided that 25,000 rupees for a construction grant and 200 rupees per month towards operating expenses would be sufficient. Their conditions were that (1) medical relief be given to all without reference to caste and creed and 'throughout the day'; (2) the Mysore Senior Surgeon could ask for periodic reports; (3) state officers could inspect the premises; and (4) the 'customs and prejudices of caste and religion shall be respected'.[24] Although the Wesleyan Methodists were critical of observing caste boundaries in other activities, Sawday accepted these conditions. Payment was authorized on 6 July 1906 when the construction was already far advanced. Maharaja Krishnaraja Wadiyar formally inaugurated the Mary Calvert Holdsworth Memorial Hospital on 21 August 1906 and announced that his mother, Maharani Vani Vilas, contributed 10,000 rupees to the hospital. She continued to contribute smaller amounts periodically.

The Holdsworth Hospital followed the pattern of other Protestant mission hospitals in its personnel. Initially its physicians were British women with M.B.B.S. or M.D. degrees from British medical schools. In January 1906 Elsie Watts M.D. arrived to head the hospital and her sister Edith Watt M.B.M.S. followed the next month as an honorary (unpaid) worker. The Wesleyan establishment provided highly trained physicians who worked for lower or even no salaries compared with similarly qualified Indian women physicians employed in princely state or colonial government hospitals where salaries might be higher and some could maintain lucrative private practices.

Around 1870 the Wesleyan Methodists and the London Missionary Society drew a line through Bangalore and the Wesleyans were to evangelize west and the LMS east. Thus the Wesleyans were responsible for four fifths of Mysore.[25] The second Wesleyan Methodist Hospital for women and children was established in 1906 in Hassan town in the western Malnad (hilly) region of Mysore. Here the Wesleyans established a church and orphanage in 1887. Illustrating missionary synergism, the Hassan orphanage sent four girls, funded by the Mysore Branch of the Dufferin Fund, to the Lying-in Hospital in Madras for one year of training as midwives.[26] When they returned to Mysore, these two women briefly worked at the state-supported

Maharani Hospital before going to outlying municipalities.[27] These midwives and their successors indicate the long trajectory of private-cum-public health initiatives in Mysore.

Reverend Ernest W. Redfern who came to Hassan district in 1893 initiated the campaign to build a hospital but he died in 1904 before it was a reality. On 7 September 1906 Reverend H. Halliday Newham, his successor, asked the chief secretary of Mysore state for a building grant for 20,000 rupees and a monthly grant of 200 rupees. Citing the lack of any hospital for women and children in the Hassan district, he promised that the missionary institution would provide women physicians from Britain who had the 'highest medical qualifications', train nurses and launch a travelling dispensary to villages. Like earlier missionary suppliants, he assured the Mysore Durbar that the hospital would be open to all irrespective of caste or creed.[28]

The desired site involved complex negotiations. In contrast to St. Martha's the Wesleyan mission had to purchase its site from the Hassan Municipality rather than receiving it as a grant from the Mysore government.[29] Moreover, the government declined to make any grant because 'of other demands'. The Hassan Municipal and District Boards offered only 200 rupees per year and not as requested per month. Both boards mentioned that they were already supporting the local Government Female Dispensary.[30]

Ironically in 1922 the Senior Surgeon of Mysore State observed that 'the Redfern Memorial Hospital at Hassan with its staff of Lady Doctors and complete equipment is attracting the major portion of the female patients of the town and suburbs'.[31] He surmised that Indian women would not patronize the government facilities because they did not want to be treated by male doctors and in buildings that lacked appropriate, that is separate, accommodation for women. To attract more women patients, the official recommended that the female dispensaries that had no adequate space for in-patients and no operating facilities be combined with the district hospitals with women doctors treating the women patients.[32]

Since most hospitals did not maintain archives for their institutional records, the annual reports of the Wesleyan missionaries to their boards and contributors in Britain are the principal sources on issues that confronted hospital administrators. As expected these sources were generally positive about their relations with their Indian clientele and emphasized what might be accomplished with more resources.

During the first year at Holdsworth Hospital Dr. Elsie Watts reported 4,765 new out-patients, 12,288 old and new out-patients who visited the dispensary and 166 in-patients since the opening of the wards in

August 1906. Most out-patients came from the congested area around the hospital and the in-patients included 72 Hindus (including 3 Brahmans), 61 Muslims and 33 Christians. The staff made 149 house calls including a few to high-caste Hindu officials and Muslim merchants. Evangelization consisted of an opening morning prayer in the out-patient waiting room and in the wards, 'in which many of the patients have joined'.[33] A list of contributors in Britain and India to the Holdsworth Hospital was appended to each annual report. From Britain Rev. and Mrs. J. Sewell Haworth contributed 300 pounds and Mrs. Nagle of Walthamstow contributed 500 pounds but most contributions ranged from 1 to 20 pounds. In India Maharani Vani Vilas at 10,000 rupees (calculated at 660 pounds) and Mahomed Badruddin at 1,500 rupees stood out from the other contributors who gave from 5 to 20 rupees.[34]

For 1907 Dr. Elsie Watts could report a significant increase of in-patients to 400 with 50 maternity cases as well as over 18,000 attendances by out-patients. One negative occurrence and two positive initiatives were noted. Because of an unfounded rumour that a Muslim woman and her children had been baptized in the hospital, Muslims were now boycotting it. Doctors, accompanied by an evangelist, visited neighbouring villages to provide simple care and to persuade more serious cases to come to the hospital.[35] Miss Frances Campbell organized the nursing work in Mysore and twelve Indian Christian girls were in training under her and two other professional head nurses.[36] With British nurses as pioneering leaders, mission hospitals recruited Indian converts and young girls from their orphanages and schools to train as nurses and compounders. By 1908 the Holdsworth Hospital had a separate Maternity Block with 130 deliveries, was performing more surgery and had attracted more high-caste Hindus as patients. They had so many Muslim zenana patients that the staff contemplated whether an additional ward was necessary to accommodate them.[37] A few years later Dr. Elsie claimed that two things attracted prospective Indian patients to Holdsworth: 'the knowledge that they were sure to get the very best medical skill and attention, and the certainty that whatever might happen they would receive the utmost kindness during their stay in the hospital.'[38]

In the conclusion to her report for 1908 Dr. Watts asserted that although she believed 'every member of the staff feels her responsibility for the spiritual welfare of the patients, limits of time and strength make it urgent that a missionary should be appointed, who can devote all her powers to our evangelistic work'.[39] Her request reflects the increasing tension that missionaries experienced because their medical work left little time and energy for evangelical efforts to convert Indians. Even so in 1909 the annual report related that one village welcomed an evangelist because of successful operations on two village children. Missionaries were acutely aware that officials and contributors in Britain wanted their medical work to gain more converts.[40]

In 1910 Dr. Elsie Watts described the organization of the hospital that illustrates how some missionary doctors responded to government injunctions and patient preferences. The Victoria Ward was for high-caste Hindus, of whom six out of seven were Brahmans in 1909. They could have their food brought to them or have it prepared in one of several separate, small kitchens. Muslim gosha women had their own ward as did Christians. Two large wards were for low-caste Hindus and for 'outcastes'. The maternity ward jumbled together all castes and creeds and the family wards, where the rule of one patient, one friend was not enforced were 'very popular, especially with nervous village women'.[41] Gleefully Dr. Watts related that the doctors could make more visits to villages with an automobile that a friend in India had loaned to them. British benefactors, some generous patients and friends of the mission in India provided another element of modernity – electric lights throughout the hospital.[42]

By 1911 retaining and replacing medical staff at the Holdsworth Hospital was a recurring problem. After five years of service Dr. Elsie went on furlough. Her sister Dr. Edith accompanied her to Britain and in 1912 returned married to Mr. Slater, a Methodist missionary in the enclave of Ootacamund where British officials and missionaries sought refuges during the hot season. For a few years Dr. Edith as Mrs. Slater practised there and received a small grant from the Mysore government. It was terminated in 1922 as part of a major retrenchment by Mysore and Slater seems to have ceased her practice.[43] After marriage many women physicians, whether missionaries or government employees, no longer practised medicine in an institution.[44] Meanwhile the home mission officers found no British physician to replace Dr. Elsie. More discouraging was that the Women's Auxiliary Committee could not support a doctor even if one could be found. Fortunately Mrs. W. Lisle Williams, the mother of Mrs. Holdsworth and a magnanimous donor, offered to support Dr. Miss M. Shepherd Allen who had L.R.C.P.&S. qualifications but would commit for only a year. It was equally difficult to replace Frances Campbell when she opened a small dispensary at Mandagadde in the relatively remote Shimoga district to care for Namadharis. Methodist missionaries deemed these sudhra cultivators to be more open to Christian teachings than other groups.[45] Whether Campbell's efforts reaped the desired converts is unknown.

Although Holdsworth Hospital attracted increasing numbers of patients, for example, 27,128 attended the dispensary, 356 operations were performed and 201 maternity cases were treated from 1 October 1910 to 30 September 1911,[46] surgery and maternity cases had declined dramatically for 1912 and early 1913 because of lack of staff. From 1 October 1913 to 30 September 1914 surgeries numbered only 250 and maternity cases were 155.[47] Even so in a report on women's hospitals in princely states that was frequently negative, Dr. (Mrs.) F. Mervyn Smith who had briefly supervised Holdsworth Hospital lauded it as the 'Standard on which all women's hospitals in India should be modelled'. She added that 'The operation theatre would do credit to a first class London hospital, while the bacteriological and pathological departments are fitted with the latest appliances of medical science.'[48] Despite these excellent facilities, the difficulty in recruiting women physicians from Britain provoked cautious steps towards greater Indianization of the physician staff.[49]

The Redfern Hospital in Hassan (1901, population 8,241) was in a very different geographical and political environment from the Holdsworth Hospital in Mysore city (1901, population 68,111) where the ruling family of Mysore resided. The Mysore state found it difficult to recruit and to retain medical employees in districts such as Hassan that were deemed isolated and unhealthy. A report on government hospitals and dispensaries for 1922 revealed that female dispensaries at Thirthahalli and Kallurkatte in Shimoga district in the Malnad, a fertile area with high rates of infant mortality and malaria and declining population, had to be closed for 'want of qualified hands'.[50]

The Wesleyan Mission found it difficult to attract financial support for Redfern from Mysore state retrenching financially, its local Indian population or Britons in India or at home. After the Mysore Durbar refused to fund construction or operations or to donate land, the hospital building was much delayed. In 1905 Dr. Enid Smyth arrived to take charge of the hospital and was reported as 'making excellent progress with the language'.[51] Since the hospital lacked in-patient wards, Dr. Smyth treated only out-patients in the dispensary. During 1906 most patients were Muslim, few came from nearby villages and all preferred receiving medicine to surgery. An older patient did not want Smyth to use a knife to remove her abscess so she used scissors.[52] By March 1907 the doctor herself became ill. In October she returned to Britain, never to return to or to use her proficiency in Kannada. Mrs. Newham (the wife of the Hassan Superintendent), who had trained as a nurse in Britain, treated patients intermittently at the dispensary. With an unfinished hospital building and no qualified doctors, the mission reverted to nineteenth-century medical practices. Early missionary men and women with a little or no professional training treated simple ailments from the contents of their personal medicine chests.[53] From late 1907 Miss McCann of unknown qualifications assisted first as nurse and then as doctor for three years. In 1910 Dr. C.V. Lowe M.B.B.Ch., sister of Mrs. Redfern, arrived. Three hundred pounds from the Misses Stephenson of Newcastle-on Tyne enabled work to resume on an Operation Theatre. But it was acknowledged that

> It is very doubtful whether the town of Hasan [sic] will ever furnish enough work for the Hospital to keep even the two wards and the maternity ward full: it has always been desired that the villages of the surrounding district should be the largest sharers in the benefit of our work. If this is to be so, a Travelling Dispensary is most imperatively required.[54]

Like other missionary organizations Wesleyan physicians focused on scheduled caste groups. In July 1911 Dr. Lowe began her itinerant work with four days in Hole Narsipur where she attended the Holeyas 'to whom medical relief in time of sickness is almost unknown'.[55] Other untouchables, Hindu social reformers and ethnologists considered the Holeyas as particularly degraded because of their work, personal uncleanliness and consumption of meat and alcohol.[56] Dr. Lowe sought to relieve physical suffering and to attract potential converts among this marginalized Hindu group but data on any converts is lacking.

For the year ending 31 October 1911 the Redfern Hospital had 7,492 patients at its dispensary; 1,601 were newcomers, 38 in-patients, 60 surgeries and 20 maternity cases.[57] In contrast Holdsworth had 27,128 patients at its dispensary of which 7,582 were new, 907 in-patients, 356 surgeries and 201 maternity case for a year in which the two Drs. Watts left and only one physician was in charge.[58] Children and women were the focus of the Redfern Hospital and gendered roles might influence treatment in unusual ways. In 1913 Dr. Lowe recorded that Holeya parents brought their baby who had an untreated burn that seared his upper arm and forearm together and caused his fingers to atrophy. When advised of the treatment needed, the father had refused because if the wife stayed with the child, he would have no one to cook his meals. Eventually he agreed to let his child and wife remain for eight days but no more.[59] Mysore officials acknowledged that Redfern Hospital attracted women because of its women physicians and better equipment compared to the government dispensary where male physicians attended to both male and female patients.[60]

The Wesleyan Methodists found it increasingly difficult to recruit British and Indian women physicians. It appears that British physicians found more opportunities at home, and both British and Indian women might have been attracted to the higher pay and possibly more urban opportunities in British government service. In 1936 the Medical Committee for the Mysore District of the newly formed Church of South India (CSI) formulated a programme to attract more highly educated Indian women physicians. Indian Christian women who had M.B.B.S. degrees from the Vellore Medical School were to be divided into two pay scales. Those M.B.B.S. graduates with unstated lesser qualifications would receive salaries of 100 rupees rising by annual raises of 10–150 rupees. Although missions generally provided housing and food, this salary was low compared to that for Indian women physicians in government service. If Indian M.B.B.S. graduates were prepared to meet more demanding qualifications including a vocation for Christian service, a three-year probationary period and service for at least six years and the ability to assume charge of hospitals, they would receive the same salary and academic leave as British physicians did.[61] Unfortunately, the major source for Indian women medical graduates in south India was confronting its own crisis.

In 1938 the Wesleyan Methodist authorities in Madras advised Reverend Newham that they could not provide any additional funds for the operation of the new maternity block at Holdsworth. The Vellore Medical School was in more dire financial straits and needed money to survive until hoped for American contributions arrived. Because of the lack of European doctors, Vellore graduates were particularly valuable.[62] This episode reflects the increasing cooperation across sectarian boundaries among Protestant mission groups.

Both Wesleyan hospitals survived the transition to independence. In 2014 Holdsworth Memorial Hospital in Mysore city had over 325 beds and multiple specializations. Redfern Memorial Hospital currently has 160 beds and in ratings on Google, it is still judged superior to the Government Hospital.

Church of England Zenana Mission hospitals in Bangalore and Channapatna

Separating from the interdenominational Indian Female Normal School Society to become an Anglican institution in 1880, the Church of England Zenana Missionary Society (CEZMS) was unusual in that women held some administrative posts in Britain and were in charge of individual mission stations. The CEZMS focused on evangelization. Its members visited secluded Indian women to introduce Christian ideals, educated girls and established orphanages ultimately to gain converts. Medical care was a path to evangelization. In India the CEZMS staunchly defined its constituency as Muslim women. Most of its institutions were in north India where sizable Muslim populations observed austere seclusion. In 1880 it inherited three stations in south India – one in Travancore and two in the Madras Presidency.

By 1887 CEZMS missionaries were visiting Indian women and educating their daughters in Bangalore. Four years later they established a dispensary for women and children in Bangalore and launched their campaign for a hospital. The Mysore Durbar declined to grant land or money to the CEZMS for its hospitals as it did for Catholics and Methodists. Eventually the CEZMS accumulated around 40,000 rupees from unspecified sources to construct their hospital.[63] Subsequently, their financial situation was more precarious than St. Martha's or the Wesleyan hospitals but they survived. The Bangalore Zenana Hospital opened on 31 October 1895, became the Church of South India Hospital in 1954 and currently is a hospital for women and men with about 200 beds in 2014. Irene Barnes, a CEZMS officer in England and prolific author of books on the CEZMS, emphasized that the new hospital would not only provide medical care for Muslims, Hindus and Indian Christians but keep them safe from the hands of Roman Catholic nuns (a possible reference to St. Martha's) whose 'coercion in which they were thus exposed in times of weakness'.[64] Subsequently the CEZMS opened a dispensary and a small hospital Channapatna in January 1906. Their two hospitals illustrate the varied relations of mission hospitals with the Mysore Durbar and significant gender issues within missionary organizations during the early twentieth century.

In early 1895 Dr. Amy G. Lillingston, recently graduated with an L.C.R.P.&S. degree from the highly regarded Edinburgh School of Medicine, arrived in India. Perhaps her sister Ann Lillingston, a CEZMS missionary in Bangalore, was one factor in her choice of Mysore. After studying Hindustani (Urdu) for six months, Amy Lillingston began her medical career as head of the Bangalore Zenana Mission Hospital where she would work until 1918. Besides being a bold administrator and effective fundraiser, Lillingston was professionally active in the Association of Medical Women in India (AMWI) founded in 1907. She participated in its meetings in Madras and Delhi, was commended for her prompt and informative reports and helped with government requests for British medical women to serve in its hospitals during the First World War.[65] In 1902 Dr. Dora Lockwood, with an L.R.C.P.&S. degree from London, arrived to assist Dr. Lillingston. She served until 1926. These two women reflect the increasing professionalization of women missionary physicians in the early 1900s.[66] But they were unusual since they spent their entire career at one hospital. The difficulties in retaining British doctors and nurses that began during the 1910s at the Wesleyan hospitals in Mysore would occur later in the CEZMS hospitals.

By 1918 the CEZMS began to employ Indian women physicians with respected degrees as well as those with L.M.P. (Licentiate Medical Practitioners with three years' training) degrees.[67] Dr. Mrs. Tungabhadra Kukde had an M.D. from the Women's Medical College of Pennsylvania, Dr. Mrs. Gulbai Dhunjhop Medhora, a Parsi, an M.B.B.S. degree from Bombay and Dr. Miss M.S. Gnanamuthu, an L.C.P.&S. degree from Bombay. As did British women during the 1920s, these three physicians served only for a few years. Subsequently, Kukde entered Pudukkottai state service[68] and Gnanamuthu joined Mysore state service.[69] Medhora's movement from Bangalore to Poona to Ahmedabad from 1918 to 1922 might indicate that she was moving because of her husband's work.[70] Dr. Dora Lockwood was positive about the work of these and other Indian physicians. Dr. Kukde was 'much loved', Dr. Medhora exerted 'a very good' influence on Indian nurses and Dr. Gnanamuthu, was 'very keen on her work & clever' and often revisited the hospital when she was in Mysore.[71]

As did other mission hospitals, the CEZMS Bangalore Hospital instituted a nursing school, reputedly the first in south India for Indian students. Clare de Noe Walker served as Nursing Superintendent from 1895 to 1903 when she left after marrying Reverend Edward Carr, the brother-in-law of Dr. Lillingston. Well-known for her nursing handbook that circulated widely in several vernacular languages, Walker actively tried to change the negative attitudes of Indian parents about a nursing career for their daughters by admitting only Christian girls of 'irreproachable moral character'. Frequently recruited from CEZMS schools and orphanages, the students had two years of training in general nursing and a third year in midwifery. Although most graduates worked in missionary hospitals, some went to government institutions.[72] One administered the first municipal crèche in the Civil and Military Station in Bangalore where she also served as a midwife.[73] Eventually difficulties in recruiting nurses from England to be superintendents led to the closure of the nursing school. The CEZMS also trained Indian women as midwives and compounders in the Bangalore Hospital.

Although not as successful at fundraising as Superiors at St. Martha's, in 1913 Dr. Lillingston secured a grant of 500 pounds from the Government of India (GOI) to construct an open-air ward on the roof of the Bangalore Zenana Hospital to treat female tuberculosis patients. The prevailing discourse that purdah women, especially Muslims who lived in the most restrictive seclusion, were particularly susceptible to tuberculosis might have stimulated this venture.[74] When this ward opened in January 1913, it was the only facility treating tuberculosis in Mysore state.[75] How the Bangalore Zenana Hospital came to focus on women tuberculosis patients by the early 1930s will be traced later.

The CEZMS Bangalore Hospital served another distinctive category of patients. Prefacing her letter with the comment that H.V. Cobb, the British Resident in Mysore, was unmarried and there was no official 'lady' closer than her (a significant exaggeration) to give advice, in June 1918 Lillingston wrote to Lady Chelmsford, as the President of the Dufferin Fund, to ask for assistance. She sought funds for a separate ward for venereal patients and their children and living quarters for the Indian doctor who then occupied the isolation ward. The CEZMS missionary graphically portrayed how during the past two years their 115 patients recorded as having syphilis or gonorrhoea had to be treated on mats in the corridors of the hospital. She added that the British were doing 'everything possible for the solider and sepoy' with the implication that they did nothing for the women who might have contracted venereal disease from them.[76]

The bachelor Cobb and British officials were aghast that the Resident had been ignored. However, Lady Chelmsford communicated that the hospital was doing good work and should be supported.[77] Her husband, the Governor General and Viceroy of India, agreed. In Bangalore George Gimlette, the Residency Surgeon, supported a grant acknowledging that the Lady Curzon Hospital in the C&M did not accept venereal patients and military authorities abandoned plans to build a women's hospital for such patients.[78] In November 1918 Cobb, perhaps reluctantly, recommended a grant of 10,000 rupees but with a warning to the CEZMS that it should finance itself in the future.[79] In January 1919 John Wood, the GOI Political Secretary in charge of the princely states, advised Cobb that 10,000 rupees should be granted from funds of the Assigned Tract of the C&M to the CEZMS 'for improvements in the Hospital building'.[80] This oblique reference might indicate how much the colonial power wished to distance itself from any responsibility for venereal disease among Indian women. In

1920 the CEZMS opened a 'Birthday' ward for women with venereal diseases and their children at the Bangalore Zenana Hospital.[81] The name of this ward reflects how difficult it was for missionaries to name this medical condition. Another service that the CEZMS provided at the request of the military authorities in Bangalore was to care for the 'Indian women' of the Sappers and Miners and the Madras Pioneers at their dispensary and hospital.[82]

In the late 1910s postgraduate instruction for medical women on the treatment of venereal diseases was initiated.[83] Here again the GOI and Mysore State wanted other institutions to do the work. In response to a report by the Dufferin Fund in 1920 about venereal diseases among Indian women, the GOI made a grant to this organization to provide instruction. Courses began in 1921. By 1923 M.D.s and lesser-credential medical women such as Miss E. Isaac, a Lady Assistant Surgeon from the Holdsworth Hospital in Mysore, were attending these programmes in Madras and elsewhere in India.[84] It seems ironic that medical missionaries and Indian Christian women were so prominent in providing care for Indian women who might have contracted venereal diseases from contact with British and Indian troops stationed in the Civil and Military Station. From brief references, the Birthday ward seemed a more benign refuge than the British lock hospitals. Although it had beds for men with venereal disease in its general hospitals, the Mysore state did not appoint a male doctor as a specialist in venereal diseases until 1929. Beds for women patients with venereal diseases did not exist in state hospitals. S. Subba Rao, the Senior Surgeon of Mysore state, suggested that midwives and lady health visitors should direct such women 'to attend the ante-natal section of the [Government] Maternity hospital' until wards were available.[85]

Tuberculosis was another area where the Mysore state initially left treatment to a missionary institution. In 1926 Dr. Lockwood reported that a new hospital for Muslim women in Bangalore might be attracting patients who earlier would have come to the Zenana Hospital.[86] Besides a decline in maternity patients who might pay fees, the limited tenure of British physicians at the hospital deepened the financial distress. CEZMS physicians maintained private practices whose fees were a significant source of income for the hospital. Consequently in 1926 CEZMS officers in London began to consider changing the focus of the Zenana Hospital from general medicine to tuberculosis.[87] In a report dated 1929 Dr. Margaret I. Neal, a respected member of the GOI Women's Medical Service who was deputed to Mysore, assured CEZMS committee members that there was no other hospital care for tuberculosis in Mysore. However, she highlighted staffing issues.

When only one European doctor was on staff, she argued that two Indian doctors were needed to substitute for the second European doctor usually there. Moreover, English nurses were 'necessary' for two reasons. First it was difficult to obtain reliable Indian nurses. Second, care for tuberculosis patients was strenuous and led to some nurses contracting tuberculosis, implying that English nurses were somehow sturdier than Indian nurses.[88] After an exhaustive review from 1928 to 1931 the CEZMS Bangalore Local Conference decided that the Bangalore Zenana Hospital should care for tuberculosis patients until the Mysore government or some other institution provided such care.[89] Like Neal in India, B.M. Peddar, the chair in England of the special subcommittee on this issue, expressed her concern that it would be difficult to recruit English physicians and nurses for this institution and to secure the needed funding.[90] Despite the reluctance of some CEZMS physicians to terminate their focus on 'general' medicine for women, the CEZMS Bangalore Hospital became a tuberculosis hospital for women. In 1953 it transitioned into a Church of South India general hospital with wards for men and women.

The CEZMS Zenana Hospital in Channapatna (1901, population 10,425) was the mofussil outpost of the Bangalore (1901, population 159,046) CEZMS Hospital as the Redfern Hospital in Hassan was of the Wesleyan Methodist Hospital in Mysore city. Around 1904 some Muslim men asked the CEZMS women in Bangalore to establish a hospital in Channapatna to serve Muslim women since the nearest hospitals were in Bangalore and Mysore city, a distance of about 40 miles in either direction. This CEZMS Hospital opened in 1905 but it closed in 1918. Few patients occupied the 10 beds, staff was transitory and funds were minimal.[91] In 1921 in the Mysore Representative Assembly Abdul Rasheed argued that a zenana hospital was needed in Channapatna as did a local Muslim organization in the following year.[92] In 1922 the CEZMS dispatched funds to reopen its hospital and dispensary.[93] By 1929 the Channapatna staff was operating an infant and maternal clinic at Maddur for which the Mysore State Rural Health Unit was 'indebted'.[94] Thus the Channapatna hospital is yet another example of how Mysore state and Christian missionaries would cooperate to provide medical services in geographical areas which state employees found unattractive.

In 1932 the Channapatna hospital again confronted closure supported first by CEZMS women in Bangalore and then male missionary officers in Madras. Their CEZMS superiors in London wanted to close their mission in Mysore city but 'the Bangalore ladies' indicated that they preferred to close the hospital at Channapatna. While some CEZMS physicians such as Dr. Lockwood, now retired and in England, campaigned to keep it open, Canon R.M. Peachey, the CEZMS secretary in Madras, approached Reverend Newham of the Wesleyan Mission to ask if his group would take over the CEZMS Hospital that bordered the Methodist compound in Channapatna. Peachey subsequently reassured Newham that the price should be nominal since the Methodists would continue the work. The CEZMS officer added 'Please don't tell the CEZMS ladies this.'[95] If and when the women missionaries knew of this exchange or their reactions is unknown. But the negotiations between the Anglican priest and the Methodist minister reveal the gender hierarchy that existed within missionary organizations, despite the authority that women held in CEZMS institutions.

The CEZMS women continued to struggle. In January 1934 Edith Potter, the Secretary of the CEZMS Local Council in Bangalore, indicated that the CEZMS wanted 3,000 rupees or not less than 1,000 rupees for its hospital property. The Methodists withdrew when two donors to the Channapatna Hospital would not transfer their endowments to them.[96] E.W. Legh, the CEZMS Secretary in Madras, lamented that no Indian woman with an L.M.P. degree applied for a position and that buildings needed significant repairs. Still he asked the CEZMS to continue their work.[97]

After receiving a report about the cost of needed repairs to the industrial home in early 1935, the CEZMS officers in London proposed closing their institutions in Channapatna. Now Legh made a strong case to retain both the hospital and the industrial home. No other hospital still existed between Bangalore and Mysore city, a distance of 80 miles and no other industrial home was closer than Madras. Dora Lockwood, now retired and living in England, made a passionate plea to retain the hospital at Channapatna. She emphasized that CEZMS missionaries knew Hindustani so could communicate with Muslim women but other missionaries knew only Tamil or Kannada. Although she realized that the 'need of the Hindu non-castes is tremendous', 'it is a need recognized by every Protestant Missionary Society working in India and by the Indian Church.'[98] Lockwood implied that other missionary societies would not be able as they were to care as well for Muslim women as did the CEZMS. Unfortunately, the available documents of the CEZMS, the reports of the Dufferin Fund and the Mysore state, and the pages of the *Journal of the Association of Medical Women* do not mention the Channapatna hospital after 1936. There is a small Church of South India hospital in Channapatna, but its relationship to the CEZMS is not clear.

Conclusion – differences, similarities and Mysore state policies

The Sisters of the Good Shepherd, the Wesleyan Methodist Mission and the CEZMS in Mysore state shared some features but differed significantly. Confronting similar challenges, they took and did whatever seemed necessary to establish their institutions. All groups requested and received varying financial support from governmental agencies. While the hospitals of the two Protestant groups focused on women and maternal care, St. Martha's maintained an equal number of beds for men and women and did not specialize in maternal health.

What was similar among the women missionaries who founded and struggled to maintain these hospitals? First, they were flexible negotiators. When seeking grants from the Mysore Durbar, district municipalities and prominent citizens, they emphasized their work with underserved populations. In order to secure funding they all agreed to respect caste practices and religious affiliations. Their hospitals had separate wards and kitchens for castes – usually one each for Brahmans, other castes and 'untouchable'/scheduled castes and for Muslim women. This concession ignored the often-furious debates within missionary societies about whether any caste distinctions were to be observed in their institutions or rituals. Although the CEZMS did not want to employ any Roman Catholics, even ayahs, by 1936 they were allowing Catholic priests to visit patients.

Second, the women missionaries were persistent negotiators. They did not meekly accept negative responses. The Superiors of the Good Shepherd established the pattern. When the British Resident refused to transfer a grant to the Pettah site, Mother Mary Visitation appealed to the public and through unrecorded channels ultimately gained 21 acres for St. Martha's and monthly grants for operation from the Durbar and the Municipal Council. For the Wesleyan hospitals, their male superintendents secured grants of land and operating funds. But women in India and Britain provided significant contributions. Possibly because of a less affluent base, CEZMS medical women were the most tenacious. Amy Lillingston's strategy was to ask the GOI for funds to serve particular populations without access to state institutions. Her first success was a grant for a tuberculosis ward. In her second major venture of building a ward for women venereal patients, she followed Sister Visitation's strategy of first approaching the wife of an influential official before requesting money from the governmental authority.

Biopolitics, that is the relationship between health and governance, has been a major analytic focus of recent research on hospitals. One strand has examined how hospitals discipline their patients and physicians. The Wesleyan and CEZMS institutions established disciplinary elements such as counting patients, prescribing allopathic medication and introducing more radical surgeries. However, they were willing to accommodate meaningful relationships of their patients. They had caste wards and sometimes even kitchens that preserved indigenous Hindu social relationships. They provided separate wards for Muslim women. Family members were permitted to bring food and to stay with patients.

Perhaps biopolitics is more useful to analyze the relationship between the religiously conservative Hindu Mysore rulers and the Christian missionaries. Missionary medical women were willing to serve populations that lacked minimal or no access to government hospitals. All three missionary groups had their principal hospital in one of the two capitals of Mysore's. Martha's, a general hospital, and the CEZMS Zenana Hospital were in Bangalore while Holdsworth Women's Hospital was in Mysore city. They focused on lower-class Indians who might not have felt comfortable or even wellserved (because of their caste or class status) in government hospitals. Although Reverend Redfern initiated Wesleyan Methodist 'mofussil' Hospital in Hassan, the CEZMS responded to the request of Muslim men when they sent to Channapatna. Thus at least one group of Indian men requested the medical aid of missionary women.

The Good Shepherd sisters, the Wesley Methodists and the CEZMS all had increasingly limited resources during the twentieth century. Consequently, they solicited support from municipal, district officials and Durbar ministers in Mysore and occasionally from the British GOI. The Mysore Durbar provided land and monetary grants for buildings and operation because the missionaries were serving populations and geographical areas that the state could not successfully penetrate. The British allotted money for medical areas it chose to ignore. The rulers of Mysore and the GOI were pragmatists. Their collaboration with Christian missionaries helped to spread disciplinary institutions to more populations – women – and regions. Still, the missionary hospitals and their training of nurses and midwives might be one factor contributing to the more favourable infant and maternal mortality rates in present-day Karnataka than in some other areas of India.

Notes

1 David Hardiman, 'Introduction', in David Hardiman (ed.), *Healing Bodies, Saving Souls: Medical Missions in Asia and Africa*, Amsterdam: Editions Rodopi B. V., 2006, 40.

2 Antoinette Burton, 'Contesting the Zenana: The Mission to Make "Lady Doctors for India"', 1874–1885', *Journal of British Studies*, 35 (July 1996), 368–97; Ruth Compton Brouwer, *Modern Women Modernizing Men: The Changing Missions of Three Professional Women in Asia and Africa, 1902–69*, Vancouver: UBC Press, 2002, especially Chapter Two on Dr. Chone Oliver; Rosemary A. Fitzgerald, 'A "Peculiar and Exceptional Measure": The Call for Women Medical Missionaries for India in the Later Nineteenth Century', in R. Bickers and R. Seton (eds.), *Missionary Encounters: Sources and Issues*, London: Curzon Press, 1996, 174–97; 'Rescue and Redemption: The Rise of Female Medical Missions in Colonial India during the Late Nineteenth and Early Twentieth Centuries,' in A.M. Rafferty, J. Robinson and R. Elkan (eds.), *Nursing History and the Politics of Welfare*, London: Routledge, 1996, 64–79; Rosemary Seton, *Western Daughters in Eastern Lands: British Missionary Women in Asia*, Santa Monica: Praeger, 2013.

3 After the British assumed control of the Mysore government in 1831, Bangalore was divided into the British-controlled Cantonment while the maharajas of Mysore presided over the Pettah, the Indian area. The maharajas of Mysore continued to reside in Mysore city. After the British rendition of control to the Mysore maharaja in 1881, the princely rulers continued to reside in Mysore city but the Mysore state administrative institutions remained in Bangalore. The British retained control over the Cantonment that became the Civil and Military Station.

4 *Down the Arches of the Years, St. Martha's Hospital Bangalore, Centenary Souvenir, 1886–1986*, n.p., n.d., 14–15.

5 Convent of Good Shepherd to Diwan of Mysore, 9 June 1883, *Arches*, 55–6.

6 S. Sreenivasa Charlu to Madam (Mother Mary Visitation), no date but between documents dated 9 June and 10 July 1883, *Arches*, 56.

7 Sister Mary Supress (sic), Convent of Good Shepherd, to J.B. Lyall, Resident in Mysore, 25 February 1884, National Archives of India, New Delhi (NAI), Mysore Residency Records (MRR), 536/1885, Serial Nos. 29–62. The Sisters of Charity of St. Joseph of Torbes also served as nurses in the Bowring Hospital in the Civil and Military Station. In 1887 they received 120 rupees for three sisters and 50 for their house rent, 22 September 1887, Serial Nos. 29–62.

8 Sister Mary Superioress, Convent of Good Shepherd to Major W. Macintyre, President, Pettah Municipality, Bangalore, 23 October 1883, Om Prakash, *St. Martha's Hospital: A Tribute*, n.p.; Bangalore, 1986, 9–11.

9 Sister Mary Supress (sic), Convent of Good Shepherd, to J.B. Lyall, Resident in Mysore, 25 February 1884, NAI, MRR, 536/1885, Serial Nos. 29–62.

10 Lyall to Lady Superior, 29 February 1884, MRR, 536/1885, Serial Nos. 29–62.

11 Sister Mary Visitation, 22 March 1884, *Down the Arches*, 58 and Prakash, *St. Martha's Hospital*, 13–14.

12 A.H. Macintire to Lady Superior, 28 July 1884, *Arches*, 59.

13 Extract from memorandum of 31 October 1883 by Dr. J. Henderson, *Arches*, 57.

14 Extract from letter of 15 November 1883 from Mother Mary Visitation to Dr. J. Henderson, *Arches*, 57.

15 Camp Nos. 228–32, Mysore 28 November 1892, Order signed by Ananda Rao, Chief Secretary, Mysore Government, *Arches*, 64.

16 Prakash, *St. Martha's Hospital*, 20–1.

17 Sister M. Breda, 'A Chain of Remembrance', *Arches*, 33.

18 Sister Emphani (spelling is not clear) to Mrs. McGann, 24 May 1913, Karnataka State Archives (KSA), General & Revenue (G&R) Medical, File No. 230 of 1912, Serials 1–2.

19 Decision of Council of Mysore on 9 August 1913, signed by M. Visvesvaraya, Diwan, KSA, File No. 230 of 1912, Serials 1–2.

20 *Report of the Wesleyan Mission in the Mysore Province for 1905*, 53, United Theological College Library, Bangalore, Ecclesiastical Archives (UTCL, EA); *Tales from the Inns of Healing of Christian Medical Service in India, Burma and Ceylon*, Nelson Square, Nagpur: Christian Medical Association of India, Burma and Ceylon, 1942, 47.

21 George W. Sawday to B. K. Venkata Varadiengar, Chief Secretary to the Government of His Highness the Maharaja of Mysore (GHHMM but further cited as Mysore State) 14 September 1905, KSA, GR-Medical, File No. 85 of 1905, Serial Nos. 1–2.

22 The Mysore Council approved the terms of this grant on 29 November 1905 and the maharaja sanctioned it on 23 December 1905. The terms were in an order dated 8 January 1906 and signed by B.K. Venkata Varada Iyengar, Secretary in File No. 85 of 1905, Serial Nos. 1–2.

23 KSA, GR-Medical, File No. 85 of 1905, Serial Nos. 1–2.

24 KSA, GR-Medical, File No. 85 of 1905.

25 G.G. Findlay and W.W. Holdsworth, *The History of the Wesleyan Methodist Missionary Society*, Vol. V, London: Epworth Press, 1924, 284–5.

26 Percy H. Benson, M.B., Honorary Secretary, Mysore, 31 December 1887 in the Third Report of the Central Committee, Countess of Dufferin Fund of 1887, dated January 1888, 102, NAI.

27 Benson, Annual Dufferin Report for 1888, Mysore, Report of Dufferin Fund, 1888, 104–5, NAI.

28 Rev. T. Halliday Newham to Chief Secretary, Mysore State, 7 September 1906, KSA, GR-Medical, File No. 86 of 1906, Serial Nos. 1–6.

29 *Report of the Wesleyan Mission in the Mysore Province*, 1904, UTCL, 67–8. The Hassan Circuit had asked the Mysore Durbar for a grant of the desired land but that property had multiple claimants and owners so the Mission had to purchase it from the Municipality.

30 The Hassan Municipal Board approved its grant on 13 October 1906 and the District Board did likewise on 10 December 1906, KSA, GR-Medical, File No. 86 of 1906, Serial Nos. 1–6.

31 Senior Surgeon, Mysore State to the Secretary Mysore State, Revenue Department, 17–18 April 1922, KSA, G&R-Medical, File No. 120 of 1921, Serial No 1 in Serial Nos. 1 & 3.

32 KSA, File No. 120 of 1921, Serial No 1 in Serial Nos. 1 & 3.

33 *Report of the Wesleyan Mission in the Mysore Province for 1906*, UTCL, 52.

144 *Barbara N. Ramusack*

34 *Report 1906*, 52.
35 *Report of the Wesleyan Mission in the Mysore Province for 1907*, UTCL, 35.
36 *Report 1907*, vii.
37 *Report of the Wesleyan Mission in the Mysore Province for 1908*, UTCL, 57–8.
38 Report 1908, 49.
39 Report 1908, 59.
40 Report 1908, 44.
41 Report 1908, 36–8.
42 *Report of the Wesleyan Mission in the Mysore Province for 1910*, UTCL, 38.
43 'Medical Department', *Mysore Blue Book Journal*, 6, 6 (May–June 1922), 572. Seen at the Mythic Society, Bangalore. This decision to terminate the grant to Mrs. Slater's Hospital was part of a major retrenchment of expenses by the Mysore government in 1922.
44 Although some physicians such as Dr. Mary O'Brien Beadon of the Women's Medical Service and Dr. Rose Fairbank Beals of the American Marathi Mission continued to practice after marriage, many did not.
45 Findlay and Holdsworth, *The History of the Wesleyan Methodist Missionary Society*, Vol. V, 296–7.
46 *Report of the Wesleyan Mission in the Mysore Province for 1911*, UTCL, 50.
47 *Report of the Wesleyan Mission in the Mysore Province for 1913*, UTCL, 48.
48 *Journal of the Association of Medical Women in India* (JAMWI), Vol.V, No. 13, February 1917, 13–14. Dr. F. Mervyn Smith had a B.Ch. as well as B.A. and M.A. degrees and was not a missionary. Around 1917 she was in Rampur, United Provinces, ibid., 41, and then subsequently in Ranchi, *JAMWI*, Vol. VII, No. 1, February 1919, 54. A married woman, she appears to function as an itinerant physician who was available to substitute for physicians on leave and to report on various medical issues.
49 'It seems impossible to get a doctor from England, so we are looking out in India', *Report of the Wesleyan Mission in the Mysore Province for 1914*, 48.
50 Report on the Working of Hospitals and Dispensaries in the State for the Year 1922, Statement A. Received from the Senior Surgeon with letter dated 24–30 July 1923, KSA, Mysore, GR-Medical, File No. 24 of 1923, Serial Nos. 1–5.
51 *Report of the Wesleyan Mission in the Mysore Province for 1905*, 57.
52 *Report of the Wesleyan Mission in the Mysore Province for 1906*, 37.
53 *Report of the Wesleyan Mission in the Mysore Province for 1907*, 40–1. In *Diagnosing Empire: Women, Medical Knowledge, and Colonial Mobility*, Farham, UK: Ashgate, 2011). Narin Hassan discusses how British women and men assumed authority over indigenous people in the Middle East by providing medical aid from their medicine chests.
54 *Report of the Wesleyan Mission in the Mysore Province for 1910*, 41.
55 *Report of the Wesleyan Mission in the Mysore Province for 1911*, 54.
56 Susan Bayly, *Caste, Society and Politics in India from the Eighteenth Century to the Modern Age*, New Cambridge History of India, IV, 3. Cambridge: Cambridge University Press, 1999, 184–5, 255.
57 *Report of the Wesleyan Mission in the Mysore Province for 1911*, 56.
58 *Report 1911*, 50.
59 *Report of the Wesleyan Mission in the Mysore Province for 1913*, 55.

60 Senior Surgeon to Revenue Secretary, Mysore Government, 17 April 1922, KSA, G&R, Medical, Mysore, File No. 120 of 1921, Serial Nos. 1 & 3.

61 The Employment of Indian Women Doctors, UTCL, Church of South India, Karnataka Central Diocesan Materials, (CSI-KCDM, XLV-Mysore), Box 62, Mysore District Medical Committee (MDMC), 1915–1956.

62 Mrs. Leith to Rev. H.H. Newham, UTCL, 21 April 1938, Box 62, MDMC, 1915–1956.

63 Irene H. Barnes, *Between Life and Death: The Story of the C.E.Z.M.S. Medical Missions in India, China and Ceylon,* 240. Barnes was the Deputation Secretary 1895–1898 and then the Editor and Superintendent of Publication Department 1898–1901 of the CEZMS in London.

64 Barnes, *Between Life and Death,* 240.

65 *JAMWI*,Vol. V, No. 14, May 1917, 2–4. Her reports were on abnormal pregnancies and abdominal surgery, specifically laparotomies that could be either exploratory or preliminary before further procedures. Lillingston also went to Simla in July 1917 to consider how the AMWI could respond to government requests for women physicians to work in their hospitals. *JAMWI*, Vol. V, No. 16, November 1917, 20.

66 Church of England Zenana Mission Society Archive (CEZMSA), Section I, East Asia Missions, Part 4, CEZ/G, EA 2/1B, Reel 86, Note by Dr. Dora Lockwood, 6 June 1929. This note is very informative on the institutional history and personnel of the CEZMS hospitals in Mysore and more measured than the glowing account by Irene Barnes.

67 Lockwood, 6 June 1929, CEZMSA, Reel 86.

68 Lockwood, 6 June 1929, CEZMSA, Reel 86.

69 Lockwood, 6 June 1929, CEZMSA, Reel 86, Gnanamuthu succeeded C.M. Robb, M.B. as head of Redfern Hospital (18 beds) in Hassan for a few years (Dufferin Report for 1922, NAI, 146) and then joined Mysore state service where in 1930 she was in charge of the female dispensary at Tarikere (Dufferin Report for 1930, NAI, 78).

70 In 1918–19 Medhora was listed in the *JAMWI* as employed at the CEZMS Hospital in Bangalore, *JAMWI*, Vol. VII, No. 1, February 1919, 50; by 1920 she was at the Sasson Hospital in Poona, *JAMWI*, Vol. VIII, No. 1, March 1920, 44 and in 1922 she had no institutional affiliation in Ahmedabad, Dufferin Fund Report for 1922, NAI, 158.

71 Lockwood, 6 June 1929, CEZMSA, Section I, Part 5, Reel 86, CEZ/G EA2/1B.

72 Lockwood, 6 June 1929, CEZMSA, Reel 86.

73 *JAMWI*, Vol. VI, No. 2, May 1918, 25–6.

74 Maneesha Lal, 'Purdah as Pathology: Gender and the Circulation of Medical Knowledge in Late Colonial India', in Sarah Hodges (ed.), *Reproductive Health in India: History, Politics, Controversies,* Hyderabad: Orient Longman, 2006, especially 97–108. Dr. Arthur Lankester, a missionary physician who later joined GOI service, was a prominent publicist of the opinion that purdah contributed to tuberculosis among Indian women as in a paper delivered at a meeting of the Association of Medical Women in India in New Delhi, 28 December 1917, *JAMWI*, Vol. V, No. 16, November 1917, 20.

75 Dr. Amy G. Lillingston to Lady Chelmsford, Vicereine and President of the Dufferin Fund, 25 June 1918, NAI, GOI, Home-Medical, January 1919, Part B, Pro. No. 71.

76 Lillingston to Chelmsford, 25 June 1918, GOI, Pro. No. 71.
77 H. Austen Smith, Surgeon to Viceroy Chelmsford, to Sir John B. Wood, Political Secretary, 11 July 1918, GOI, Pro. No. 71.
78 Undated note by Colonel Gimlette, Residency Surgeon, GOI, Pro. No. 71.
79 Cobb to J. B. Wood, 14 November 1918, GOI, Pro. No. 71.
80 J.B. Wood to Cobb, 7 January 1919, GOI, Pro. No. 71.
81 Lockwood, 6 June 1929, CEZMSA, Section I, Part 5, Reel 86, CEZ/G EA2/1B.
82 Lockwood, 6 June 1929, CEZMSA, Reel 86.
83 *JAMWI*, Vol. VIII, No. 3, November 1920, 29.
84 *JAMWI*, Vol. XI, No. 2, June 1923, 37.
85 S. Subba Rao, Senior Surgeon, to Officiating Chief Secretary of Mysore Government, 17 July 1929, KSA, Mysore, G&R, File No. 24 of 1929, Serial Nos. 1–9.
86 *JAMWI*, Vol. XIV, No. 3, August 1926, 52.
87 CEZMSA, Section I, Part 9, Reel 182, CEZ/C AD 4/1. This file includes extensive minutes of meetings in London, three different proposals for the Bangalore hospital, a trial period as a tuberculosis hospital and then the decision in 1931 that it will be a specialist hospital. This file is particularly difficult to use since the documents are not filmed in chronological order and there is no pagination of the documents filmed.
88 Medical Report by M.I. Neal, April 1929, CEZMSA, Reel 182.
89 Resolution Passed by Bangalore Local Conference, 14 April 1930, signed by Edith M. Potter, Honorary Secretary, Bangalore Local Conference Brief History and Financial Position, CEZMSA, 182.
90 Letter from B.M. Peddar to Rev A.J. Mortimore, Clerical (General) Secretary, (1930–1939) CEZMSA, London, 25 November 1930, Reel 182, CEZ/C AD 4/1.
91 Government Review on the Medical Report for 1918, *The Mysore Blue Book Journal*, Vol. IV, No. 3 (1919–20), 326. Read at The Mythic Society Library, Bangalore.
92 Abdul Rasheed, 18–21 June 1921, KSA, Mysore Representative Assembly, Printed Proceedings (MRA, PP) 1921, 44. Address of Anjuman-e-Mahdaviah Islam, Channapatna, 2–10 October 1922, KSA, MRA, PP, 1922, 17.
93 Correspondence between Clerical Secretary of CEZMS in London and Local Governing Body of CEZMS in Madras from December 1921 to 7 November 1922, UTCL, Bangalore, CEZMS, Vol. 3. Address of Anjuman-e-Mahdaviah Islam, Channapatna, 2–10 October 1922, KSA, Mysore Representative Assembly, Printed Proceedings, October 1922, 17.
94 Annual Report of the Mysore Health Department for 1929, 15, submitted July 1930 from J.V. Karve, Director of Health, to N. Madhava Rao, Chief Secretary to the Government of Mysore, M 47, Karnataka, Division Archives Office, Mysore city, Karnataka. CEZMSA, Section I, Part 5, Reel 90, CEZ/G EA5, 5D.
95 R.M. Peachey to Mr. Newham, 4 July 1932, UTCL, CSI-KCD, XXXV-Channapatna, File No. 1.
96 Peachey to Edith Potter, Secretary, Bangalore Local Conference, CEZMSA, 20 January 1934, UTCL, Channapatna, File No. 1.

97 Letter and Report on Channapatna from E.W. Legh, Corresponding Secretary of Madras CEZMS, to Rev A.J. Mortimore, 6 May 1936, CEZMSA, Section I, Part 5, Reel 90, CEZ/G EA5, 5D. The L.M.P. degree was designed for doctors who were to practice mainly in rural areas. The Bhore Report of 1946 recommended that it be terminated.

98 Lockwood to Miss Smith, Honorary CEZMS Secretary Foreign and Candidates, London, 12 October 1936, CEZMSA, Reel 90.

7 The epidemiological, health and medical aspects of famine

Views from the Madras Presidency (1876–78)

Leela Sami

The medical aspects of famine constitute an exciting area of research which has not received as much attention in the Indian as in the Irish contexts.[1] Our aim in this chapter is to open up this area through a study of the famine of 1876–78 in the Madras Presidency. We chose this episode for a variety of reasons, but the most important of these was the relatively better quality and quantity of the demographic and medical information available.[2] Although this data has been examined by social, economic and demographic historians, there remain fresh insights to be culled from an examination of this information.[3]

Here, we discuss two aspects. First, what did people suffer from and die of during the famine? Several studies have suggested that climatic and social factors were more important than nutritional ones in explaining mortality in south Asian famines.[4] We attempt to show that people *starved to death* during this famine – an almost axiomatic statement, but one that ironically needs reiteration.[5] We then look at medical responses to famine-related disease and mortality to examine their impact on the suffering of the famine stricken.

I: Starvation or disease? Explaining famine mortality

We begin by looking at the causes of famine mortality through an examination of death statistics taken from the Annual Reports of the Sanitary Commissioner of Madras Presidency during the years 1876 through 1878. Table 7.1 shows the distribution of deaths by cause over the years 1871–78. Of these, the famine years 1877 and 1878 saw the highest number of deaths, although there had been a steady upward climb since 1875.

In the first year (1877), 'other causes' dominated the returns. In 1878, 'fevers' overtook 'other causes'. Cholera constituted the third-largest cause of deaths in 1877. In 1878, there were relatively few cholera

Table 7.1 Deaths by cause 1871–78

Years	Total deaths	Cholera	Smallpox	Fevers	Bowel complaints*	Injuries	Other causes
1871	444,371	17,656 (3.9%)	20,823 (4.6%)	192,469 (43.3%)	38,928 (8.9%)	15,323 (3.4%)	159,172 (35.8%)
1872	508,182	13,247 (2.6%)	39,034 (7.68%)	214,148 (42.1%)	39,387 (7.75%)	15,150 (3%)	187,176 (36.8%)
1873	513,232	840 (0.16%)	51,784 (10.08)	222,843 (43.4%)	36,392 (7.09%)	14,251 (2.77%)	187,124 (36.4%)
1874	521,329	313 (0.06%)	48,343 (9.27%)	226,220 (43.3%)	37,993 (7.28%)	13,065 (2.5%)	195,395 (37.4%)
1875	641,260	94,546 (14.7%)	24,775 (3.86%)	252,042 (39.3%)	37,484 (5.84%)	12,421 (1.93%)	219,992 (34.3%)
1876	680,384	148,193 (21.7%)	23,469 (3.4%)	230,092 (33.8%)	38,176 (5.61%)	11,175 (1.64%)	229,279 (33.6%)
1877	1,556,312	357,430 (22.9%)	88,321 (5.67%)	469,241 (30.1%)	133,366 (8.5%)	16,460 (1.05%)	491,494 (31.5%)
1878	810,921	47,157 (5.8%)	56,360 (6.9%)	374,443 (46.1%)	48,083 (5.93%)	15,007 (1.85%)	269,861 (33.2%)

Source: Annual Reports of the Sanitary Commissioner of Madras 1871–78. (The title of the series varies from year to year.)

Note: * Prior to 1875, this was divided into dysentery and diarrhoea.

deaths. Deaths from smallpox, the fourth-largest registered category, reached their highest point in 1877. In 1878, the absolute number of smallpox deaths declined, but its contribution to total deaths nearly doubled. Bowel complaints caused 8.5% of all deaths in 1877, whilst the following year, this proportion reduced to just under 6%. Finally, deaths from 'injuries' also increased sharply in 1877 and 1878.

Monthly distribution of deaths from each cause

The monthly distribution of deaths is represented in Table 7.2 and graphically in Figure 7.1.[6]

Phases of famine mortality

Figure 7.1 indicates that there were four phases of famine mortality.

Phase I: 'Other Causes', Fevers and Cholera, March to November 1876.

The general death rate began to rise from March 1876, peaked in July 1876, and fell again until November 1876. It was led by 'other causes', fever and cholera. A fall in cholera deaths from July to November 1876 led to a dip in the general death rate.

Phase II: 'Cholera', November 1876 to April 1877.

From November 1876, a sharp rise in cholera deaths forced up the general death rate. Cholera deaths peaked in January 1877, and then slowly declined.

Phase III: 'Other Causes', April to October 1877.

The connection between cholera and the general death rate lost strength dramatically. Yet, the general death rate began to rise sharply from April 1877, led by 'other causes', which peaked in September. *Phase III was the most lethal in the entire course of the famine, with August 1877 registering the maximum deaths.* Thereafter, the general death rate declined, but began to rise again in October 1877.

Phase IV: Fevers, October 1877 to December 1878.

The fourth phase of famine mortality began from October 1877, when 'fever' deaths, which had been increasing from May 1877, overtook 'other causes'. The general death rate peaked again in December 1877. This was the highest absolute number of deaths from a single cause in any month. *Yet, fever deaths caused a smaller peak than that of 'other causes' in August/September 1877.* This was because the December 'fever' peak was neutralized to some extent by falling death rates in other categories.

Table 7.2 Monthly distribution of deaths by cause 1876–78

Causes	Jan-76	Feb-76	Mar-76	Apr-76	May-76	Jun-76	Jul-76	Aug-76
Cholera	14,607	11,683	8,299	10,834	11,463	14,681	18,641	10,363
Smallpox	2,038	2,889	3,517	2,460	1,750	1,462	1,398	1,244
Fever	21,118	18,898	16,660	16,166	17,036	17,953	19,778	18,687
BC	3,563	2,966	2,367	2,582	2,950	3,355	3,802	3,430
OC	19,705	18,065	15,763	16,271	17,566	18,368	20,963	20,339
Total mort	61,962	55,432	47,537	49,244	51,696	56,750	65,513	54,994

Causes	Sep-76	Oct-76	Nov-76	Dec-76	Jan-77	Feb-77	Mar-77	Apr-77
Cholera	5,265	3,280	7,894	31,183	58,712	51,211	43,753	31,005
Smallpox	1,192	1,150	1,551	2,812	4,989	6,863	9,653	8,837
Fever	17,959	18,216	22,671	24,950	21,556	18,713	21,801	21,404
BC	2,931	2,827	3,170	4,233	6,087	4,994	4,841	4,274
OC	19,387	18,649	20,314	23,918	23,479	21,564	22,232	22,241
Total mort	47,665	45,053	56,511	88,027	116,195	104,717	103,652	89,133

Causes	May-77	Jun-77	Jul-77	Aug-77	Sep-77	Oct-77	Nov-77	Dec-77
Cholera	37,139	25,921	27,353	31,737	24,501	10,390	8,416	7,292
Smallpox	6,849	6,014	6,324	6,798	7,392	8,302	8,034	8,266
Fever	25,670	31,418	44,366	49,034	49,085	49,226	65,683	71,275
BC	5,400	7,677	17,670	22,129	19,826	16,155	13,180	11,173
OC	27,656	36,115	53,634	62,863	65,818	56,177	51,708	47,973
Total mort	104,086	108,517	150,719	173,933	167,994	141,622	148,393	147,351

(Continued)

Table 7.2 (Continued)

Causes	Jan-78	Feb-78	Mar-78	Apr-78	May-78	Jun-78	July-78	Aug-78
Cholera	4,439	1,985	2,981	2,726	4,160	5,368	8,343	7,525
Smallpox	7,200	7,546	8,693	7,524	6,221	4,681	3,873	3,051
Fever	54,363	34,373	30,769	23,914	21,695	22,147	26,429	28,209
BC	7,989	4,855	3,929	3,055	2,867	3,185	3,788	4,623
OC	35,002	23,292	20,509	17,316	17,834	18,724	20,302	25,359
Total mort	110,243	73,301	68,131	55,785	54,027	55,355	63,985	70,017

Causes	Sep-78	Oct-78	Nov-78	Dec-78
Cholera	5,432	1,659	983	1,556
Smallpox	2,558	2,024	1,376	1,613
Fever	29,433	31,605	32,142	39,364
BC	4,643	3,538	2,945	2,666
OC	24,536	22,424	20,834	21,656
Total mort	67,852	62,590	59,530	68,105

Source: Annual Reports of the Sanitary Commissioner of Madras 1871–78

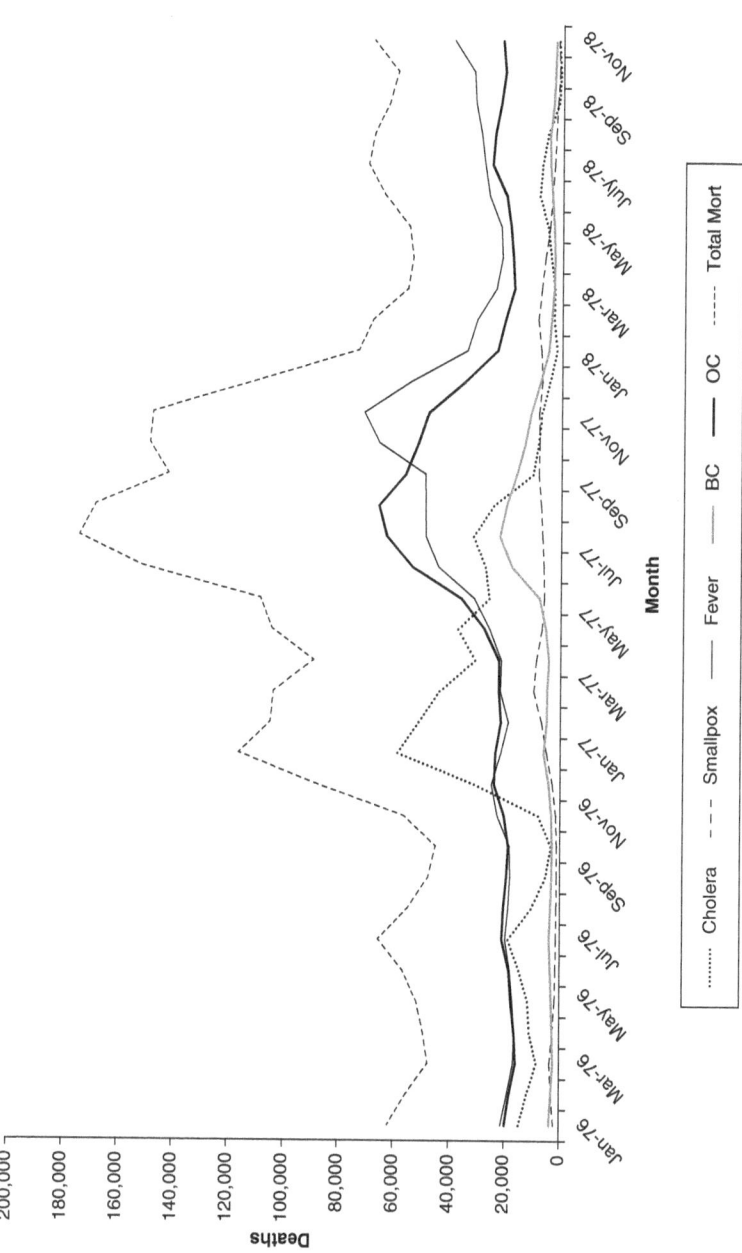

Figure 7.1 Monthly movement of death 1876–78

Source: Annual Reports of the Sanitary Commissioner of Madras 1871–78

Thereafter, the total death rate declined, although there was another minor peak in August 1878, which was due to 'fevers'.

Interpreting categories of death-causes during the 1876–78 famine

How do we interpret these data? We need to remember that a huge number of deaths were classified under four or five crude categories. Starvation never appeared in the statistics as a matter of course. The mortality data were collected by mortuary and crematorium officials at the time of burial or cremation and passed on to heads of villages or towns. The village heads passed their monthly totals on to the district collector, in whose office the data for all the villages in a district were collated. Finally, the data received from each individual district were compiled in the provincial Sanitary Commissioner's office. They were then published in an annual report which was sent to the Government of India.

Despite the high likelihood of under-registration of deaths, the returns were believed to be a fair approximation of general trends.[7]

'Other causes'

Medical officials at the time believed that most of this category's increase in the most lethal phase of famine consisted of starvation deaths. Dr. Alexander Porter, Principal of the Madras College, conducted autopsies on the bodies of 459 famine victims in Royapettah Hospital between November 1876 and May 1878. Porter wrote of his investigations:

> Many cases were suffering from no appreciable disease. These were generally returned under debility, privation or atrophy . . . they (were) all grouped under 'other causes'.[8]

In all the bodies he had seen in the postmortem room, 'the most notable feature was emaciation'. Fully 86% of men and 83% of women whose bodies he saw between November 1876 and May 1878 had wasted to the point where they had reached two thirds of their normal weight.[9]

Dr. William Robert Cornish, the Sanitary Commissioner of Madras, apprehended that government's order to village officials that 'no person was to be permitted to die from want of food' would prevent these officials – also responsible for registering deaths – from recording the truth. Cornish wrote:

> the fear of getting into trouble with the authorities would . . . have the effect of making these servants record mortality as due to 'old age', 'fever', or any other head of classification, rather than to the proper heading 'chronic starvation'.[10]

It appears likely that the huge increase in 'other causes' must have been composed largely by the effects of starvation.

Fevers

The correspondence between the term 'fevers' and malaria as we know it today – with its symptoms of spleen enlargement and hot and cold phases – appears not to have been watertight. 'Malarial fevers' was used in the sanitary reports to represent a class of diseases thought to be caused by poisoning both indirectly through exposure to contaminated air, and directly through emanations from decayed vegetable matter. *It did not always refer to a specific disease entity.*

Alexander Porter's investigations between November 1877 and May 1878 also indicate that 'fevers' referred to a variety of syndromes, and that pneumonia accounted for a large proportion of these:

> I have no doubt that many of these . . .(fever death statistics in the Sanitary Report, compiled from village and district level death returns) . . . were deaths from pneumonia, present in a large proportion of famine sick; in fact in the post mortem room pneumonia . . . was found in one case in every four.[11]

'Fever' was mentioned as a *cause of death* in only 7 out of Porter's 459 autopsies. It was mentioned as a *symptom* in numerous cases where the cause of death was recorded as *pyaemia, phthisis pulmonalis,* acute pneumonia and hepatic abscess.

There *was* a fever epidemic 'not during the time of greatest famine pressure, but after the rainfall following on prolonged drought . . . and . . . after the worst pressure of famine had been relieved'.[12] It affected 'all classes . . . even the European officials'.[13] But the likelihood of *death* was much higher amongst those who were starving. The most common fever – 'an ordinary malarious ague' – occasioned 'very little mortality with the strong and well-to-do', but with the 'weakly and half-starved victims of famine, it was very fatal'.[14] Cornish reiterated:

> The relation of the fever mortality to the famine appears to be this, that a vast number of people had been so debilitated by want that they (were unable) . . . to withstand a disease which, in ordinary years, is not very fatal.[15]

Cholera and bowel complaints

There was a cholera epidemic in late 1876 and early 1877, which appears to have been partly due to scarce and contaminated water supplies and consumption of rotten or indigestible food.[16] Yet, it seems likely that very many deaths registered under cholera and bowel complaints consisted of starvation cases. Early in 1877, there was a dispute between the Government of India and the Madras Government over the adequacy of wages for labourers on famine relief works. The Imperial Government, desperate to minimize expenditure, insisted that one pound of grain per person per day was sufficient to maintain the health of famine-stricken labourers on the works. The Provincial Government of Madras strongly protested that anything less than a pound and a half would starve people. It was backed by its medical officials, especially Cornish, who fervently believed that a large proportion of the deaths occurring in the Presidency from late 1876 onwards were caused by starvation.[17] The dispute between the two governments became more acrimonious, and there was a series of written volleys between Cornish and the Government of India's delegate Sir Richard Temple, who was sent to Madras in January 1877 with specific instructions to reduce expenditure on relief.[18]

Cornish and his team noted that there was both inadvertent and deliberate mis-representation of excess deaths, particularly since the Government of India informed local revenue officials – responsible for registering deaths – that they would be held responsible for any starvation deaths occurring within their jurisdiction.[19]

FAMINE DIARRHOEA AND CHOLERA

In February 1877, Cornish noted the presence of 'diarrhoea of a very severe type' amongst inmates in the relief camps in Madras. A week later, having come across it frequently, he termed it 'famine diarrhoea'. He soon came to believe that it was a sign of irreversible starvation.

Some of its symptoms appeared similar to those of ordinary infectious dysentery and cholera:

> The sick lie on the ground, in extreme weakness, curled up like a ball, the thighs drawn up against the abdomen, the head bending forward on the chest, and the arms folded close against the body. The surface of the body appears to be below the normal temperature, and the pulse is weak and barely to be felt. The motions are mostly of a dysenteric character, and if they do not contain blood, the bright green tint of the matters passed, betoken *blood* in an *altered* condition.[20]

Famine diarrhoea appears frequently to have been confused with cholera by administrators of relief camps. For example, Surgeon B.R. Thompson reported that in a hospital attached to a relief camp in Madras town:

> All the thousand odd patients admitted with symptoms of cholera were found later to be suffering from pathological changes in the digestive functions consequent upon starvation.[21]

Errors of diagnosis were common and attributed to the lack of medical training amongst administrators. Dr. Gray from Chingleput district mentioned, 'Cases of irritative dysentery and diarrhoea (are) being put down as cholera'.[22] Another official in Cuddapah wrote that 'some coolies supposed to have cholera . . . were all cases of famine-diarrhoea'.[23]

Yet others noted a wilful mis-recording of deaths. In Nellore district, a journalist interviewing the *tahsildar* of the Gudur *talook* reported that, according to the tahsildar, no-one in the *talook* was starving. When the journalist asked if the weekly mortuary returns did not indicate starvation, the *tahsildar* answered that they 'did not and could not, for in the event of an emaciated corpse being picked up, the village *munsiff* . . . whose duty it was to report (deaths) would not attribute the death to starvation but would say cholera, or dysentery, "or some usual disease" '.[24]

BOWEL COMPLAINTS

'Bowel complaints' was a category introduced in the death returns in1875 by the Indian Medical Department to refer to deaths from bowel discharges other than cholera.[25] It was likely that this category understated deaths in the best of times, and particularly so during famine periods. Cornish wrote that 'deaths from bowel complaints are not representative of the entire amount of fatal diarrhoea and dysentery'.[26]

Like cholera, the great increase under this category was probably partly due to the consumption of contaminated or poisonous food and foul water. Yet it was also closely allied with famine diarrhoea. The death ratio from bowel complaints in Madras city, where migrants flooded in throughout the famine period, was 38.2 per thousand as against a five-year mean of 5.0 in 1877. Cornish noted that

> Diarrhoea and dropsy of the whole body are the usual endings of four fifths of the famine stricken.[27]

Surgeon D.D. Cunningham, sent down by the Government of India to investigate famine deaths, wrote of his postmortem investigations:

> 'Famine diarrhoea' and 'famine dysentery' . . . are . . . morbid changes and degenerations dependent on malnutrition. Many cases . . . are complicated by the supervention of other diseases such as acute diarrhoea, dysentery (and) pneumonia . . . although in the majority of such cases the conditions leading to true 'famine diarrhoea' may be distinctly detected, yet the fatal termination is caused, or at all events, accelerated by the complications.[28]

Famine diarrhoea was thus a physiological phenomenon involving irreversible changes in the digestive tract, rather than an infective condition. It was also extremely fatal. In February 1877, Surgeon Lancaster reported to Cornish that, 'when I see it I always think the case hopeless.'[29] An officer visiting a relief camp in Salem district in April 1877 noted that patients were unresponsive to feeding, eventually dying after weeks or months:

> Some of the children came into the camp in very bad condition . . . they cannot assimilate the rice and broth . . . they had been tried with *ragi*, with rice and *cholum*, and . . . with sago, but nothing would bring them around.[30]

More recent research also substantiates the non-infectious and often irreversible character of famine diarrhoea. In the European concentration camps in the 1940s, bacteriological research 'failed to reveal any causative organism in famine diarrhoea . . . amongst extremely emaciated patients, (it) was refractory to any treatment and death was the usual outcome'.[31] W.R. Aykroyd also emphasized that 'infective organisms have rarely been isolated in famine diarrhoea; the condition is primarily due to wastage and ulceration of the intestinal walls'.[32] Similarly, biologists J.P.W. Rivers and Nevin Scrimshaw concluded that famine diarrhoea was a sure portend of death in severely malnourished people.[33]

Smallpox

The total number of deaths from smallpox increased significantly in 1877 and remained high in 1878. These deaths began to rise from November 1876 and peaked in March 1877. There was another (minor) peak in December 1877 and yet another in March 1878. In the early stages, when people crowded to relief centres, smallpox deaths were very numerous. Once the measures for famine relief were in place, the deaths remained high but stable. After March 1878, they declined. Cornish noted:

> The condition of the population was such as to be eminently favourable to the spread . . . of smallpox . . . thousands . . . wandered away from their homes to the nearest towns or markets or to relief works and camps, so that the people got herded together in large crowds.[34]

Injuries and accidents

While the number of suicides due to mental depression rose during the famine, the abnormally high levels of urban trade in grain also contributed to deaths under this category.[35] In 1877, deaths from injuries and wounds in Madras city alone amounted to 1,066, nearly a tenth of the entire number of deaths from this cause. Cornish reported:

> Nearly all the rice brought by sea was removed to the railway goods station, nearly two miles distant, by carts drawn by men, and very frequently the wheels of heavily laden carts caught the naked heels of the pullers. This crushing of the heels generally led to great sloughing and constitutional disturbance, and frequently tetanus supervened.[36]

In 1878, deaths from ulceration and 'sloughing' of wounds were common. Medical professionals ascribed these deaths to the effects of general weakness on healing processes.[37]

Who dies? Starvation, poverty and famine mortality

In his work on famine in Darfur, Alex de Waal suggested that personal habits and cultural factors determined the likelihood of death to a much greater extent than poverty.[38] In Madras, however, socioeconomic indicators *were* indeed accurate predictors of who died during the famine. The great majority of Alexander Porter's 'sample' were agricultural labourers from the Pariah and Palli castes, as well as several weavers and potters.[39] Landownership and caste – both strong predictors and indices of social and economic status in nineteenth-century Madras – greatly determined the chances of life or death during the famine of 1876–78. This is corroborated by data from the census of 1881.[40]

II: Medical responses to famine and famine mortality

In connection with medical involvement in famine, two questions have been asked by previous scholars. The first pertains to the content of their work and its efficacy: what did they do and did it work? Joel Mokyr and Cormac O'Grada have suggested that medical and popular ignorance of infectious disease causation and prevention was the main reason for the high mortality during the Irish famine of 1846–51. Had doctors and lay persons understood the ways in which infectious diseases are caused and transmitted, much might have been done to prevent or cure at least half of all deaths between 1846 and 1850.[41]

The second question pertains to motives and effects. David Arnold has argued that the nineteenth-century Indian famines 'constituted one of the few occasions when Indians became the focus of state medical concern' at 'a time when colonial medicine in India still remained closely tied to the needs of the European population and the army'.[42] Because of the risk of contracting infectious disease from the famine-stricken people, Arnold suggested, colonial medicine was forced to move towards 'a more general system of public health for the people of India'.[43]

Content and efficacy

The most striking feature of medical responses to famine and famine disease in Madras was indeed complete helplessness in saving the sick. Alexander Porter wrote:

> The only effective treatment of famine diseases is the prevention of famine, or, if this be impossible, the efficient organization of

famine relief. This to be efficient must be early in the famine, before the famine-stricken have begun to suffer from the disorganization of the tissues of the alimentary canal.[44]

Remedies for starvation

The work carried out by the Madras Medical Department during the famine was mostly palliative. This included the provision of food to restore the patients and remedies to calm pain. While possibly relieving some discomfort, much of it appears in retrospect to have been useless, if not dangerous, although European medical practitioners reported early treatment to be fairly successful. Famine diarrhoea was treated with liquid diets containing milk and soups. Mixtures containing cod liver oil, dilute sulphuric acid, opium, nitric acid, chlorodyne, ipecac and morphine were also administered.[45] Dropsy or swelling, characteristic of starvation, was treated by administering diuretics and sudorifics, which probably hastened fluid loss. In some hospitals, coconut oil was massaged into the skin to soothe the itching of characteristic dry 'famine skin'.[46] At others, the burning thirst of cholera patients was treated by giving them a mixture of dilute sulphuric acid in water. For acute pneumonia, 'a stimulating treatment of bark and ammonia, brandy and egg mixture and broths' was believed to be effective.[47] It is uncertain whether these 'worked' in the sense of forestalling death, although there might have been some relief from secondary symptoms.

Indigenous medical practitioners and their therapies were incorporated into famine relief efforts sporadically.[48] During this famine, however, *Vythians* were employed by the Collectors of Madurai and Coimbatore districts for the reason that '(they) treat successfully those maladies which are now so rife, diarrhoea and dysentery . . . we cannot cope with disease which is now carrying off so large a percentage of our population'.[49] However, we hear little else about them in the official reports.

Sanitary arrangements and the control of disease

Sanitary arrangements – particularly the provision of pure water supplies, for relief camps and relief works – might have been beneficial in curbing some of the death and disease from cholera after the first few months of 1877. Yet, municipal and local budgets were severely stretched during the crisis. Several municipalities reported that want of funds had impeded any sanitary or conservancy works, while in others, these consisted largely of works which could be carried out as famine relief works.[50] Sources of water supply became scarce and contaminated. In Cuddapah district in 1877:

> owing to the drought, most of the drinking water was taken from a public well fed by springs from the bed of the river, or from holes in the river bed. These sources were liable to constant pollution.[51]

In Madras town:

> the reservoir supplying the town . . . ran so low that the water had to be pumped into the delivery channel . . . and was very much the consistency of green pea soup, offensive to smell and taste.[52]

A Special Health Establishment funded jointly by the Madras Municipality and the Provincial Government toured Madras town from February 1877 to December 1877. Starving people were taken to relief camps and kitchens, or to infectious disease hospitals. Vaccinations were performed and dwellings were cleansed. Though the towns were better provided for, the urban death rates were exceedingly high: in Madras town, the death ratio was 118 per thousand population, while in other towns they ranged from 99 to 252 deaths per thousand population.[53]

In the countryside, innumerable deaths occurred outside the purview of state institutions – on roads and highways, in ditches and riverbeds. The disposal of the dead created a sanitary problem of massive proportions. A civil servant, Mr. Oldham, described a road in the Adoni *talook* of Bellary as covered with the dead and dying so that it 'resembled a battlefield'.[54]

Smallpox vaccination had been known and performed by vaccinators employed by local administrations in the Presidency since the turn of the nineteenth century.[55] It was carried out with great persistence during the famine, despite fears that it would further weaken starving people. A reporter remarked of the relief camps in North Arcot,

> Vaccination, of all things, had been scrupulously attended to, and I noticed several emaciated children and diarrhoea patients with marks of recent vaccination on their arms. This, I have been told at the Madras relief camps, is very wrong . . . no-one is to be vaccinated who is not in a tolerably sound condition of body.[56]

From 383,067 in 1875–76, the number of the vaccinations doubled to 787,730 in 1877–78. Yet, as we saw in Table 7.1, smallpox deaths increased manifold in 1877.

Institutional arrangements, overcrowding and disease

A common observation made by nineteenth-century administrators was that 'the strength of prisoner (population)' was 'an index of distress among the population'.[57] Economic distress was usually accompanied by high crime levels and enlarged prison populations. In 1877, there certainly was an enormous increase in the number of prisoners confined in the jails of Madras. In Bellary central jail, in ordinary times, 400 prisoners could be accommodated, while on 2 October 1877, there were 2,988 prisoners confined.[58]

Jail mortality in 1877 and 1878 was appalling. The average death ratio for jails in the famine districts (Bellary, Chingleput, North Arcot, Cuddapah, Madras, Madurai, Nellore, Salem, South Arcot, Trichinopoly) was 216 per thousand population, while the average for all other jails was 68.3 per thousand population in 1877.[59] (The general death rate was 53.2 per thousand population in the districts, though this masked wide variations between different districts and rural and urban areas.)[60]

However, overcrowding was not the only – or even the main – cause of high mortality. Although jail authorities struggled to maintain basic sanitation in the face of an influx of starving, emaciated prisoners, most inmates admitted in 1877 were far gone by the time they were imprisoned.[61] The Collector of the Salem District reported in 1877 that 'the jails and their compounds were often . . . overflowing . . . but there was little or no mortality which could be traced to overcrowding'.[62] This is borne out by Table 7.3, which shows jail mortality in relation to length of confinement across the Presidency.

Those imprisoned in the late 1876 and early 1877 had a much higher likelihood of dying than did those who had been in jail for a longer period. Of the deaths registered amongst prisoners, 1,668 out of 3,593 were due to 'dysentery and diarrhoea' while 480 were due

Table 7.3 Length of imprisonment and mortality in 1877 in the jails of Madras

Length of imprisonment undergone	No. of deaths 1877	Rate of mMortality
Under 6 months	2,212	30.34
6–12 months	642	14.55
1–2 years	301	10.80
2–3 years	150	7.30
3–7 years	211	7.79
Above 7 years	77	5.38

Source: Report on Administration of Jails 1877, p. 29

to 'anaemia and general debility'; 516 were due to cholera; 437 were from 'other diseases'; 169 from respiratory diseases; 118 from intermittent fever; 116 from ulcers and boils; 35 remittent and continued fever; 27 scrofula and phthisis pulmonalis; 18 smallpox; 1 suicide; 8 jaundice.[63] Starvation appears to have been the most important factor in the appalling prison mortality in these years.

Hospitals

Government hospitals were also crowded. The number of patients admitted to the 165 institutions across the Presidency rose steeply. Thus, in 1875–76, the total number of in-patients was 28,968; in 1876–77 it was 38,751, and in 1877 it was 82,820.[64] In Bellary, the Inspection report stated that 'the hospital building has been, and is now, much overcrowded. The sick are put everywhere – in the verandah, bathroom, and wherever a covered corner can be found'.[65] Yet, as in the case of jails, the deaths in these institutions were probably related more to starvation and social dislocation outside them rather than to overcrowding within. Of the diseases which were treated in 1877–78, the maximum were treated for dysentery, diarrhoea and injuries. The mortality rate for dysentery and diarrhoea was 77 per thousand population (dysentery) and 72.5 per thousand population (diarrhoea).[66]

As Arnold points out in the case of prisons, if people did seek out state institutions for sustenance and survival, then this strategy was sadly miscalculated.[67] These institutions were stretched to their utmost by the crisis. Where starvation had indeed gone too far, even the provision of food, rest, cleanliness, medicine and shelter could not prevent death.

Thus, knowledge about preventing the spread of disease through sanitary precautions would probably have been limited when the means were often scarce and disease was far advanced. Until famine relief policy became able to prevent large numbers of people from sliding down the ladder into irreversible starvation, such knowledge would have had limited success in saving the people of Madras.

Motives and effects

Although they were powerless to prevent or cure famine diseases, medical officials in Madras observed and recorded the symptoms of starvation and starvation-related disease in detail and attempted to communicate them to a general and medical audience.

This intense inquiry appears to have been motivated by more complex motives than simply protecting the armies and European settlements from infectious disease, as David Arnold has suggested.[68] Indeed, European civil and military health was left almost untouched by famine, despite contact with the starving population. Cornish remarked in his annual report for 1877 that:

> The British soldier could not take his walks abroad without encountering the victims of smallpox and cholera, and running the risk of personal infection; but we shall see how little these circumstances have affected a body of men, provided with wholesome food and drink . . . whose domestic situation was thoughtfully cared for by the State.[69]

This immunity was also reflected in the death rates of different sections of the population, as seen in Table 7.4.[70]

Why, then, did doctors like Cornish and Porter pay so much attention to recording the symptoms and conditions of the famine-stricken? Administrators had begun to recognize the need to planning for famine prevention and relief in the future as a part of general governance from the 1860s onwards. By the end of the famine – which affected southern and western India in 1876–77 and northern India in 1877–78, there were concerted efforts to evolve an effective crisis management system, which would straddle the tension between state responsibility for human lives and concerns over 'extravagance' in famine relief. There had been disputes between the Imperial and Provincial Governments over this issue throughout the mid-1870s, and a standard of nutritional support for workers was at the heart of many of these discussions. Determining the point at which starvation became irreversible was central – indeed vital – to Imperial attempts to control Provincial expenditure and Provincial attempts to defend its expenditure on famine relief. Medicine was thus staking a claim for

Table 7.4 Death rates amongst different sections of the population

Section of population	Deaths per 1,000 population
European army	17.25
Native army	15.2
Jail population	175.4
General population	53.2

Source: Annual Report of the Sanitary Commissioner of Madras for 1877

greater involvement in future governance by virtue of its expertise in recognizing irreversible starvation.

The weight test of nutritional adequacy

In March 1877, the Government of Madras sanctioned a regular and periodic inspection of workers and of people on relief camps and works by officers of the Indian Medical Service deputed to famine duty. They were to note their observations on the prevalence of a number of signs and symptoms of starvation, including the prevalence of anaemia, wasting, emaciation, physical and muscular development and whether the prescribed diet was being given to people on works and in camps.[71]

Whilst all sections of people were observed, those of the relief works received the most attention, because their physical condition was central to resolving the dispute between Madras and India over the adequacy of famine wages. The weighing of labourers on the famine wage was conducted in four places (Nellore, Chittoor, Palaveram and Poonamallee) from March 1877. The 'scientific' conduct of these macabre weighings was crucial to arguments that the Government of Madras was justified in providing more liberal scales of relief.

Sustained observation of the same cohort was almost impossible, due to the paucity of weights and scales, the highly mobile population and rumours amongst the population that they were being weighed in preparation to be deported (in the final scenario, 'the first weighing was also the last').[72] Yet amongst the one cohort which was regularly weighed, doctors found that between March and June 1877, workers on the Imperial (lower) wage lost weight. The condition of the people on the lower wage deteriorated rapidly, and the Madras Government abandoned the wage in May 1877 in favour of a higher one.[73]

The paradox of helplessness and expertise: the effects of medical inquiry

European medicine was helpless, in its curative and preventive aspects, in dealing with famine disease and famine mortality because most famine-stricken people were too far gone by the time they reached the doctors. Yet, at the same time, the importance of determining a nutritional standard of state support allowed doctors at the time to claim expertise in developing a *medical* body of knowledge regarding starvation. This paradox of helplessness/expertise is summarized in Cornish's lament in December 1877:

> A very large proportion of those applying for relief are so far reduced in frame that the expert can at a glance say of but too large a number, 'these *must* die'.[74]

Claims to expertise were strengthened by scientific recognition of their findings outside of the famine area. Surgeon D.D. Cunningham published a treatise on starvation, based partly on his investigations on famine diarrhoea, in Calcutta shortly after the famine.[75] Alexander Porter's work on famine diseases in Madras was published by a London firm in 1889.[76] Cornish's work on famine dropsy was recognized as pioneering by later medical writers.[77] While their work did not immediately lead to scientific investigations on nutritional standards, it did inform the development of a system of state intervention in famine relief, as embodied in the Famine Codes of the 1880s.[78]

Conclusion

Starvation played a far more important role in causing deaths during the Madras famine of 1876–78 than has been recognized by earlier studies, which focused overwhelmingly on climatic sequences and social displacement. A careful weighing of the evidence leads to the conclusion that starvation and its companion, famine diarrhoea, were the real culprits.

Because of the irreversible physiological effects of long continued starvation on the bodies of the famine-stricken, European medical responses to famine were characterized by the paradox of helplessness and expertise. While much of the preventive, palliative and curative work of the Madras Medical Department was ineffective in stalling, reversing or curing the famine-stricken, detailed inquiries into the signs and symptoms of irreversible starvation created the space for medical men to claim expert status in the prevention and management of famine disease. These concerns were increasingly important to the interventionist state in the decades following the famine.

Notes

1 See for example L.A. Clarkson and E. M. Crawford, *Famine and Disease in Ireland*, Vols. I–V, London: Pickering and Chatto, 2005.

2 See T. Dyson, 'On the Demography of South Asian Famines Part I', *Population Studies*, 45, 1 (1991), 7.

3 Earlier references include B.M. Bhatia, *Famines in India: A Study in Some Aspects of the Economic History of India*, London & New Delhi: Asia Publishing House, 1967, 93–6; I. Klein, 'When the Rains Failed: Famine, Relief and Mortality in British India', *Indian Economic and Social History Review* 21, 2 (1984), 185–214; R. Lardinois, 'Famine, Epidemics and Mortality in Southern India: A Re-Appraisal of the Demographic Crisis of 1876–78', *Economic and Political Weekly*, 20, 11 (1985), 454–65; E. Whitcombe, 'Famine Mortality', *Economic and Political Weekly*, 28, 23 (1993), 1169–79; M. Davis, *Late Victorian Holocausts: El Nino Famines and the Making of the Third World*, New York: Verso, 2001; L. Brennan, 'The Development of the Indian Famine Codes: Personalities, Policies and Politics', in B. Curry and G. Hugo (eds.), *Famine as a Geographical Phenomenon*, Dordrecht: Reidel 1984; D. Hall-Matthews, 'The Historical Roots of Famine Relief Paradigms', in H. O'Neill and J. Toye (eds.), *A World Without Famine? New Approaches to Aid and Development*, Basingstoke: Palgrave Macmillan. See also S. Hodges, ' "Looting" the Lock Hospital in Colonial Madras During the Famine Years of the 1870s', *Social History of Medicine*, 18, 3 (2005), 379–98.

4 See Dyson, 'On the Demography of South Asian Famines Part 1'; Whitcombe, 'Famine Mortality'; D. Arnold, 'Social Crisis and Epidemic Disease in the Famines of Nineteenth Century India', *Social History of Medicine*, 6, 3 (1993), 385–404.

5 For a more detailed discussion, see L. Sami, 'Starvation, Disease and Death: Explaining Famine Mortality in Madras 1876–78', forthcoming, *Social History of Medicine*, 24, 3 (2011), 700–19.

6 The annual sanitary reports did not contain monthly figures for deaths registered under the category 'other causes' or 'injuries and accidents'. But by first subtracting the monthly deaths from cholera, smallpox, fevers and bowel complaints from the total number of deaths for each month, we arrived at the combined monthly total for 'other causes' and 'injuries'. The monthly average of deaths from injuries was obtained by dividing the yearly total for injuries by 12. This average was then subtracted from the monthly combined total for injuries and other causes. What remained was the monthly total of deaths from 'other causes'. Although this method tended to smooth out the monthly or seasonal variations in deaths from injuries by using a flat average, we justify its use on the grounds that the number of deaths from injuries was a very small proportion of the total (between 1.05% and 1.85% of all deaths). This would not disturb the monthly variation in the combined total of 'other causes' and 'injuries' to a great extent.

7 *Annual Report of the Sanitary Commissioner of Madras for 1866*, 161. See also Cornish's remarks in *Annual Report of the Sanitary Commissioner of Madras for 1877*, 75.

8 A. Porter, *Diseases of the Madras Famine*, London: H.K. Lewis, 1889, 104.

9 Ibid., 201.

10 *Annual Report of the Sanitary Commissioner of Madras for 1877*, 147.

11 Porter, *Diseases of the Madras Famine*, 131.

12 *Annual Report of the Sanitary Commissioner of Madras for 1877*, 141.

13 Ibid., xxviii.
14 Ibid., 142.
15 Ibid. See S. Zurbrigg, 'Hunger and Epidemic Malaria in Punjab 1868–1940', *Economic and Political Weekly*, 27, 4 (1992), PE 2–PE 26.; and A. Maharatna, 'Famines and Epidemics: An Indian Historical Perspective', in T. Dyson and C. O'Grada (eds.), *Famine Demography: Perspectives from the Past and Present*, Oxford: Oxford University Press, 2002, 137.
16 *Annual Report of the Sanitary Commissioner of Madras for 1877*, 103.
17 The literature cited in note 3 contains several accounts of this debate. The original sources are contained in Correspondence between the Secretary of State for India and the Government of India on the Subject of the Threatened Famine in Western and Southern India Parts 1, 2, 3, 4 in the Oriental and India Office Collections in London (henceforth Famine Correspondence).
18 Letter from the Secretary to the Government of India to the Hon. Sir Richard Temple, Bart, K.C.S.I., Lt. Governor of Bengal (on a Special Mission), dated Calcutta the 16th January 1877. (Famine Correspondence 2.)
19 *Annual Report of the Sanitary Commissioner of Madras for 1877*, 141.
20 Ibid.,188.
21 Ibid.
22 W.R. Cornish, 'The Sanitary and Medical Aspects of Famine', in *Annual Report of the Sanitary Commissioner of Madras for 1877*, xxvi.
23 Ibid.
24 W. Digby, *The Famine Campaign in Southern India*, London: Longmans Green and Company, 1878, 103–4.
25 Prior to 1875, 'diarrhoea' and 'dysentery' had been registered separately.
26 Proceedings of the Government of Madras in the Public Department dated September 14th, 1877, No. 32–4, TNSA.
27 *Annual Report of the Sanitary Commissioner of Madras for 1877*, 143.
28 Letter from Surgeon D.D. Cunningham, to Surgeon Major S.C. Townsend, Officiating Sanitary Commissioner with the Government of India, dated Calcutta, 18th June 1877 (Famine Correspondence 4, OIOC).
29 Cornish, 'The Sanitary and Medical Aspects of Famine', xxxv.
30 Memorandum by C.E. Bernard on relief affairs in the worst part of Salem district in April 1877 dated Morapet, 16th April 1877, Famine Correspondence 4, OIOC.
31 A. Keys, *The Biology of Human Starvation*, Vols. 1–2, Minneapolis: University of Minnesota Press, 1950, 588–89.
32 W.R. Aykroyd, 'Definition of Different Degrees of Starvation', in G. Blix, Y. Hofvander and B. Vahlquist (eds.), *Famine: A Symposium Dealing with Nutrition and Relief Operations in Times of Disaster*, Uppsala: Almqvist and Wiksell, 1971.
33 J.P.W. Rivers, 'The Nutritional Biology of Famine', in G.A. Harrison (ed.), *Famine*, Oxford: Oxford University Press, 1988, 63, 78; N.S. Scrimshaw, 'The Phenomenon of Famine', *Annual Review of Nutrition*, 7 (1987), 1–21, 7.
34 *Annual Report of the Sanitary Commissioner of Madras for 1877*, 137.
35 The increase in suicides and depression had been noted in earlier Indian famines as well. See J.C. Geddes, *Administrative Experience Recorded of Former Famines: Extracts from Official Papers Containing Instructions for Dealing with Famine*, Calcutta: Government of Bengal, 1874, 187–88.

36 *Annual Report of the Sanitary Commissioner of Madras 1877*, 145.
37 It was reported in 1878 that fatal abscesses and gangrenous ulcerations were unusually prevalent amongst the poor (*Annual Report of the Sanitary Commissioner of Madras for 1878*, 135). This was also the case during the second year of famine in Bengal in 1943–44. (Famine Inquiry Commission, *Final Report on Bengal*, Usha, Calcutta, 1945.)
38 A. De Waal, *Famine That Kills: Darfur, Sudan 1984–1985*, Oxford: Oxford University Press 1989, 182.
39 Pariah and Palli were untouchable castes, members of which performed various forms of agricultural labour, owned almost no land and were at the bottom of the economic and social stratum throughout the Presidency. See D. Kumar, *Land and Caste in South India: Agricultural Labour in the Madras Presidency During the Nineteenth Century* (First published 1965); reprinted New Delhi: Cambridge University Press, 1992.
40 *See Imperial Census of 1881: Operations and Results in the Presidency of Madras*, Vol. I, The Presidency of Madras Government Press, Madras, 1883, 109 and 115.
41 J. Mokyr and C. O'Grada, 'Famine Disease and Famine Mortality: Lessons from the Irish Experience, 1845–50', in T. Dyson and C. O'Grada (eds.), *Famine Demography*, Oxford: Oxford University Press.
42 Arnold, 'Social Crisis and Epidemic Disease', 404.
43 Ibid.
44 Porter, *Diseases of the Madras Famine*, 209.
45 'Remedial Measures Ordered to be Adopted in Connection with the High Death Rate in Madras Town Due to Cholera', Proceedings of the Government of Madras in the Public Department, Nos. 68–9 dated 13th February 1877, TNSA. Porter reported that diarrhoea was concealed by patients in hospital for fear that they would be put on a bland diet of milk and soup and deprived of 'curry'.
46 Cornish, 'The Sanitary and Medical Aspects of Famine', xv.
47 Porter, *Diseases of the Madras Famine*, 210.
48 During a previous famine in Ganjam district in 1866, the Madras Government made an attempt to lay the foundations for 'schooling' them in biomedicine.
49 Letter from A. Wedderburn, Esq., Collector of Coimbatore, to C.A. Galton, Esq., Acting Secretary to the Board of Revenue dated 21st August 1877, No. 319, Proceedings of the Madras Board of Revenue, September 3, 1877, TNSA.
50 *Annual Report of the Sanitary Commissioner of Madras for 1877*, 160–78.
51 Ibid., 118.
52 Ibid., 103.
53 Ibid., 84.
54 Ibid., 121.
55 *Manual of Administration of the Madras Presidency, in Illustration of the Records of Government and the Yearly Administration Reports*, E. Keys, Great Britain,1885–1893, 511.
56 Report by the Special Correspondent of the Friend in India, dated March 16, reproduced in Digby, *The Famine Campaign in Southern India*, 100.

57 Dr. G.S. Sutherland in Report of the Indian Jail Conference, Calcutta 1877, quoted in Arnold, 'Social Crisis and Epidemic Disease', 396.
58 Proceedings of the Government of Madras in the Judicial Department dated 30th March 1878, Nos. 164–6, TNSA.
59 *Annual Report of the Sanitary Commissioner of Madras for 1877*, 69.
60 Ibid., 83.
61 Ibid.
62 H. Le Fanu, *Salem District Gazetteer*, Government Press, Madras, 1918, 307.
63 Ibid, 27.
64 *Annual Report on Civil Hospitals and Dispensaries for 1877–78*, 5.
65 Ibid., 17.
66 *Annual Report on Civil Hospitals and Dispensaries in Madras for 1877–78* and *Annual Report on Civil Hospitals and Dispensaries in Madras for 1878*.
67 Arnold, 'Social Crisis and Epidemic Disease', 396.
68 Ibid., 404.
69 *Annual Report of the Sanitary Commissioner of Madras for 1877*, 17.
70 Figures taken from *Annual Report of the Sanitary Commissioner of Madras for 1877*.
71 *Annual Report of the Sanitary Commissioner for Madras for 1877*, 203.
72 Ibid.,221.
73 Letter from Secretary of State to Government of India, No. 43, dated India Office, 10th May 1877, No. 251, Famine Correspondence 3 (OIOC).
74 'Remedial Measures Ordered to be Adopted in Connection with the High Death Rate in Madras Town Due to Cholera,' Proceedings of the Government of Madras in the Public Department, Nos. 68–9, dated 13th February 1877, Nos. 68–9, TNSA.
75 D.D. Cunningham, *On Certain Effects of Starvation on Vegetable and Animal Tissues*, Office of the Superintendent of Government Print, Calcutta, 1879.
76 A. Porter, *The Diseases of the Madras Famine*, London: H.K. Lewis, 1889.
77 See J.A. Nixon., 'Famine Dropsy and Pioneer Work in India', *Proceedings of the Royal Society of Medicine Section of the History of Medicine*, 14 (1920–21).
78 On the making of the famine codes, see Brennan, 'The Development of the Indian Famine Codes', and K.S. Singh, 'The Famine Code: Context and Continuity', in J. Floud and A. Rangasami (eds.), *Famine and Society*, New Delhi: Indian Law Institute, 1993.

8 Gender and insanity

Situating asylums in nineteenth-century Bengal

Debjani Das

The Western medical practice and the medical care of the late eighteenth and early nineteenth centuries was primarily meant for the maintenance of the army's troops. Hence, military considerations were the prime concern for the establishment of several medical institutions of the time, which included general hospitals and fever hospitals, other than the military hospital: all meant for the cure and well-being of the army. Insane hospitals were also built during the period to treat those soldiers who were diagnosed with mental illnesses. The European Insane Hospital in Calcutta was the oldest asylum and dated back to the 1780s. Its social composition was limited to European military personnel and the institution was primarily concerned with the treatment of physically and mentally unfit soldiers. Initially this asylum was maintained by the Military Department; later when European women were also admitted into the asylum, its social composition changed and thereafter it came under the superintendence of the General Department.[1] This asylum located at Calcutta in Bhawanipur was built to temporarily detain insane Europeans who were eventually shipped back to Europe.

Other than one European asylum, Bengal Presidency in its lower provinces in the nineteenth century witnessed the birth of several 'native' asylums. These included those at Dacca, Moorshedabad, Patna, Berhampore, Moydapore and Russapaglah, later known as Dullunda at Calcutta. Initially 'native' asylums were meant to shelter the wanderers, deviants, vagrants and criminals, but gradually began accommodating patients who were diagnosed as mad. By the second decade of the nineteenth century, along with the establishment of several asylums in the Presidency, several definitions of madness began to be constructed by the European medical practitioners within the asylums, and means to control and cure them were also practised accordingly. Hence, the social composition of admission into the asylum began to change, and it continued to change further as the understanding and diagnosis of madness gradually evolved.

There were several differences in the characteristic features and the functioning of the European and the 'native' asylums; also treatment of the insane often differed in both places. But, the point of similarity between the two was the question of insane women, both European and non-European. Why was it so? In order to seek an answer to this question, one needs to know how women's insanity was understood by the physicians of the time and it is within this context that this chapter seeks to situate the issue of women in the asylums of Bengal in its lower provinces in the nineteenth century. Hence, it is through an exploration of the various definitions of insanity and on the issue of labour at the asylum in which both men and women were engaged that this chapter tries to argue whether there was any difference in understanding the insanity of women and that of men and also how labour used as a therapeutic strategy was universal. It was labour that cuts across the definitions of women's insanity and places the European and non-European women on a similar basis.

At every stage of their practice in the asylums of Bengal, European physicians not only followed the current medical literature of England and Europe but also tried to implement it. This transformation of practices ranged from the duties and qualifications of a superintendent to the changing perceptions and definitions of insanity. They often made comparisons between asylums of Bengal and those of Europe and England. This was reflected in their definitions of insanity and the method of treatment for the malady. Until the mid-nineteenth century, the medical practitioners appointed at asylums were not specialized in the treatment of mental diseases as insanity was yet to be recognized as a disease. Physicians engaged with the cure of the insane dealt with their general illnesses. Therefore, definitions and classifications of insanity varied from one asylum to another, which often led to a much generalized, non-professional or non-specialized treatment of insanity. In most of the cases bodily diseases were dealt with, which ranged from general weakness to treatment of diseases like cholera. Various English and European physicians, many of whom were also the superintendents of those asylums, constructed the different forms, causes and effect of insanity. While the medical professionals defined its causes amongst men in terms of their physical weaknesses, women's insanity was often defined in terms of their emotional expressions, behaviours and manners. Before going into the reason for this difference, it is necessary to look at the social composition of women admitted in the asylums.

Social composition of women in 'native' asylums

Women admitted into the 'native' asylums of Bengal mainly included beggars, coolies, cultivators, labourers, fisherwomen, housewives and prostitutes, and by the 1870s, there were also references of insane women who prior to their admission worked as domestic servants, washerwomen, shopkeepers and weavers. Of the different women admitted in the European Lunatic Asylum, wives and daughters of European soldiers were predominant. The difference in admission procedures among women into the 'native' and European Lunatic Asylum was that in the former asylum women were often picked up from the streets by the police officers and admitted into the asylum with the permission of the magistrate, whereas in the latter instance, women were admitted by the members of their families, friends or relatives. Although the government partially funded the maintenance of European lunatics, the asylum at Bhawanipur mainly ran on a private ownership, where the individual patient's family had to pay for their maintenance at the asylum. The situation was different at the 'native' asylums where the Company and later the Crown were responsible for their maintenance. This continued until the end of the nineteenth century when to reduce the increasing number of patients in the 'native' asylums, the medical officers decided to admit paying patients only.

In 1862, A. Fleming, the Official Civil Surgeon of the Moorshedabad Lunatic Asylum, stated that institutionalized lunatics mostly belonged to the poorer classes of the community.[2] He further stated that women were usually not sent into the asylum at Moorshedabad, other than women who wandered the streets as friendless *faqueer*, bazaar girls and criminals. According to the official records, the majority of the lunatics, either male or female, admitted in the asylums of Bengal were from the 'lowest and least educated classes'. This class composition of the lunatics continued to be the same throughout the nineteenth century. For instance, even after a decade later amongst the patients admitted into the Moydapore Asylum by 1872, the male population mainly consisted of cultivators whereas beggars made up the female population.[3] The social composition of women continued to be the same when in Dullunda in 1875, there were two beggars, five coolies, one fisherwoman, one housewife, eight prostitutes, three domestic servants, one washerwoman among female inmates and twenty-two cases were 'unknown'. Similarly, at Dacca there was one beggar woman, two *grihisti* or housewives, one domestic servant and one case was 'unknown'. Amongst women admitted at Patna, there was one beggar, three cultivators, one labourer, one prostitute, one domestic servant, one shopkeeper, one weaver, one from another occupation and five cases were unknown. At Cuttack in the same year, an insane woman was a coolie before she was admitted. At Berhampore, there were four cultivators, one labourer, two domestic servants and one from some other occupation.[4] At Dullunda in 1885, there were two beggars, one maid servant, one potter, one prostitute and one teacher. Eight women were not engaged in any occupation, and in case of one woman lunatic there was no prior history. At Dacca there was one beggar, seven cultivators and one Christian missionary. At Patna there were five beggars, two cultivators, two labourers and two undertakers. At Berhampore there was one beggar, one cultivator and the case histories of three women lunatics were not known.[5] Medical officers faced difficulties in registering the accurate details of an insane person's age and previous history of illnesses. According to James Wise, a wandering lunatic picked up by the police could hardly give any account of himself or herself. At the same time, relatives were so 'ignorant and unobservant of dates' that exact details were impossible to procure.[6]

At a time when there were very few insignificant references of the social background of women admitted in the asylums, the official reports on lunatic asylums complicated the situation by introducing the term 'unknown'. This category of 'unknown' was a hindrance for the asylum physicians because they found it difficult to acquire knowledge of the prior case histories of those who fell into this category and many did. Prior case histories were significant because it often helped the asylum physicians to begin with the treatment of lunatics as soon as they were admitted into the asylums, but in its absence lunatics were put under observation and treated accordingly. It, therefore, often delayed not only the initialization of the treatment, but also chances of their recovery. In order to understand women's insanity, therefore, it is also necessary to know how the medical officers defined insanity.

Women in the European Lunatic Asylum

The condition of women in the European Lunatic Asylum was different from that of the 'native' women. This difference was not based on an understanding of their 'deranged state of mind', but rather on class divisions. In the European Lunatic Asylum, women of upper, middle and pauper classes were admitted. They were usually maintained by their friends, relatives or acquaintances, unlike in the 'native' asylums where lunatics were kept at the expense of the government. Some of the case studies regarding women in the European Asylum showed how, in several situations, they underwent difficulties due to this transfer from the upper- to the lower-class rooms of the asylums. This transfer was often due to lack of funds, particularly in instances where the families, friends or relatives of the upper-class patients refused to pay for the lunatic's further maintenance in the asylum. Therefore, European women faced several problems on admission, other than their physical and mental illnesses, which had already reduced their physical strength. They also had to become accustomed to their new place of confinement. A change of lifestyle caused by the shift from upper to lower class worsened their situation.

The number of women admitted at the European Lunatic Asylum was not only less in comparison to the number of men admitted but was also far less than the number of women admitted in the 'native' asylums. This was because of the obvious reason that there were many 'native' asylums while, on the contrary, there was only one European Lunatic Asylum in Bengal. Another reason, as stated by R. Bird, the Superintendent of the Asylum, was that the number of European men in India was much greater than European women.[7] This comparison between numbers of men and women in the asylum showed that although fewer women were admitted, insanity was in no way a rare occurrence amongst European women in India.

Causes of insanity: an attempt to understand the difference between male and female insanity

Intoxication was considered one of the most significant causes of insanity among men but the asylum report also mentioned that it was a cause of insanity among women, albeit not a major one. For instance, in 1835 at the Dacca Asylum in the case of most of the male lunatics, insanity was found to originate in 'dissipation', especially in the habitual and excessive use of intoxicating liquors and drugs. There were instances of relapses amongst such patients. Official records cited a case in which a man who had been discharged after being perfectly sane for several months in the asylum returned in a state of raging insanity three or four days afterwards due to the re-consumption of *bhang* or *ganja*.[8]

The cause of insanity amongst both men and women, according to the Superintendent of Moorshedabad Asylum in 1842, was physical.

> That was when one or more of the mental powers or manifestations were abysmal owing to the derangement either organic or functional of the cerebral centre on which that manifestation depend.[9]

A similar view of the physical causes of insanity was taken in 1842 by the Superintendent of the Dacca Lunatic Asylum. The physical causes of insanity at the asylum in order of 'frequency of occurrence' were *ganja*, opium, epilepsy, intemperance and heredity.[10] The Superintendent assumed that since women were less addicted to *ganja* smoking than males, their numbers were fewer, and also because almost 'no females excepting such as belong to the lower classes would generally be allowed to visit a public hospital'.[11]

The medical officers had repeatedly expressed their discontent with the fact that it was exceedingly difficult to obtain correct information on the causes of lunacy among those admitted in the lunatic asylums because lunatics were seldom accompanied to the asylum by anyone who had any knowledge of the matter.[12] This was true for both men and women. But throughout the nineteenth century, in various medical reports, the medical officers asserted that this situation was more frequent in women. Superintendent A. Payne stated that it was more difficult to assign the causes of insanity amongst asylum inmates in India than in England. He observed reluctance amongst the patients to speak of their hereditary background and to disclose the habits which had preceded the onset of the problem. Therefore, he was apprehensive of the fact that error might arise from mistaking those practices as causes of insanity, which were otherwise only its 'first manifestations'.[13]

The Superintendent of the Patna Lunatic Asylum stated that women lunatics admitted into the asylum suffered from chronic symptoms, which often resulted in a state of dementia. He, too, considered physical illnesses as the cause of insanity but what he found problematic was the fact that such illnesses increased with age, rendering mental disease less tractable. In cases where 'organic disease was often present, . . . they were less curable as regards their mental condition'.[14]

As far as European women were concerned, there was a growing belief that their illnesses were due to their particular sensitivity to climate. W.J. Moore, for example, pointed out that many suffered from 'uterine disease' due to 'climatorial influences'.[15] In Moore's view, 'young females' during their long voyages to India got emotional on leaving England and their home, and this was followed by 'excitement consequent on a succession of new scenes, and sea sickness, before the menstrual function'.[16] In addition to this he further stated,

> there is frequently exposure to chilling winds and moisture, neglect of suitable clothing, the tedium and fatigue of a long march up country, and, lastly, the early marriages so constantly negotiated, all powerful agents to disturb the uterine, nervous, and vascular system.[17]

The 'mental emotion and vomiting' that accompanied such disturbances led to the delay in 'established or un established catemenial flow'.[18] Amongst 'native' women, he stated, early marriages before the 'thorough development' of the sexual organs often led to diseases of the womb. This illustrated that European physicians established the onset, even or uneven flow of menses as a significant reason associated with mental illnesses among women. The lack of discussion on women's mental health in the nineteenth century by European medical practitioners in India means that it is impossible to know their opinion on the association of the menstrual cycle and female insanity. Indeed, Moore pointed out that 'the influence of tropical climates on the rise and progress of uterine disease does not appear to have received that attention, which the subject demands from Indian medical authors'.[19] This explained the attempt to impose similar views in understanding mental illnesses amongst both European and 'native' women.

In 1835, in a report on the Insane Hospital of Dinajpore, J. Marshall, the Superintending Surgeon, expressed his doubts about reaching any accurate conclusion as to the comparative frequency of insanity amongst men and women. According to him, the 'middle life period of women was most obnoxious to insanity'. He was of the opinion that puerperal[20] mania was common in India. According to medical reports, women usually faced this problem after laborious and difficult childbirth. There were very few references to puerperal mania in the asylums of Bengal. According to the medical officers, it was more frequent among women in the European Asylum than among those in the 'native' asylums. According to the English physician James Reid,

> the term puerperal insanity is not only understood to imply aberration of the mind, or derangement of the cerebral functions in the puerperal state itself, but to include those attacks which occur sometimes during the period of gestation, as well as those which we more frequently meet with few months after parturition, whilst the patient is suckling her infant.[21]

Thomas A. Wise, Surgeon of the Dacca Lunatic Asylum, also believed that 'the variety of mental derangement incident to women soon after parturition seems to be less common in Bengal than in Europe'.[22] According to the Superintending Surgeon, as no 'decent' family permitted their women to be confined in a public asylum, he was frequently consulted by the local people of Dinajpore to treat their female relatives at home. This indicated incidents of women suffering from puerperal fever outside the asylum as well. The Superintendent found it difficult to conclude the extent of such cases in Bengal, because amongst those who were admitted into the asylum it was infrequent and he treated few such cases outside the asylum. According to Yannick Ripa, women with puerperal fever and or mania either suffered from 'intense depression or acute frenzy'.[23] Pointing to the frequent occurrence of puerperal insanity in England, Elaine Showalter has claimed that 'it seemed to violate all of Victorian culture's most deeply cherished ideals of feminine propriety and maternal love'.[24] But the issue of puerperal mania went beyond the question of maintaining or breaking the norms of femininity. It also raised questions about the treatment of women's illnesses: for instance, what led to so many cases of puerperal mania or fever? Was it related to hygiene? Did women give birth in an unhygienic condition? Puerperal mania questions both her reproductive and mental health conditions. Therefore, this particular cause of women's insanity questions both her reproductive and mental health. While much was done about women's reproductive health, with the aid of the Dufferin Fund towards the end of the nineteenth century, the issue of women's mental health was never taken into serious consideration by the European medical practitioners of the time.

Of the other causes mentioned by the physicians, the consumption of *ganja*, hereditary, epilepsy and puerperal fever were categorized as physical causes, whereas grief or domestic problems were classified as moral causes. Anger, passion, melancholy, acute mania and intemperance were classified as emotional causes of her insanity. By 1865, the causes of insanity amongst women lunatics of Dacca remained largely 'unknown' other than a few instances of anger, passion, grief, loss of property, epilepsy, *ganja*, hereditary and congenital tendencies. The diseases from which they suffered were mainly chronic mania and dementia. Reasons for complications among the remaining lunatic women were syphilis in two, paralysis in one and 'cachexia' in the rest.[25] According to Superintendent James Wise, 'cachexia' was a general deterioration of health, recovery from which was uncertain, especially when combined with the other diseases an inmate was susceptible to in an asylum. Therefore, the practice was to take into account the most prominent disease on admission into hospital and enter it in the monthly register. In the course of the illness the patient could be affected by other diseases and the one under which the patient was admitted was probably not the reason for the lunatic's death.[26]

Another disease which often caused the death of women lunatics was known as 'asthenia'. The report of the number of women admitted at the Dullunda Asylum in 1865 reflected maximum death amongst women was due to 'asthenia'. Superintendent A. Payne explained that it was a condition in which an inmate died of physical exhaustion without assignable organic cause and unattended by marked anaemia or other evidence of blood disorder.[27] By 1871, according to James Wise, melancholia was very common among 'natives'. Males, he further stated, were more subject to it than females.[28]

The cause of insanity due to consumption of intoxicating substances, particularly *ganja*, was contested by medical professionals throughout the nineteenth century. Until the establishment of the Indian Hemp Drug Commission in 1893, the medical officers had serious misgivings about the relationship between *ganja* and insanity. An interesting conundrum about *ganja* smoking, which the medical officers could not solve, was whether it was reasonable to suppose that excessive *ganja* smoking was due to insanity, or insanity was due to excessive use of *ganja*.[29]

Although the European medical officers mentioned certain cases of insanity among women which were due to the consumption of intoxicating substances like *bhang*, *ganja* or *charas*, some of them argued that the consumption of intoxicating substances generally was not the main cause. In 1886, A.J. Cowie, Inspector General of Civil Hospitals, Bengal, in his annual report on the insane asylums stated that women 'did not acquire the *bhang*, *ganja*, or *charas* habits and for *obvious* (italics mine) reasons'.[30] Instead, he pointed out that the majority of the cases of intoxication admitted into the asylum included young or middle-aged men. He pointed out that it was a social taboo for a woman to consume such substances. This was an attempt to guard the notion of a righteous woman who would not indulge in such activities. They tried to refer to the norms of feminine behaviour by putting forth such ideas. During the period when women's insanity was not much discussed and not many women were admitted into the asylum, cases of insanity among women due to substance consumption complicated the issue. It broke the pattern of visualizing women as an epitome of moral values. Colonized people were understood in terms of these Victorian norms and values which cut across class divisions. Women admitted in the 'native' asylums by and large belonged to the 'lower' classes of society, whereas the officers tried to implement the values of upper-class Victorian women on them. In 1884, in the report on the lunatic asylums of Bengal, the causes of insanity were mainly attributed to the use of *ganja* and spirits. In this context the Inspector General remarked,

> One woman is set down as having suffered from the effects of bhang (Dullunda), while opium is alleged to have caused mental

disease in another (Patna). Yet opium is said to be extensively consumed by both sexes in some districts. Spirits as a cause of insanity is largely represented. No mention, notwithstanding this, is made of 'alcoholism' or 'delirium tremens' in any of the returns.[31]

By the end of the nineteenth century with the progress in the treatment and understanding of insanity, the Inspector General of Hospitals was often critical of the Superintendents' views. It was a time when doubt had been cast on the earlier belief in the strong relationship between hemp and insanity. He also doubted the correctness of assigning so many cases to excessive drinking. Hence, he considered such analyses of the causes of insanity by the Superintendents to be mere 'guess work'.[32] Therefore, over time the method of classifying different forms of insanity underwent revision with the object of securing some uniformity of classification. But, as pointed out by the Inspector General, it was impossible to expect absolute accuracy and uniformity, since the diagnosis depended almost entirely on the views held by individual Superintendents. It was well known how prone some persons were to ascribe *ganja* as a cause of insanity, while others considered it an innocuous stimulant.[33] Regarding *ganja* smokers or other inebriates, A. Payne stated that 'their resort to a stimulant was an effect and not a genuine cause of mental failure'.[34]

In 1872, according to the Inspector General of Hospitals, the proportion of acute insanity was lower among females than among males. According to him, mental depression, resulting in suicide, was very common among both Muslims and Hindus. This was because 'natives' functioned mostly under the influence of emotions, unlike Europeans.[35] According to the Superintendent of the Dacca Lunatic Asylum, James Wise, depression was very common among 'natives' and often resulted in suicidal tendencies. Among those treated during 1871, one Muslim female, three Hindu males and one Hindu female had attempted to commit suicide before admission. Two Muslim males and three Hindu males attempted to commit suicide since they came to the asylum.[36] He further stated that grief over the loss of children or parents, and anxiety was the most frequent moral causes of insanity among 'natives'. Sixteen women out of a total of forty-six women admitted at the Dacca Asylum during the year were reported to be mad due to the loss of family members. Only thirty-three out of two hundred and fourteen males were affected in a like manner. Even by 1872 debauchery was understood as a moral cause of insanity. James Wise by 1872 stated that intoxication alone was not the cause of insanity; instead insanity was the result of a combination of causes.

> The wild, reckless, and irregular life, and the feeling of self degradation, was probably more to do with the production of insanity than the sensuality and depravity of their lives.[37]

In 1872, in the European Lunatic Asylum, the moral causes of insanity included pecuniary difficulties and domestic troubles. Four patients admitted in the asylum during the year (three men and one woman) were said to be suffering from insanity induced by moral failure. Five of the other female inmates died during childbirth and the rest of those admitted during the year were instances of puerperal mania and imbecility. However, it was clear that there was great uncertainty over the etiology of their diseases. As the Superintendent admitted:

> It was not to be understood that all cases could be so strictly classified with accuracy; for it was difficult in many cases to decide what name the disease should bear, and this for the reason, that the manifestations of the disease in many persons are characteristic of more than one variety. For instance, it was not easy to say in many cases whether the disease was chronic mania, or acute mania, for the time comparatively quiescent; chronic mania or dementia; chronic mania, with fixed delusion or melancholia, liable to lapse into mania. The nomenclature, in most instances, was only approximately correct.[38]

Insane women vs. insane men: an issue of comparison or contest?

The physicians of the asylums constantly made comparisons and came to the conclusion that the number of women at the asylums of Bengal was always lower than the number of men. In 1835, at the Insane Hospital of Calcutta, the average age of males when admitted was 25 years while that of women was 20 years. The number of women as compared to men was 1 to 3 or 4. Based on these records reflecting on the proportion of sexes, the Superintendent Surgeon stated that insanity in reality was more frequent amongst males than amongst females of the country.[39] Four decades later, the proportion was very similar; women constituted 21.5 per cent of the admissions in the asylums of Bengal by 1871, against 23.6 of 1870 and 20.8 of the five preceding years.[40] In 1871, J. Campbell, the Inspector General of Hospitals, stated that in the asylums of England the population of insane women generally exceeded the number of males, whereas in Bengal, the number of women admitted in asylums constituted only 22 per cent of the total. The number of female patients treated in the hospitals (not mental hospitals) and dispensaries of Bengal contributed to 26 per cent of the population. As the number of women treated for their illnesses outside the asylums was higher than of those in the asylum, he presumed that

> whatever the relative amount of male and female population of Bengal, or the relative number of lunatics among males and females, the people are more loath to send females to asylums, and contrive to manage them at home.[41]

This, according to him, was because the 'custom of the country (India) was opposed to sending women either to hospitals or asylums'.[42] The number of females admitted to the Moorshedabad Asylum in 1842 was not above 1/6 or 1/7 of the male numbers, while in Europe the former predominated.[43] Insanity due to substance consumption like liquor or hemp was categorized as having a moral cause. In Europe men were more subject to such influences than women. At Dacca by 1835, the proportion of males to females was 4 to 1, respectively. But certain circumstances made this deduction 'doubtful', according to the Superintendent. He condemned the 'habits' of the 'natives', and believed that insanity was as common among women as it was among men.[44]

According to J. Fullarton, writing in 1876 of the moral causes of insanity in the asylums of Bengal, grief, particularly amongst women, was the principal factor. Next in 'order' were anger, religion, poverty and love, which were also considered as particularly important reasons for insanity among women. Of the total number of women treated in the asylums of Bengal, 45.73 per cent suffered from insanity caused by physical causes, 7.93 per cent from moral causes and 46.33 per cent from unknown causes.[45] According to Superintendent Payne of Dullunda Asylum, dysentery, fever, diseases of the nervous system and phthisis covered 60 per cent of the total admissions amongst the male patients, while amongst the women, diseases of the nervous system, dysentery, cholera and fevers contributed to more than half the admissions.[46]

John Haslam, who was in charge of several madhouses in England, stated that insanity was more frequent in men than amongst women.

Women, according to him, were more frequently prone to insanity because of certain natural processes such as menstruation, parturition and preparing nutriment for the infant, often while suffering from other diseases common at those periods of life.[47] But his view was refuted by J. Swiney of the Medical Board in India. According to him, Haslam's theories were applicable to female insanity in England, but it could not be assumed that they would be so in the case of the 'native' women of India. He further stated that

> our want of more general seclusion of females adopted in this country precludes our getting correct information or making an accurate comparison upon this point but the females who are admitted into our presidency insane hospital are few in number as compared with the males.[48]

Furthermore, in England, case histories of patients after admission were regularly maintained and most were admitted with a prior case history. But in India this was not possible. Most of the lunatics admitted in the 'native' asylums of Bengal belonged to the poorer sections of society. They were not necessarily admitted by their friends, family or relatives. In most of the cases they were picked up from the street by *chowkidars* or police. Therefore, it was difficult to state whether insanity was more frequent amongst men than amongst women in India. Swiney did not look at insanity as only a consequence of pain or mere suffering, but as one, which was an 'independent and associated effect of the general diseases'.[49]

The proportion of female admissions to lunatics in the asylums in England was always higher than that of men and data collected for England and Wales by the Royal Commissioners in Lunacy suggested that institutionalized women outnumbered men in 1880, a difference of about 7,000. The total number of women was 39,027 and that of men 32,027.[50] This was not the situation in India and particularly in Bengal. For instance, in 1865, out of fifty-six Hindu patients, forty-seven were male and only nine were female; amongst fifty-eight Muslims, there were fifty-one males and seven females.[51]

According to Waltraud Ernst,

> the phenomenon that women are more likely than men to be diagnosed as mentally unstable has become part of feminist orthodox in the West.[52]

In 1862, the Superintending Surgeon of Moorshedabad, after judging the reports of the lunatic asylums in England, concluded that women there were as much, and even more, subject to this malady than males. But according to him, this increase in the proportion of women lunatics in England had no correlation with the admission of women in the asylums of Bengal.[53] Elaine Showalter in her book *The Female Malady*[54] pointed out that in England insanity was a more popular diagnosis than it was in India and, 'alongside the English malady, nineteenth century psychiatry described a female malady'. She further stated that 'even when both men and women had similar symptoms of mental disorder, psychiatry differentiated between an English malady, associated with the intellectual and economic pressures on highly civilised men, and a female malady, associated with the sexuality and essential nature of women'.[55] In India and particularly in Bengal not only could the term 'female malady' not be applied to specifically define female madness, the number of women admitted was considered far lower than what it was in England.

In Bengal, insanity was common among both men and women. In the mental hospitals of England and Europe, proper records with case studies were maintained of the number of lunatics admitted. In India or in Bengal many women were not sent into the asylum because insanity was considered a social stigma. Women inmates existed only as numbers in the statistical records with hardly any references to their case histories, except in a few rare instances. Therefore, it is difficult to conclude that insanity was regarded as a specifically female malady in India. Rather, insanity was said to be of common occurrence. But the complexity of the problem lay in the definition and in the understanding of the term 'insanity'. However, it is difficult to ignore that a gendered definition of insanity was gradually constructed in which women's insanity was explained more in terms of their emotional states, which at times was described as melancholic and distressed while at other times it was represented as violent and outrageous. The official understanding of female insanity was often related to emotional exuberance, for instance, ways of laughing, singing or talking to oneself. It seemed that the medical officers assumed that women in general had no control over their emotions, which often caused insanity. Hence, they were more prone to it.

Labour: occupational therapy

Labour was another important issue in the asylum, and this too was gendered. The division of labour among men and women was specific, more so, for if an insane person, irrespective of gender, was considered able to work, it called into question the very definition of insanity.

During their temporary stay at the asylum, European women were also made to work, but European men were not engaged in labour. Robert Gardiner Hill, who specialized on the treatment of insanity, was a member of the Royal College of Surgeons and Resident Medical Superintendent of the Lincolnshire County Asylum; he stated that no patients, either male or female, should be compelled to work. Instead, they should voluntarily make themselves useful and industrious.[56] However, it was difficult to put such theories into practice. In Bengal, asylum physicians stated that they did not apply force and labour was done by lunatics voluntarily, but every mode of labour was directed and controlled by the administrators. The various kinds of hard labour, which lunatics always had to perform while they were suffering from various maladies, were dreadful. This strongly suggests that force was applied, as few people who were mentally or physically ill would voluntarily perform such activities. Or else, very few of those admitted in the asylums were actually insane.

In 1835, lunatics of the Insane Hospital of Calcutta were employed in gardening, and the convalescent patients in gardening, digging, weeding and other 'gentle'[57] exercises. The insane were also made to whitewash the asylum, do repair work, including plastering as well as constructing the *machans* on which they slept.[58] At the Dacca Lunatic Asylum, under the Civil Surgeon G. Lamb, lunatics were also employed in gardening and other similar activities. He complained about getting women lunatics to do any work in the asylum while at the same time employing them in *soorky* or brick pounding,[59] which actually involved a lot of physical strength. Brick pounding increased in the asylums with the expansion of the Public Works Department. Women did not voluntarily do the job of *soorky* pounding.

John Connolly, who specialized on the treatment of insanity without mechanical restraint and was also a Fellow of the Royal College of Physicians, London, pointed out that sedentary labour was less conducive to the recovery of patients than active labour and further stated that

> More women get well who are employed in the kitchens, laundries, and wards than in the workrooms; and more men recover who work in the gardens and on the farms than in the tailors' or shoemakers' shop.[60]

This outlook towards a gendered division of labour was also enforced in the asylums of Bengal. As James Mills has pointed, 'the gendered division of labour was intended to reinforce sex identities that the British thought proper'.[61] For instance, according to the Surgeon of the Patna Lunatic Asylum, 'women were particularly good hands at the shelling and picking of the seed'.[62]

Women in the asylums of Bengal were employed more in indoor activities like spinning, weaving and threading, while men did gardening, brick pounding and fetching water for the asylum. But even indoor labour, such as *soorky* pounding, required a lot of strength. According to James Wise, it was carried on in the asylum in two ways. Women were provided with a wooden lever or *dhenki* fixed in the centre. They had to press it with their feet, which crushed the brick placed underneath the hammer fixed at its end. Men did the same job in a different way; they were provided with iron pestles. They pounded the bricks between it and a large stone.[63] Both involved a strenuous process. Therefore, it was not a question of indoor or outdoor labour, and who was engaged in which labour; rather, it was about laborious manual labour in which both were involved and affected equally. The asylum officials of Bengal repeatedly stated that women were employed in less strenuous jobs and were mainly engaged in indoor activities. But they chose to overlook the fact that those indoor activities also required a lot of hard work.

In 1841, lunatics of the Dacca Asylum were also employed in *soorky* pounding for the construction of the roads, in gardening, carrying water from the tank in order to wash the wards and cells, cooking and repairing the straw mattresses on which they slept. There was no respite from work for any of the lunatics. Often, they were engaged in construction and maintenance work of the asylum where they were admitted as patients. The physicians considered it necessary to make them work, as a part of moral treatment. They anticipated that an involvement with labour would work as therapy. Even inactive lunatics were forced to work. According to the Civil Surgeon of Dacca, those patients who were not active were put to make twine and mattresses, mend clothes and blankets.[64] Female patients in the Dacca Asylum were employed in making *soorky*, cleaning cotton and spinning thread.[65] By 1852, according to the Superintendent of the asylum, Alexander Wise,

> The difficulty of finding occupation for the women was greater than for the men, as it had never been exacted from them compulsorily; and their love and habit of inactivity, prevented many from exerting themselves.[66]

There was always an uneasiness among the Superintendents and the medical officers of the asylum about making lunatics work, irrespective of the fact that they were daily employed in asylum labour. In the Dacca Asylum, women worked for an hour before breakfast, and about four hours afterwards. Every morning, some of them washed the wards, while others cleaned the cotton. Spinning, knitting, sewing and other domestic occupations were particularly introduced in the asylum for women lunatics. The Superintendent claimed that he found it easier to employ men for work like gardening, cultivating the soil, digging, weeding, fetching bricks from the town in small carts and pounding those, or other even heavier activities, because most of them worked as cultivators before their admissions.[67] He probably overlooked the fact that many of the women lunatics admitted in the asylum were also labourers or cultivators or were employed in similar jobs before their admissions.

In 1861, at the Moydapore Lunatic Asylum, lunatics were employed to manufacture their own clothes and also the *morah*, or small cane stools. Considerable profit was realized from the sale of both products, which according to the Superintendent Surgeon, was used to obtain additional comforts for the lunatics, such as blankets and new clothes. In certain cases a sum of 3 or 4 rupees was also given to those lunatics on their discharge, especially to those who had no relatives or friends, so that they could sustain themselves for a few weeks after release.[68] Similar instances were also prevalent in Moorshedabad Asylum during the same year. The profit made from the sale of articles manufactured by the lunatics, as per order of the Secretary of State, was used to procure 'little indulgences for the patients themselves'.[69]

Medical officials always emphasized the noble intentions of work without coercion, as well as its healing aspects. The therapeutic ideology behind this was that if lunatics were removed from work, they would become more unruly and difficult to control. Lunatics were made to labour under all circumstances, because the medical officials believed that the symptoms of insanity often subsided under industrial occupation.

Officials were also at pains to point out that lunatics were not engaged in labour to profit the authorities but for the treatment of their malady and to provide them with additional comforts. But deriving profit from asylum labour was as important for the officers as it was for the lunatics. Yet asylum officials differed in their views about whether such labour could make an important contribution to the running costs of the asylum. One official of the Patna Lunatic Asylum believed that profit could not be derived from lunatics, whereas the Superintendent of the Dacca Lunatic Asylum employed the idiotic, imbecile and more intractable lunatics in the task of *soorky* pounding, earthwork, gardening and in the oil mill for pressing mustard seeds. In the employment of such cases, there was clearly no therapeutic rationale.

In 1869, the Deputy Inspector of Hospitals, G. Saunders, visited the asylums of Bengal and commented on the kind of labour and its impact on treatment. His observations on the European Lunatic Asylum revealed that labour was not a significant part of asylum management there. According to him, the situation at the Bhawani-pore Lunatic Asylum was different from the 'native' lunatic asylums because, although labour helped to cure different forms of mental diseases, the inmates were hardly engaged in any kind of labour. It seemed there was considerable difficulty in organizing any kind of work at the asylum because lunatics were only there for a short while. Soldiers, who constituted an important part of the population, hardly worked because they were soon returned to England, whereas women lunatics were engaged in delicate activities like needlework and croquet stitching.[70] Dr. Bird, Superintendent of the European Asylum, in 1872 stated that the question of getting lunatics to work was easier at a place where they spent almost their entire life, unlike in the European Lunatic Asylum where lunatics stayed for a shorter period, before they were sent off to England.[71] Waltraud Ernst has pointed out that the reason why employment was not an important task for the European Lunatic Asylum was that Europeans of any social class considered it inappropriate to debase themselves by carrying out tasks which the 'natives' could do.[72]

G. Saunders's moderate observations on labour at 'native' lunatic asylums were different from the views of superintendents and other medical officers. According to him, the object with which 'native' asylums were established was to give shelter and medical aid to 'poor creatures'[73] who, due to their mental illness, could neither take care of themselves nor could their relatives provide for them. Therefore, it was 'most desirable that no occupation should be allotted to them'.[74] But he also stated that if it was considered necessary to engage lunatics in asylum labour as a 'curative agent', the profit of the industrial fund should not be 'brought forward or exhibited as a means of lowering the expenses of attendant on the support of the institution'.[75] More-over, he considered machine work as a better alternative to manual labour and introduced looms and other similar occupations at the Patna Asylum,[76] which he thought were less laborious than manual work like *soorky* pounding or manufacturing oil.

In order to engage patients in a regular occupation, they were both persuaded and encouraged, but in no instance was 'compulsion or harsh treatment' enforced.[77] Lunatics worked in the garden, wove their own clothes, stitched blankets for themselves and also prepared the strip of sack on which they slept at night. Women spun thread, cotton and woollens. During summer, male patients were encouraged by the Superintendent to make bricks.[78] By 1871, asylum labour constituted the principal feature in the management of Bengal asylums.[79]

Conclusion

Towards the end of the nineteenth century, asylum physicians began to recognize insanity as a mental disease which could be medically treated. Women were as prone to insanity as much as men. The gendered definition of madness arose from both biological differences and imagined psycho-social factors, particularly the view of women as unsettled and prone to emotional exuberances. As insanity was muddled with women's 'natural' emotions, asylum physicians were unable to clearly define the reasons for female insanity. Although women in 'native' asylums were not classified on the basis of class as in the European Lunatic Asylum, reasons for diagnosing insanity were much the same in both cases. While men in the European Lunatic Asylum were not meant to engage in labour, women in both 'native' and the European Lunatic Asylum were expected to do so, as labour was considered as an important strategy for the treatment of lunatics while also being an important factor in their internal economy.

Notes

1 Letter sent to President and Member of the Hospital Board from Mr. Dick, Surgeon to the Hospital for Insane, dated Calcutta15 October 1796. Medical Board Proceedings 27 October 1796, National Archives of India (Henceforth NAI).
2 Report on the Moorshedabad Lunatic Asylum for the year 1862. A. Fleming, Officiating Civil Surgeon, Moorshedabad, Superintendent. NAI.
3 Report on the Moydapore Lunatic Asylum for the Year 1872 by Superintendent J.M. Coates, *Annual Report on the Insane Asylums of Bengal for the Year 1872*, J. Campbell Brown, Inspector General of Hospitals, Indian Medical Department to Secretary to the Government of Bengal, dated Fort William, 20 June 1873. Calcutta: Calcutta Central Press Company Limited, 1873. NAI.
4 Annual Report on the Insane Asylums of Bengal for the Year 1876, J. Fullarton Beatson, Surgeon General, Indian Medical Department. Calcutta: Bengal Secretariat Press, 1877. NAI.

5 Home, Medical, Number 131, July 1886. NAI.
6 Report on the Dacca Lunatic Asylum by Superintendent James Wise. Annual Report on Insane Asylums of Bengal for the Year 1871, J. Campbell Brown, Inspector General of Hospitals, Indian Medical Department. Calcutta: Bengal Secretariat Press, 1872. NAI.
7 Report on the Bhawanipore Lunatic Asylum by Superintendent R. Bird. Annual Report on the Insane Asylums of Bengal for the Year 1872, J. Campbell Brown, Inspector General of Hospitals, Indian Medical Department to Secretary to the Government of Bengal, dated Fort William, 20 June 1873. Calcutta: Calcutta Central Press Company Limited, 1873. NAI.
8 Medical Board Proceeding, Number 7, 9 November 1835. Letter sent to James Hutchinson, Secretary Medical Board from Mr. Lamb, Civil Surgeon Dacca, dated 31 December 1835. NAI.
9 Medical Board Proceedings, May 1842. Annual Reports on the Insane Hospital in Moorshedabad, 26 March, 1842, NAI.
10 Medical Board Proceedings, May 1842.
11 Medical Board Proceedings, May, 1842. Letter sent to G. Bushby, Secretary to the Government of India from A. Kean, Civil Assistant Surgeon, dated Moorshedabad 12 November 1841. NAI.
12 Medical Board Proceedings, May 1842. Annual Reports on the Insane Hospital in Moorshedabad, 26 March, 1842. NAI.
13 *Annual Report of the Lunatic Asylum, 1879* by Arthur J. Payne, Surgeon General for Bengal. Calcutta: Bengal Secretariat Press, 1880. NAI.
14 Report on the Patna Lunatic Asylum for the Year 1862, John Balfour, Deputy Inspector General of Hospitals, Dinapore Circle. *Annual Report on Asylums of Bengal, 1862.* Calcutta: Calcutta Gazette Office, 1863. NAI
15 W.J. Moore, *A Manual of the Diseases of India*, London: John Churchill, 1861. National Library [Henceforth NL].
16 *A Manual of the Diseases of India*, 129 [NL].
17 Ibid., 130 [NL].
18 Ibid.
19 Ibid., 128 [NL].
20 Peurperal, Origin L. Peurpera, a lying-in woman; peur child+parere to bear: cf. F. Puerperal. Puerperal fever is a postpartum sepsis (the presence of organisms in blood) with a rise in fever after the first twenty-four hours following the delivery, but before the eleventh postpartum day.
21 James Reid, 'On the Symptoms, Causes and Treatment of Puerperal Insanity', reprinted from *Journal of Psychological Medicine and Mental Pathology*, 1 and 2, edited Forbes Winslow, in John Charles Bucknill (ed.), *Asylum Journal*, 2 (1855–56), Welcome Library [Henceforth WL].
22 Thomas A. Wise, 'On the Principal Remarks on Insanity as It Occurs Among the Inhabitants of Bengal', *The Monthly Journal of Medical Science*, (August 1852). WL
23 Yannick Ripa, tr. by Catherine du Peloux Menage, *Women and Madness: The Incarceration of Women in Nineteenth Century France*, Minneapolis: University of Minnesota Press, 1990.
24 Elaine Showalter, *The Female Malady: Women, Madness and English Culture, 1830–1980*, London: Virago, 1987, 58.
25 Report on the Dacca Asylum for the Year 1865, W.B. Beatson, Dacca Lunatic Asylum. *Annual Report on the Asylums for the Year 1865*, W.A.

Green, Officiating Principal Inspector General, Medical Department. Calcutta: Military Orphan Press, 1866. NAI.

26 Report of the Dacca Lunatic Asylum for the Year 1871 by Surgeon James Wise. *Annual Report on Insane Asylums of Bengal for the Year 1871*, J. Campbell Brown, Inspector General of Hospitals, Indian Medical Department. Calcutta: Bengal Secretariat Press, 1872. NAI.

27 *Annual Report on Insane Asylums of Bengal for the Year 1871*. NAI.

28 Report on the Dacca Lunatic Asylum for the Year 1870 by Superintendent H.C. Cutcliffe, *Report on the Lunatic Asylums, Vaccinations, and Dispensaries in the Bengal Presidency for the Year 1870*, Assistant Surgeon K. Macleod, Officiating Secretary to the Inspector General of Hospitals, Indian Medical Department. Calcutta: Bengal Secretariat Press, 1872. NAI.

29 Home, Medical, Number 195, June 1893. NAI.

30 Home, Medical B, Numbers 130–1, July 1886. Report on the Lunatic Asylums, Bengal 1885. NAI.

31 Home, Medical, Number 100, September, 1885. NAI.

32 Ibid.

33 Home, Medical, Number 10, January 1892. Report on the Lunatic Asylums of Bengal by H.H. Risley, Officiating Secretary to the Government of Bengal. NAI.

34 *Annual Report on the Lunatic Asylums of Bengal for 1880*, A.J. Payne, Surgeon General for Bengal, Calcutta: Bengal Secretariat Press, 1880. NAI.

35 *Annual Report on the Insane Asylums of Bengal for the Year 1872*, J. Campbell Brown, Inspector General of Hospitals, Indian Medical Department to Secretary to the Government of Bengal, dated Fort William, 20 June 1873. Calcutta: Calcutta Central Press Company Limited, 1873. NAI.

36 *Annual Report on the Insane Asylums of Bengal for the Year 1872*. NAI.

37 Report on Dacca Lunatic Asylum by Superintendent James Wise. *Annual Report on the Insane Asylums of Bengal for the Year 1872*, J. Campbell Brown, Inspector General of Hospitals, Indian Medical Department to Secretary to the Government of Bengal, dated Fort William, 20 June 1873. Calcutta: Calcutta Central Press Company Limited, 1873. NAI.

38 Report on the Bhawanipore Lunatic Asylum by Superintendent R. Bird, *Annual Report on the Insane Asylums of Bengal for the Year 1872*, J. Campbell Brown, Inspector General of Hospitals, Indian Medical Department to Secretary to the Government of Bengal, dated Fort William, 20 June 1873. Calcutta: Calcutta Central Press Company Limited, 1873. NAI.

39 Medical Board Proceeding, Number 8, 26 March 1835. Enclosure to letter sent to James Hutchinson, Secretary to the Medical Board from Mr. Swiney, Second Member Medical Board also Superintendent Surgeon Presidency. NAI.

40 *Annual Report on Insane Asylums of Bengal for the Year 1871*, J. Campbell Brown, Inspector General of Hospitals, Indian Medical Department. Calcutta: Bengal Secretariat Press, 1872. NAI.

41 *Annual Report on Insane Asylums of Bengal for the Year 1871*. NAI.

42 Resolution, Judicial Department, Medical, Calcutta, A. Mackenzie, Officiating Secretary to the Government of Bengal, dated 4 October 1872.

Annual Report on Insane Asylums of Bengal for the Year 1871, J. Campbell Brown, Inspector General of Hospitals, Indian Medical Department. Calcutta: Bengal Secretariat Press, 1872. NAI.

43 Medical Board Proceedings, May, 1842. Letter sent to G. Bushby, Secretary to the Government of India from A. Kean, Civil Assistant Surgeon, dated Moorshedabad 12 November 1841. NAI.

44 Medical Board Proceeding, Number 7, 9 November 1835. Letter sent to James Hutchinson, Secretary Medical Board from Mr. Lamb, Civil Surgeon Dacca, dated 31 December 1835. NAI.

45 *Annual Report of the Insane Asylums of Bengal for the Year 1876*, J. Fullarton Beatson, Surgeon General, Indian Medical Department sent to the Secretary to the Government of Bengal, Judicial Department. Calcutta: Bengal Secretariat Press, 1877. NAI.

46 Ibid.

47 Medical Board Proceeding, Number 8, 26 March, 1835. Letter sent to James Hutchinson, Secretary to Medical Board from J. Swiney, Second Member in Charge of Superintendent Surgeon Office Presidency, dated 24 March 1835. NAI.

48 Ibid.

49 Ibid.

50 Waltraud Ernst, 'Feminising Madness-Feminising the Orient: Madness, Gender and Colonialism in British India, 1860–1940', in Biswamoy Pati and Shakti Kak (eds.), *Exploring Gender Equaltions: Colonial and Post Colonial India*, New Delhi: Nehru Memorial Museum and Library, 2005.

51 Report on the Dacca Lunatic Asylum for the Year 1865 sent to G. Saunders, Secretary to the Principal Inspector General, Medical Department from W.B. Beatson, Superintendent of Dacca Asylum. *Annual Report on the Insane Hospitals of Bengal for the Year 1865*, W.A. Green, Officiating Principal Inspector General. Calcutta: Military Orphan Press, 1866. NAI.

52 *Annual Report on the Insane Hospitals of Bengal for the Year 1865*. NAI.

53 *Annual Report on the Moorshedabad Lunatic Asylum for the Year 1862*. A. Fleming, Officiating Civil Surgeon, Moorshedabad, Superintendent. NAI.

54 Elaine Showalter, *The Female Malady, Women, Madness and English Culture, 1830–1980*, London: Virago Press, 1987.

55 Ibid., 7.

56 Robert Gardiner Hill, *A Concise History of the Entire Abolition of Mechanical Restraint in the Treatment of the Insane*, London: Longman, Brown, Green and Longmans, 1857 WL.

57 Medical Board Proceeding, Number 8, 26 March, 1835. Letter sent to James Hutchinson, Secretary to Medical Board from J. Swiney, Second Member in Charge of Superintendent Surgeon Office Presidency, dated 24 March 1835. NAI.

58 Medical Board Proceeding, Number 8, 26 March, 1835.

59 Medical Board Proceeding, Number 7, 9 November, 1835. Letter sent to James Hutchinson, Secretary to Medical Board from G. Lamb, Civil Surgeon. Dacca dated 31 October 1835. NAI.

60 John Conolly, *The Construction and Government of Lunatic Asylums and Hospitals for the Insane*, London: John Churchill, MDCCCXLVII, p. 79. WL.

61 James Mills, ' "More Important to Civilise than Subdue"? Lunatic Asylums, Psychiatric Practice and Fantasies of "The Civilising Mission" in British India 1858–1900', in Herald Fischer Tiné and Michael Mann (eds.), *Colonialism as Civilising Mission, Cultural Ideology in British India*, London: Anthem South Asian Studies, 2004, 179–90, 188.

62 Report on the Patna Lunatic Asylum, 1872 by B. Simpson, *Annual Report on the Insane Asylums of Bengal for the Year 1872*, J. Campbell Brown, Inspector General of Hospitals, Indian Medical Department to Secretary to the Government of Bengal, dated Fort William, 20 June 1873. Calcutta: Calcutta Central Press Company Limited, 1873. NAI.

63 Home Department, Public Proceedings, December 19, 1868. Letter from James Wise, Superintendent of Lunatic Asylums, Dacca to William Keates, Deputy Inspector General of Hospitals, Dacca Circle, Dated Dacca 24 June 1868. NAI.

64 Medical Board Proceeding May 1842. Letter sent to Robert Brown, Officiating Surgeon from J. Taylor, Civil Surgeon Dacca, dated Dacca 2 May 1842. NAI.

65 Medical Board Proceeding Number 18, 1843. Letter sent to Robert Brown, Superintending Surgeon Dacca by J. Taylor, Civil Surgeon, Dacca, dated 13 April 1843. NAI.

66 Alexander Wise, 'Principle Remarks on Insanity as it Occurs among the Inhabitants of Bengal', *Monthly Journal of Medical Science, Volume 15, Jule–December 1852*, p. 33. WL

67 Ibid., 32–3.

68 General Proceeding, Medical Department, Number 4, February 1862. Report on the Moydapore Lunatic Asylum for the Year 1861, dated 1 January 1862, Berhampore. WBSA.

69 General Proceeding, Medical Department, Number 5, 1862. Letter sent to Principal Inspector General, Medical Department from H. Bell, Officiating Junior Secretary to the Government of Bengal, dated 4 February 1862. WBSA.

70 Annual Inspection Report of the Bhawanipore Asylum by G. Saunders, Deputy Inspector General of Hospitals in the *Annual Report on the Insane Asylums of Bengal, 1869*, J. Murray. Calcutta: Bengal Secretariat Office, 1870. NAI.

71 *Annual Report on the Insane Asylums of Bengal for the Year 1872*, J. Campbell Brown, Inspector General of Hospitals, Indian Medical Department to Secretary to the Government of Bengal, dated Fort William, 20 June 1873. Calcutta: Calcutta Central Press Company Limited, 1873. NAI.

72 Waltraud Ernst, 'Idioms of Madness and Colonial Boundaries', *Comparative Studies in Society and History*, 39, 1 (1997), p. 158.

73 Annual Inspection Report of the Bhawanipore Asylum by G. Saunders, Deputy Inspector General of Hospitals in the *Annual Report on the Insane Asylums of Bengal, 1869*, J. Murray. Calcutta: Bengal Secretariat Office, 1870. NAI.

74 *Annual Report on the Insane Asylums of Bengal, 1869*.

75 Ibid.

76 Ibid.

77 *Annual Reports on the Lunatics Asylums for the European and Native Insane Patients at Bhawanipore and Dullunda for 1856 and 1857.*

Selections from the records of the Government of Bengal. Calcutta, John Gray, Calcutta Gazette Office 1858. NAI.

78 Home Department, Public Proceedings, December 18, 1868. Memorandum from G. Saunders, M.D., Deputy Inspector General of Hospitals, Lower Provinces, number 809, dated Dinajpore, 5 June 1868. NAI.

79 Letter Number 346 from J. Campbell Brown, Inspector General of Hospitals, Indian Medical Department to the Officiating Secretary to the Government of Bengal. Dated Fort William, 27 June 1872. *Annual Report on the Insane Asylums in Bengal for the Year 1871.* By J. Campbell Brown, Inspector General of Hospitals, Indian Medical Department. Calcutta: Bengal Secretariat Press, 1872. NAI.

9 Confining 'lunatics'

The Cuttack Asylum, c.1864–1906[1]

Biswamoy Pati

> There is, perhaps, no better established fact in British society than that of the corresponding growth of modern wealth and pauperism. Curiously enough, the same law seems to hold good with respect to lunacy. The increase of lunacy in Great Britain has kept pace with the increase of exports, and has outstripped the increase of population.
>
> —Karl Marx, 'The Increase of Lunacy in Great Britain.'
> —*New York Tribune*, 20 August 1858 (Source: marxist.org)

'A strange meeting'

> In prison Mangaraj [a tyrannical landlord/moneylender] encountered the very Dombs [outcastes] whom he had implicated in false cases . . . While pushing the oil press they would beat up and kick Mangaraj . . . Unlike nowadays, the madhouse was not located at Darghabazar [in Cuttack]. The mad people were kept as prisoners in the Cuttack jail . . . close to Mangaraj's cell. Among them was a dreaded madman who never slept at night . . . Whenever he saw Mangaraj he ran out to bite him. On that eventful day. . . [the madman] suddenly ran towards Mangaraj and bit off his nose.
>
> —Fakirmohana Senapati, 'Chamana Athaguntha' (originally written in a serialized form in the Oriya newspaper *Utkala Sahitya* in 1897 and published as a novel in 1902. I have taken these lines from Senapati's novel *Chamana Athaguntha*, Cuttack: Friends Publishers, 1990 (reprinted), chapter 27, 140–3; translation mine)

These short quotes perhaps highlight some serious points. Thus, most scholars working on the lunatic asylums or the madhouses in colonial India, even while they acknowledge the possibilities of interactions with the 'outside' world, make these appear as autonomous sites. A serious methodological question that needs to be considered

is whether such institutions could indeed have an autonomous existence. Marx was not a social historian of health and medicine but the
interactional associations observed by him hint at the broader linkages
between the Industrial Revolution and the increase of 'lunacy' in a
largely open-ended manner. Of course, madness in Great Britain, especially England in the nineteenth century, has been a serious subject of
research – Roy Porter, Elaine Showalter, Andrew Scull, Joseph Melling
and Bill Forsythe among others highlight many fascinating aspects of
the lunatic asylum in nineteenth-century England.[2]

Coming to Fakirmohana's 'Chamana Athaguntha', one can see how
it projects the creative writer's 'memories' of the Cuttack Asylum.
Originally this work appeared in a serialized form in 1897 and this
quote is from one of the closing scenes that highlight the meeting of
an ace exploiter/tyrant in the form of Mangaraj and the victims of his
machinations, including Bhagia and some Dombs, in the Cuttack Jail.
Bhagia and Saria were a weaver couple, and the 'mad man' in the Jail
is Bhagia, who had gone mad after the death of his dear wife Saria.
Mangaraj is in Jail since he has been associated with Saria's death.

Initially the 'mad' were confined within the Cuttack Jail. Moreover, even after the separation of the Asylum from the Jail in 1864,
they shared the same location, with the Asylum building being built
adjacent to the Jail. Both were located in Darghabazar, and possibly
the Asylum had a separate entrance. Consequently, the narrative ima-
gines a past that was very different from the 'present' (viz. 1897), by
which time the Asylum was situated at Darghabazar, away from the
Jail.[3] This imagined location of the Asylum perhaps also illustrates a
middle-class reformist's ideas about a change that had not really happened throughout the Asylum's existence, until it was closed down in
1906, when the space was taken over by the Jail. What needs emphasis
is that even during the Asylum's 'imagined' independent existence in
the 1890s both the Jail and the Asylum shared the same location, separated by a wall. Besides this, the blurring of the dividing line between
the 'criminal' and the 'lunatic', with the use of terms like the 'criminal
lunatic,' insofar as colonial classification strategy is concerned, needs
to be highlighted while discussing the problems that had its origin in
the Jail. Besides, 'Chamana' also demonstrates the wider links with the
colonial world that saw the decline of the traditional weaving industry
in coastal Orissa (viz. Cuttack, Puri and Balasore) and land displacements – areas that I will return to later – to argue about the process of
colonial expansion and its effect on a large mass of people.

And talking of madness in colonial India, the engagements of
scholars like Waltraud Ernst and James Mills in this area have been

particularly significant.[4] More recently, scholars such as Debjani Das, Anouska Bhattacharyya, Shilpi Rajpal and Pranjali Srivastava have added nuance through their attention to the diversity of conditions and experiences.[5] Nevertheless, some of the complexities of these institutions remain to be explored.

A typical problem in scholarship to date seems to be the hegemonic hold of Michel Foucault, with undeclared assumptions about the relevance of his work when it comes to colonial India.[6] While one cannot ignore the fact that the very meaning of madness changed with and after Foucault, it is important to emphasize that Foucault's *Madness and Civilisation* has contextual/locational specificities that can have disastrous consequences if applied mechanically to colonial India. Such attempts contradict the very core of his method.[7] One does not find any parallels in India to the end of the hysteria generated by leprosy in Europe, with madness replacing it at the end of the Middle Ages, or anything like 'The Ship of Fools' that wandered through the waterways of Europe. Besides, the obvious problem about applying Foucault's notion of a 'great confinement' to colonial India is that the exercise of power was far more complicated. While some of these themes will be examined later on, it needs to be stressed that colonial India saw the tremors generated by both madness and leprosy in the post-1860s. And, the torch-bearers of post-Enlightenment and European 'modernity', who rode the horse of 'science', were fettered by a level of unreason and unscientific barbarity in their efforts to deal with both.[8]

This chapter is a micro-study of the Cuttack Lunatic Asylum. Its focus is on certain dimensions that are intrinsically linked with the colonial context and which are rooted in the economic and social history of the region.

Orissa's colonization

Although Orissa was formally colonized after its takeover in 1803–4, the early years of this process began with the English East India Company (hereafter EIC) acquiring the 'grant of the diwani' in 1765 and the initial short-term land settlements, with the Permanent Settlement being finally put in place in 1793.[9] However, the coastal tract (comprising Cuttack, Puri and Balasore) continued to have short-term settlements until 1837, when temporary settlements were introduced for thirty years at a time. This was systematized through the Settlement of 1897 and Revision Settlement of 1927.[10] Thus imperialist intervention can be traced to a period long before Orissa's formal colonization.

Land auctions had inaugurated the problem of land displacements and dispossession, and in the initial years after the EIC took over Orissa, there was a series of revolts that challenged the EIC. The first major rebellion was the 'Paik *meli*' (Paik rebellion: the Paikas were foot-soldiers, who were feudal retainers) of Khurda (1817). This rebellion echoed some of these problems, along with the increasing price of silver in relation to the value of the cowries (traditional currency) from the closing years of the eighteenth century, which implied severe burdens on the poor and marginal Kandhas (tribals). Thus, the Kandhas 'descended' from the hills of Ghumsar and joined the Paikas in what was the first major anti-imperialist rebellion faced by the EIC in Orissa.[11] The popular rebellions of the tribals, outcastes and other marginal sections continued unabated in the western tract and the hills from the 1830s until the Great Rebellion of 1857. Occasioned by to the desire to tap resources in the hills of Orissa, these severe conflicts resulted in murderous assaults on the people and the destruction of the agrarian system and environment of western Orissa.[12]

Consequently, the early years of Orissa's colonization leading up to the mid-nineteenth century were traumatic for the entire coastal belt. There were severe droughts and the failure of crops, and the people in the Mughalbandi area lived on roots and leaves. The distress among the poor was reflected in the increase of 'simple' thefts (wherein the value of the property stolen was rarely more than 10 rupees); murder of children to steal cheap 'ornaments' of little value from their person; 'burglaries' (with the prisoners in some cases 'gladly acknowledg[ing] their crime to get comfortably fed in jail'); 'robberies' (which included attempts to 'pluck' a handful of rice, a pumpkin or a mango); cutting corn 'forcibly', 'dacoities' (e.g. in one case 30–40 people 'armed with sticks' carried away a 'great quantity' of grain); and highway robbery. Moreover, we also come across the 'cutting of embankments' to divert water, a large number of violations of salt laws along the coast and 'attacks' on salt depots, as well as instances of violence in the countryside, which included the elimination of oppressive landed elements or intermediaries that often assumed 'collective forms'.[13]

Orissa's colonization saw the process of the decline of traditional industries like the salt industry and cotton textiles. The introduction of the monopoly system from 1814 ensured a major source of revenue, and by the 1840s the EIC made nearly 18 rupees lakhs annually.[14] This meant unemployment for those who were associated with salt production. Alongside this, the coastal tract was famous for the production of cotton, which also declined over the nineteenth century, with the inflow of cheap cotton from England.[15] Thus, what needs to be stressed is the destruction of existing traditional industries. These features are major indicators that illustrate the association of the Industrial Revolution with a colony that led to the phenomenon of de-industrialization in the region. Taken together, these posed serious challenges to the new order that was being imposed by the EIC and measures had to be taken to control and prevent them.

Early colonial health concerns

Keeping these factors in mind, one needs to highlight some of the early colonial health concerns. From the beginning, two basic aspects were considered vital. One was related to a Puri-centric order that identified the city as Orissa's capital and its raja, who resided there, as Orissa's king.[16] The other aspect included a clear focus on the 'white man', especially the colonial army. These two factors determined the colonial regime's health policies in the initial years. Given Puri's importance as a major pilgrim centre that saw a demographic invasion for the annual *ratha jatra* (chariot festival), efforts had to be made to protect the colonial outpost, comprising the white population.[17] However, the logic of confining prisoners was a priority aspect that began with the initial use of the Barabati Fort at Cuttack to 'confine' political opponents associated with the rebellions. After the initial years the Cuttack Jail was built in 1810 and was ready for occupation in 1811.[18]

Proceeding forward we see that the 'lunatics' and 'criminal lunatics', along with the prisoners, were confined in the Cuttack Jail. If John Howard (1726–90), an English philanthropist who was dedicated to prison reforms and improvements in public health, had visited the Cuttack Jail as late as 1854–55 he would have been shocked to witness what he had seen over fifty years before in the European world. He would have observed work progressing to construct a 'female hospital, and also a ward for the insane containing four rooms [that were to be] . . . completed within the walls of the Jail'.[19] Needless to say, the housing of the 'insane' in the Cuttack Jail did influence their 'confined' existence with the prisoners. This can be perhaps explained by referring to areas like the level of violence and the 'prison labour' that they were exposed to. Besides hard labour, this included the very 'profitable' production of paper and spinning of thread by women that contributed to the profits earned by the jail.[20]

In this context, one needs to also mention certain ideas of philanthropy that had developed in the late eighteenth century in Europe.[21] Waltraud Ernst mentions these humanitarian reform movements and the related idea of the asylum as a retreat in the context of England.[22] However, subsequently these notions suffered a severe setback in England due to the dismantling of the old 'Poor Laws' through amendments in the British Parliament in 1834. The idea that the poor were lazy and did not want to work conditioned the way in which the state provided employment in the workhouses – which were the new prisons – to those desiring to work.[23] As for colonial India, the ideas of Utilitarianism and the missionaries highlighted a 'decadent' India and advocated reforming it.[24]

These beliefs conditioned the colonial administration and its medical establishment, and the ideas of humanitarianism did not seem to matter at all, at least as far as the insane of colonial India were concerned. Thus, the blurred worlds of the 'criminal' and the 'lunatic' were subsumed under terms like the 'criminal lunatic' that assumed serious significance, with the Jail confining both the dangerous and the unruly sections of the 'native', along with the 'lunatic'. Consequently, the need to regulate and control the colony determined the logic of confining a large section of the poor and the 'lunatics' in a crisis-ridden context that criminalized them – a phenomenon that was critiqued even by some within the colonial bureaucracy.[25] Of course, the insecurities and fears generated by the 1857 Rebellion reinforced these ideas, even as they strengthened notions of ensuring racial superiority. In fact, these formed a distinct part of the notions of governance that developed with the 'crown' taking over India in 1858. They not only influenced the enforcement of the Indian Lunatic Asylums Act of 1858, but also the setting up of asylums for both Europeans and 'natives' throughout British India in the latter half of the nineteenth century and, more importantly, codified the procedures for admitting patients. In ideological terms then the asylums were seen as sites that segregated the 'lunatics', since they were considered dangerous to the society.[26] Ernst mentions that any person charged with a crime and considered to be mentally ill had to be produced before a magistrate and jail officials for admission in the region's general mental hospital.[27] However, it perhaps ought to be added here that this provision could operate in different locations in different ways. Moreover, the 'silence' about their arrests or other repressive components in the *Reports* hardly need to be stressed as long as one bears in mind the operation of the Indian Lunatic Asylums Act in 1858. Thus, the insane person was confined for the safety of society and not for being looked after, or for her or his treatment. As Mills correctly highlights, it formed a part of the 'civilising mission' and its regulatory component.[28]

The dialectics of transition: from the jail to the lunatic asylum

Some caveats are due before exploring details of the Cuttack Lunatic Asylum. In particular, mention must be made of the Naanka Famine (1866) that devastated a far wider region beyond what received wisdom – i.e. the coastal tract comprising Cuttack, Puri and Balasore – informs us.[29] A major development was the creation of the Criminal Tribes Act (1871) that criminalized certain tribal people and then there was the Indian Forest Act (1878) that imposed restrictions on the tribal population's use of forests, affecting the livelihood of a large section of the population. Alongside this, there was continued extension of communication networks (like roads and railroads) and the recruitment of forced and indenture labour.[30] Consequently, the second half of the long nineteenth century spelt doom for the vast mass of the people in the region, with the stabilization of the economics of imperialism along with de-industrialization and de-peasantization.[31]

One needs to also bear in mind the Census operations and the Census of 1871–72. Besides providing the data on the 'insane', its classification strategy polarized identities, especially those related to caste, class, gender and religion. As will be seen, this knowledge system influenced both the perception of 'madness' and the working of the Cuttack Lunatic Asylum.

Many of these features shaped the way in which the 'lunatic' asylums – and most certainly the Cuttack 'lunatic' Asylum – were perceived in colonial India. In fact, this implied the rather predictable expansion of the Cuttack Jail to accommodate the Lunatic Asylum, with the latter developing, as it were, from 'within the womb' of the Cuttack Jail. Though we are not told anything about the labour obtained for this purpose, it would be difficult to imagine that the inmates of the Jail (viz. which included the prisoners and the 'criminal' lunatics – if not only the 'lunatics') – were not involved with the construction of the Asylum.

It is in this overall context that the Cuttack Lunatic Asylum began to function from February 1864, until it was closed on 30 March 1906. On the basis of an overview of the initial *Annual Reports* of the Asylum, we will examine the extent to which the Asylum could 'break off' from the Jail. The first *Annual Report* (1864), drafted by J.M. Coates, charted certain aspects of the jail that would characterize its operation in the coming years. It mentioned that the Lunatic Asylum comprised two double and four single wards for males and one double and two single wards for females, 'the whole form[ing] one building adjoining the jail'. It was built on 'low ground, so low that water floods the compound in the rains, and does not run off by the only drain' that was at a higher level than the Asylum. This made half the Asylum compound 'very damp' and 'somewhat unhealthy'. The wards 'have . . . very high floors, and so are dry and healthy. . . [and] well ventilated'. As for 'conservancy, the same disgusting arrangement that occurs in the Jail Female Hospital and Male Lachar Kathri has been followed in the Asylum Wards. The patients defecate in these rooms, and the faeces are, or were supposed to be, washed out through a hole in the wall on a level with the floor, into a gamla placed under this hole on the outside. Thus each ward becomes nightly a privy, and the unfortunate insanes have to sleep alongside their own defecations. The day privy is a good one, but very inconveniently constructed, both for males and females.' It seems that the Mihtarani (viz. sweepress) cleaned the ward at about 4 P.M. the next day.

> The diet is the same that is issued to Jail labouring prisoners, plus what I [viz. Coates] choose to give in addition to those requiring extra allowances. The water is not good; it is the same as that used by the prisoners. When the wells were being dug they were not dug deep enough. . . [consequently] the water is not pure . . . but unhealthy surface water. There has been scarcely any illness; the patients are treated easily in their wards; there is no special hospital for them, nor in one required as. . . [they] are as yet too few.

As Coates put it, no labour was extracted prior to his taking charge, 'excepting a few men who worked at twine and a woman at cotton spinning'. The compound was cleared of bricks and roads and paths were constructed and grass was 'encouraged to grow . . . by watering the soil'. Since gardening was 'most agreeable to the insane' it was encouraged. It helped save money that would have been spent to buy vegetables from the bazar. Gardening helped the men stay 'physically healthy and morally happy', and it helped 30 per cent of the inmates to recover. The female ward had a male guard, who was replaced with a female guard. Coates suggested some steps to help the 'recovered lunatic'. These included issuing a certificate to them that would help in procuring a subsistence allowance from the Magistrate, and providing them with clothing in case they did not possess any by the Superintendent. These, he felt, would ensure that they did not steal on their return journey and remained protected from nature.[32]

Moving on, the *Annual Report for 1865* referred to three 'criminal lunatics' who were admitted for the first time, along with the Inspection

Report of F.J. Mouat (Inspector General of Jails) which referred to the 'cell's' in the Asylum.[33] We are also told about nine inmates who 'had been transferred from the Jail Asylum Cells'. In terms of numbers, 20 per cent of the inmates were 'criminal lunatics'. Twine-making and cotton spinning continued in the usual way, and as mentioned no one was 'coerced into working'. The 'real profits' jumped from 10.14.0 rupees in 1864 to 94.4.10 rupees in 1865, along with the value of 'lunatic' labour – from 17.2.0 rupees to 623.10.6 rupees. A typical phenomenon noted was the allegation of a 'friendless insane woman' being forced to part with her gold and silver ornaments by a Police Sub Inspector before she was taken to the Asylum. This was found to be correct after an enquiry, and led to the recovery of some of the stolen ornaments.[34]

The *Annual Report of 1866* did refer to the Naanka Famine and categorically stated that all the insanes were employed in some work 'with salutary effect'. As mentioned earlier, the price of grain was high and the cost of each insane inmate had increased. The *Report* mentioned the admission of three 'criminal lunatics', which amounted to 'ten percent of the total admissions'. Even in this context, the Asylum 'profits' increased to 136.14.6 rupees, and the value of 'lunatic labour' increased to about 782 rupees.[35]

The *Annual Report of 1867* for the first time referred to the necessity of having a separate (small) place to accommodate Europeans. This was occasioned by the fact that Bunkall, the Inspector of Irrigation, who had been in charge of 'important assignments' and also had an estate at Cuttack needed treatment. He was shifted to Bhowanipore for treatment, away from 'an asylum in which no provision. . . [was made] for European cases'. In fact, it identified the rapid progress of a new building for 'Europeans' that was being built as an 'improvement'. In a repeat of what had happened in 1865, Bustam Das had complained that many of his belongings were not returned after his recovery. He had been picked up and put into the Soro police station. After his complaint Das's belongings were auctioned and the proceeds (100 rupees) returned to him.[36] And finally, the *Report for the Year 1868*, besides outlining the 'profits' made, mentioned that the inmates performed 'coolie work' in the 'Statement of Profit of Labour'.[37]

Even a superficial analysis of these four *Reports* illustrates how the Cuttack Jail haunted the Asylum 'like a nightmare'.[38] Its location, the living conditions of the criminalized inmates, the transfer of 'criminal lunatics' from the Jail to the Asylum, the absence of a woman guard for the female ward, the environment and even drinking water and food supplied were clearly on the lines of the Cuttack Jail. As clearly asserted, a hospital was not required for the Asylum and that labour was not being extracted forcibly. In a narrative which admitted that some forms of 'labour' were acceptable even to the inmates, the silence on the labour needed to clean up the area, 'develop' roads and paths and the growth of grass – or even 'coolie labour' – seems particularly striking, unless of course all these are assumed to be different aspects of 'gardening'. The connection made between gardening and the recovery of 30 per cent of the 'lunatics' is indeed incomprehensible. Here the ideas about the poor being lazy and the therapeutic component associated with work – a point that was repeated over the years – need to be noted.[39] One can also refer to the inmates being made to push the oil press that seems to have existed from the early years, though the first reference to it is from the *Report for the Year 1877*.[40] Popular imagination distinctly associated this as a punishment meted out to prisoners in the colonial Jail, and as already delineated at the outset, Fakirmohana mentioned it in the 1890s. One needs to also refer to a rather irresponsible suggestion to use the route via the river Mahanadi to ensure a trouble-free transportation of the 'lunatics' from Sambalpur district to the Cuttack Asylum.[41]

The consistent references to the Asylum 'profits', the 'value of labour', along with how gardening helped to reduce the money spent on vegetables, provide a picture that matches with that of the Jail. It seems that the government hardly had to spend anything for maintaining the Asylum – a very significant aspect of the 'civilising mission'.

The repressive and coercive components are of course visible when it comes to the reference related to 'coolie' labour, the Police Sub Inspector helping himself to the ornaments of a woman before she was admitted to the Asylum or the functioning of the Soro police station. Although the colonial administration could have defended itself by pointing its finger at a brown subordinate (viz. Police Sub Inspector) who was involved with this crime, or the Soro police station actually returning Bustam Das 100 rupees, these had deeper implications. After all, they reflected the way in which a 'lunatic' was perceived in a context that criminalized her or him and the virtually non-existent/fluid boundary between the Jail and Asylum.[42] These notions continued and were reinforced even in the case of the 'recovered lunatics', who were provided meagre resources based on philanthropic ideas, but especially to also ensure that they – being poor – did not steal and pose any danger to the public on their return journey. And, in the context of the existing conditions the question of admitting Bunkall – a white man – into the Asylum could not have been even imagined as a possibility, given the logic of race and class – but especially race associated with a colonial power. After all, a white man going 'mad' threatened to undermine the power and *prestige* of the empire.[43]

The ideas of reform that had intrinsic connections with the 'civilising mission', however, could never be abandoned altogether and this perhaps led to the setting up of the James Clark Enquiry to examine the working of the fourteen Asylums, which included the Cuttack Lunatic Asylum in 1868.[44] Significantly the official discourse, as is evident from the response to the questions related to the Enquiry of James Clark, mentioned that the Cuttack Lunatic Asylum was situated next to the Cuttack Jail, and that it was originally designed for a Lunatic Asylum. Nevertheless, if visualized in terms of what has been already delineated, the footprints of the Cuttack Jail remained clearly inscribed on the very existence of the Cuttack Lunatic Asylum. Further, it mentioned that the Asylum housed only 'native patents', comprising 33 males and 7 females, who were separated with a 'partition wall'. Each 'patient' was provided with 47 'superficial feet' of space.[45] Although not mentioned, the Asylum had reached its full capacity by 1868.

In response to the question related to 'Treatment', it *denied the use of 'mechanical restraint'*, even as it referred to its use when a patient became violent or assaulted other inmates, or was likely to inflict self-injury. Similarly, even while it mentioned that there were *no cells for solitary confinement*, as it was seldom necessary, it acknowledged how the smaller cells were used to confine 'violent patients' and that within the 'last half-year' three persons were confined in this way for two to three days 'at a time', though 'not continuously'.[46] In response to the general queries, it was stated that gardening was a 'favourite occupation', and added the 'pumping of water for bathing and Asylum purposes generally', spinning, weaving, stone breaking, sewing and matting to this list.[47] The silence on the extraction of 'coolie labour' (that had been observed in the *Report of 1868*) is particularly striking. Moreover, considering that the clothing for all the inmates were manufactured by the 'lunatics themselves' in 1869, it is very likely that the system had emerged earlier, especially if one goes by the manufacture of all the ancillaries needed for the purpose in the Asylum.[48]

The response went on to state that the Puri and Balasore 'Jail Hospital' 'detained' the 'suspected insane' for a day or two until the Medical Officer reported their cases, after which they were transferred to the Cuttack Asylum. In fact, if the 'insane' were found to be disturbing the peace in the 'country' (viz. the rural areas) then they were taken by the police 'at once' and sent to the nearest Magistrate.[49] Of course, there is no need to deconstruct the silence about their arrest or other repressive components, as long as one bears in mind the operation of the Indian Lunatic Asylums Act, 1858. Thus, even though the response to Clark referred to the inmates as 'patients', it hardly needs any reiteration that the colonial order located them not as people who were ill or needed treatment, but as criminals.[50] In many ways, then, the geographical location of the Asylum and its 'architecture' typifies an ideological position related to the logic of space that was supposed to be assigned to it.[51] It is interesting to note that Clark's Enquiry suppressed much more than what it revealed when it concluded that things were by and large fine as far as the working of the Asylum was concerned. The type of questions posed – which did not provide any space for responses related to the actual living conditions of the inmates who slept with their defecation – the data supplied to Clark and their selective usage, together made Clark's cover-up effort relatively easy.[52]

Of course, it needs to be added that the official discourse that stood by the planning, setting up and the working of the Asylum was itself strangely divided about the location of the Asylum. How else does one explain the efforts to discuss the alternative sites where the Asylum could be shifted to? This seems to have had its origins in the need to take care of Bunkall (1867), and was followed by a murderous assault, leading to the death of an inmate (1868). M.J. Mouat, the Inspector General of Jails, Lower Provinces, mentioned that the Asylum needed more space, and also separated from a 'crowded town'. He considered the extension of the Asylum towards the Jail 'undesirable' as it was bad for both.[53] T.E. Ravenshaw (Commissioner Orissa) advocated the removal of the Asylum to a more favourable site and added that neither the Jail nor the Asylum could be 'extended without affecting the other'. However, he also speculated whether the Jail should be included with the Lunatic Asylum or the vice versa.[54] The problem of 'insufficient space' for the inmates in the Asylum and the extension of the Jail were also noted by A.J. Payne, the Superintendent of Asylums at the Presidency.[55] Besides, the solution to avoid overcrowding in the Asylum was to ensure that the district officers detained 'their lunatics' in their respective jails,[56] which implied that they could languish in these jails for years. Thus, in the light of our discussion it is hardly surprising that the official discourse related to the need for more and a 'suitable' space of the Asylum consistently invoked the Jail in some form or the other, with the latter emerging almost as a 'historic bloc'. However, nothing was done about it.

The Cuttack Asylum faced the problem of overcrowding almost since its inception, though it began to be accepted in official reports from the 1870s. Thus, as delineated by W.D. Stewart (Surgeon) in 1874 the Asylum was 'built in 1864 to accommodate 31 males and 12 females'.[57] However, in 1864 itself, 30 inmates had been admitted; and in 1865 along with the remaining 18 inmates, 30 others were admitted.[58] As outlined, in 1866 the accommodation had been 'increased' to have 38 inmates, which coexisted with a 'high mortality rate'. The mystery about the elasticity of space – between 1864 and 1866 – seems difficult to reconcile to, especially if we take into account the fact that there were 48 inmates in 1865 and 69 inmates in the Asylum in 1872.[59] However, W.D. Stewart's *Report of 1874* resolves the mystery by mentioning the steps taken to 'relieve' the pressure of overcrowding. This included making 12 inmates sleep in the verandah, a part of the 'female ward' being 'set apart' to put up some males at night and five inmates being accommodated in the 'European Ward', which was most probably never used at all.[60] Needless to say, some of these methods were perhaps tried earlier and logically later on as well. After all, it had to be shown that the Asylum was never overcrowded, and as A.J. Payne asserted in the *Report of 1880*: 'From the figures it would appear that the Cuttack Asylum was overcrowded . . . It was not so.'[61]

At this point it is worth exploring some of the alternative sites for the Cuttack Lunatic Asylum in order to see how far the imagination of the official discourse could transcend the 'historic bloc' that has been mentioned earlier. H. Calley, the Superintendent of the Asylum, summarized the various proposals for the site. Here he mentioned the old 'Mahratta Fort'. This was not found suitable as it was close to the regiment parade ground and as felt the noise from the shooting practices would be injurious to the 'lunatics'. Besides, there was no space in between the European 'station' and the military cantonment to add a new building. Moreover, the Fort was unhealthy as it was surrounded by swamp and stagnant water. He also referred to the Tulsipore area – outside and adjacent to the Fort – which had not been objected to. Nevertheless, as observed, this part of the Station had no 'practical advantages' and the area had swamps and stagnant ponds which were 'malarious' and 'unhealthy', and hence considered risky.[62]

Chowliagunje, in which the cavalry barracks was located, was the next site considered.[63] It was rejected as it was very far away (3 kms) from the 'main part of the Station' and would prevent the Civil Surgeon from looking after the Asylum and also attend to his duties. In Calley's opinion, the Mungalabag compound was the 'best of all', as it was well drained and was 'first rate garden land'. However, he promptly added that there could be objections 'as land was more valuable' here and would mean an expenditure of 12,000 to 15,000 rupees. The last site he mentioned was the tract between the new Hospital (next to Munglabag) and Jobra, as it was open and well 'exposed to prevailing winds', and the well water was 'good' and 'abundant'. Although the soil was sandy and would prevent developing a garden that aided the 'treatment of lunatics', he mentioned that trees could be planted. As he put it, this was the 'best site'.[64] T.E. Ravenshaw clearly approved a 'small asylum' of a 'cheap' and 'semi-cutcha' character that could accommodate 80–100 patients at Jobra, even as he advocated the transfer of the existing Asylum buildings to the Jail 'for use as a female ward'.[65] However, an 'Official Note' in 1876, which stated that, 'The construction of a new asylum at Cuttack has been postponed merely on financial ground but will be taken in hand as soon as funds are available', clearly ended the 'search'.[66] Ironically, the *Report of 1876* mentioned the inspection of the Presidency Circle Deputy Surgeon General (2 December) who found everything to be *'satisfactory'* with the Asylum, along with a 'Resolution' which categorically stated that its condition was *'unsatisfactory'*, that it was 'over-crowded', and that it had an exceptionally high *'death rate'* (16.75 for males and 28.57 for females). It also wondered about the necessity of having an Asylum at Cuttack when regular steam connection had been established between False Point (near Kendrapada) and Calcutta, where there were alternatives.[67]

Beyond these contradictory pulls, ambiguities and cover-ups, some basic features are observable. For one, the insecurities posed by the 'criminal lunatics' perhaps explains the manner in which the official discourse was dominated by the Cuttack Jail, even in discussions related to the search for alternative sites for the Asylum. The reference to the Fort as a site was in itself a part of this imaginary. As has been already mentioned, it had a history of confining prisoners; besides, by this time the military parade ground and cantonment stood close by. The idea behind the other locations that were discussed was to either retain control over the Asylum by keeping it within a specified distance especially from the troops stationed at the Fort – viz. Mungalabag and Jobra – or to shift it away from urban areas altogether – viz. to Chowliagunje, near the cavalry barracks. Beyond all this, the data provided by the Census of 1871–72, though inaccurate, quantified the number of the 'insane' and this indicated the absence of any real threat from them:[68]

1872 Census	
Total population	*Total population of insanes and 'idiots'*
Cuttack 1,494,784	377 (255 + 122)
Balasore 770,232	95 (53 + 42)
Puri 769,674	202 (140 + 62)
Orissa states 1,283,309	329 (175 +154)

Consequently, the insignificant numbers of the 'lunatics' in the region diluted the fears of the colonial establishment and accounts for the government's directive in 1876 about not admitting 'harmless insanes' and incurables who had friends to take care of them.[69]

The official discourse of the 1870s, that had expressed its lack of interest in spending any resources on the Asylum or the treatment of the 'lunatics,' was clearly conditioned by the type of people who were 'confined'. After all, it was not a simple coincidence that the European overseer was removed to cut costs in 1871.[70] This particular aspect is evident from a superficial survey of the social origins of the inmates over the period.

At this point, one needs to throw some light on the inmates in the Cuttack Asylum. The *Reports* over the period suggest that it included Hindus and Muslims, along with some Christians. The inmates from the 'jungles' of the 'tributary mahals' (i.e. princely states) – most probably tribals – were clearly stereotyped as the 'Other' in the way that three of the 'criminal lunatics' who had committed murder and an insane person were described in the *Report of 1865*.[71] As for the other features, the *Report of 1864* mentioned the details of the 30 inmates, out of whom 22 were males and 8 were women. Most of them were from among the marginalized sections of the poor – viz. 5 beggars (3 males and 2 females), 5 housewives, 4 farm labourers (males), 3 messengers (males), 3 fishermen, 1 cheroot-maker (male), 1 shoe-maker (male), 1 spirit-seller (male), 1 bird-catcher (male) and 1 prostitute (female). It would be difficult to locate the two sepahis, a writer, a shopkeeper and a priest (all males) among the inmates as affluent people. Thus, the sipahi could have well been associated with the 1857 Rebellion that lasted in some parts of western Orissa until 1864 (viz. the Sambalpur tract); most probably the priest and the writer did not have regular or stable employment; and, finally it would not be possible to consider a rural shopkeeper as an affluent person.[72] The *Report of 1865* mentioned rather clearly that most of the inmates had 'no regular or settled employment' and the details of the 30 inmates who were admitted broadly match the details outlined in the *Report of 1864*. Thus, there were 6 'fukirs', 5 cultivators (which included 4 men and 1 woman), 3 shopkeepers (2 females and 1 male), 1 prostitute (woman), 1 cobbler (Mochi – male), 1 cowherd (Goala – male), 2 weavers (Tanti – 1 male, 1 female), 1 'coolie' (female), 1 Hadi (outcaste) woman, 1 Brahmin (priest ?), 4 Muharir (petty clerk), 1 constable, 1 carpenter, 1 petty trader (male) and 1 person (male) about whom nothing was known. In terms of caste, they were mostly from among low/outcastes.[73] Over the 1860s these trends continued, with one exception – thus the Report of 1868 mentioned the presence of a zamindar among the inmates, though remaining silent about where he was actually accommodated in the Asylum.[74]

Although similar trends are visible, a marginal shift is observable as one proceeds to explore the 1870s. Thus, the *Report of 1876* lists 2 beggars (males), 3 coolies (2 males and 1 female), 2 cultivators (males), 2 goldsmiths (males), 2 shopkeepers (males) and 6 (males) who had 'other occupations' 2 (males) whose occupation was 'unknown'. Needless to say, most of them were from among low/outcastes. Alongside, it mentioned that 15 males were transferred from the Cuttack Asylum to the Dullunda Asylum due to reasons of space, and perhaps for the first time there was a reference to a relatively poor 'paying patient', whose 'friends' could 'only afford' to pay 4 annas a day for him.[75] This trend of having 'paying patients' continued. The *Report for 1877* put the amount paid by the 'paying patients' at 169.14.3 rupees even as it mentioned clearly that the majority of the inmates either did not have any relations, or if traced, were very poor and could not afford to pay for them.[76] The *Report for 1878* mentioned that there were 66 inmates in the Asylum, out of whom 16 were admitted and 3 others were re-admitted. It contained a reference to 4 'paying patients' (whose relatives together paid 253 rupees), among whom was most probably a zamindar – a clear exception. The 3 other inmates were perhaps some relatively well-off people, possibly from among the urban sections.[77]

One observes the same trend in the 1880s. Thus, the *Report of 1884* while outlining the details of the 23 inmates mentioned that there was a barber (male), 2 beggars (males), 2 boatwo/man (1 female and 1 male), 1 brick-maker (male), 1 carpenter (male), 1 constable (male), 4 cultivators (males), 1 fisherman, 1 goldsmith (male), 2 milk-sellers (1 male and 1 female), 2 priests (males), 1 peon (male), 1 shopkeeper (female), 1 talookdar (male), 1 washerwoman and 1 writer (male).[78] One sees identical trends over the 1890s as well. Thus, out of the total 12 inmates, the *Report of 1894*, for example, listed 1 barber (male), 2 beggars (males), 2 coolies or labourers (males), 3 cultivators (males), 1 sepoy (male), 1 shopkeeper (male) and 1 sweeper (male).[79] Consequently, the affluent sections did not perceive the Asylum as an alternative space for 'treatment'. After all, the insecurities and fears posed by 'lunacy' led to its stigmatization among them as well as the urban population, who could not even think of admitting their relatives to the Asylum.

As regards the original areas of the inmates, the *Report of 1864* mentions that a large number of them were from Cuttack, Puri and Balasore and some were from the Garjats.[80] Besides, a few inmates were from faraway places like Oudh, Benaras, Sarun, Nagpur, Madras, Mysore (1864), Muzaffarnagar (1865) and Nepal (1866).[81] This latter aspect can be explained if one bears in mind the 'pilgrim traffic' associated with Puri. Similar trends are visible in 1881, and besides being from different parts of Orissa, a few of the inmates were from Meerat, Gwalior and Bombay.[82] Over the 1880s there was a notable absence of inmates who were from outside Orissa. The absence of separate reports on individual Asylums, together with the truncated/ merged nature of the available *Reports* over the 1890s and the table-oriented *Reports* from 1900, make it difficult to say anything clearly on this matter.

The search for a new location might have started with some reformist notions that had coexisted with the idea of retaining control and confining the lunatics more effectively. Classification of the insane on the basis of 'Religion' and 'Castes' assumes significance if seen along with the fears and insecurities of the colonial administration of the 'mobile people' like the mendicants, the Fakirs and the low castes/ untouchables or tribals. However, the small number of the insane population in the region, coupled with their predominantly poor social origins (as was also clear from the details of the inmates of the Asylum) over the nineteenth century[83] accounted for its low priority insofar as investment was concerned. After all, class/caste mattered. It is also abundantly clear that most the inmates were adept at working in the garden and the cotton/cloth manufacturing since they were associated with agriculture and the cotton textile industry, as delineated earlier.

Explaining 'madness'

At this point one needs to explore how 'madness' was explained in the nineteenth century. Let us begin by focusing on the 'irrational' and 'unscientific' world of the tribals which had complex connections with 'madness' as far as tribal society was concerned. The tribal world emphasized the human angle and its interactions with the shifts and changes taking place to explain madness. The Santals, for example, connected it with a *bonga* (evil spirit) which had fallen in love with the affected person.[84] The Mundas believed that it was caused by one's own *bhoot* (spirit) which struck back when offended.[85] The Hos connected it to the *bonga* (ghost) which struck back through it when injured and insulted, especially due to indiscriminate choice of places to eject human waste – viz. excreta and urine. More significantly, perhaps, it was seen to be a result of the desecration of the sacred groves, through the cutting of trees (*jahira*).[86] Insanity was also seen as a hereditary disease. The Kandhas, for example, saw it as a result of excess bile in the head which was hereditary and a child inherited this from her or his parents. The cure included the cooling of the head as a major component.[87] What is thus witnessed is a complex set of ideas that explained insanity as a problem related to the head and which touched upon major shifts and changes taking place in the nineteenth century to explain 'madness'. Thus, if seen closely, the association of 'madness' with the *bongas* or the *bhoots* indicates the levels of dislocation faced by tribal society, including the manner in which these impacted their lives, habitat and environment. This assumes a clearer form if the cutting and desecration of the forests are seen as metaphors related to the violence inflicted on tribal society, dispossession, the recruitment of forced labour, its movement that was intrinsically a part of the process of Orissa's colonization, especially in the second half of the nineteenth century.[88] Interestingly, from the James Clark Enquiry we get a reference to the Raja of Kanika being 'a monomaniac for four years – the result of his own wicked excesses'. The way in which these articulations are linked, along with the reference to the 'natives' of Kanika and a 'native' revenue official believing in the connection, blurs the labels – viz. 'crude' and 'superstitious belief[s]' of the 'natives' through which they explained the Raja's madness. After all, these were a part of the belief systems that he interacted with.[89]

Unfortunately, research related to areas of the social history of health and medicine is at an elementary stage as far as Orissa is concerned. This remains a major problem and one is ignorant about the prevailing Unani and Ayurvedic systems of Orissa and the way they located 'madness'.

Of course, the *Reports of the Cuttack Lunatic Asylum* over this period, starting with the *Report of 1864* outlined a scientific, colonial explanation of madness. Starting with 'Ganjah and Dissipation' (listed under 'Physical causes') leading to the insanity of 12 of the inmates (out of 30), ganjah was repeated as a cause routinely in most of the *Annual Reports*. The list contained factors that explained insanity by mentioning: 'Physical Causes' – 'Hereditary' (2); 'Jungle fever' (1); 'Moral Causes' – 'Jealousy' (3); 'Religious excitement' (3); 'Loss of property' (2); 'Grief' (1); 'Fright' (1); 'Family quarrel' (1); and 'Unknown causes' (4).[90] *The Report of 1865* echoed this trend. Thus, out of 48 inmates, 'Ganjah' was deemed to be the cause of insanity in 21 inmates; 'Opium' (2); whereas 'Masturbation' was left blank (though the 'Annual Register' contained 2 entries under this head) and 'Dissipation' included 1: 'Religion' (3); 'Grief' (6); 'Loss of crops' (10); 'Poverty' (1); 'Unknown causes' (6); and both 'Hereditary' and 'Congenital' did not have any entries.[91] The *Report of 1866* held 'Intoxicating Drugs', especially 'Ganjah', responsible for causing insanity among 23 (out of 52 inmates – viz. 46.5 per cent); it connected 'Religion' to the insanity of 4 inmates; and left columns like 'Debauchery' and 'Heredity' and 'Loss of crops' blank; and attributed 'Starvation' to the insanity of 3 inmates. It touched upon masturbation leading to 'madness'.[92]

As for the connection between ganja, opium, liquor and 'madness', what needs emphasis is that along with the super profits related to the 'unofficial' drugging of China, one witnesses an increase in the consumption of opium and liquor in Orissa over the nineteenth century. In fact, ganja accounted for two-fifths of the Abakari (excise) revenue of Puri, and the use of opium had 'greatly increased' in Balasore by 1859 itself. There seems to be an increase in the excise revenue over the 1866–1905 period with the increasing consumption of both opium and liquor.[93] The links between 'madness' and ganja assumed the form of a knowledge system, and as Mills puts it, by 1873, cannabis was linked to most of the factors generating colonial anxieties that ranged from sexual immorality and chronic indolence to violent and disorderly behaviour. The Asylum Reports from India provided the basis for assumptions that were reproduced in medical journals that reinforced these ideas, and led to the setting up of the Hemp Drug Commission (1894).[94]

Coming to the association between masturbation and insanity, the myth of 'masturbatory insanity' had its origins in Europe in the eighteenth century, and survived until the middle of the twentieth century.[95] Interestingly, the first reference to masturbation as a cause of insanity appeared in England in 1828.[96] Efforts to see this in noninteractional terms has led some scholars to locate its origins in the metropolitan world that was mechanically reproduced in Indian (viz. Bengali) periodicals.[97] Though this formulation needs to be probed further, the idea of the 'sexual obsession of the Hindus' was a typical colonial stereotype or construct that developed since the early years of the nineteenth century that focused on practices like child marriage and masturbation. The interaction of these notions with developments in England provided a 'scientific' veil to explain insanity in colonial India, to which the colonial establishment also added, even as it reinforced some, specific features. Thus, the *Report of 1864* mentions this crucial link between ganja and dissipation, and explains this as the 'cause' of insanity of 7 men and 1 woman – a prostitute – in the Cuttack Asylum.[98] Of course, masturbation was also seen as an independent cause of insanity. Thus, the *Report of 1865* refers to two 'non-criminals' – Munia, a fakir (Rajput) from Oudh and Bissun, who was associated with agriculture (Dholee caste) from the garjat – whose 'cases' were supposedly complicated due to their indulgence in masturbation.[99] The *Reports of 1866* repeated the references to these cases.[100]

The rather few references to masturbation in the Cuttack Asylum and the preference for the term 'dissipation', along with the dominant association of both masturbation and dissipation with the male body, seems striking and rooted in a logic that only women who were prostitutes consumed ganja and masturbated. Moreover, women were supposed to be 'less in control' than men and liable to more 'fiercer excitement' and 'more frequent paroxysms'. Besides 'one woman giving way to her impulses, acts more injuriously on her fellows in similarly exciting them, than occurs among the male lunatics'. These points were connected to prove statistically that they made 'recoveries among the women less frequent than among the males'.[101] One also witnesses the effort to connect 'lunacy' with 'heredity' in the case of women.[102] Alongside, some new 'heads' were introduced over the 1890s to explain insanity among women which included 'menstrual disorder', 'childbirth' and defective 'uterine function'.[103] One can clearly see the way in which patriarchal, upper-caste notions interacted with Victorian morality to generate a discourse that influenced the colonial medical and administrative establishment.

The entries under 'unknown causes' in the *Reports* assume significance especially since they echo dimensions associated with popular culture and the manner in which it explained madness by connecting it with bhoots. Ironically, the colonial health and administrative establishment that was critical of this was itself quite comfortable with leaving certain areas unexplained. It is perhaps this dimension that provided a liminal space to some of the marginal sections of the society to subvert the colonial order that criminalized 'lunacy' in order to gain access to the Asylum that ensured a shelter and a regular supply of food. One can cite as examples the presence of a leprosy-affected person in the Asylum in 1866 for two years after which he died,[104] and the case of a woman inmate delivering her baby twenty-seven days after she was admitted.[105] Even though the details of their 'madness' are not mentioned, it is probable that whereas the leprosy-affected person got food, shelter and some medical attention in a context when the colonial establishment had no idea about the disease and the threat that it posed for the public, the Asylum provided a safe and secure place for the woman to deliver her baby.

Thus, as is clear the colonial medical establishment had no clues about 'insanity'. This was explained through a host of meaningless terms that veiled its ignorance – viz. monomania, mania, melancholia, dementia and amentia – that were repeated mechanically.[106] I am not discussing details related to the treatment methods beyond what has been already touched upon. The reference to 'Bazar medicines' in many of the *Reports* of the period is intriguing, especially as it is not explained if they were procured to treat the inmates for 'madness' or other ailments. It is indeed striking that although the crisis facing the agrarian world, poverty, hunger and starvation 'entered' the *Asylum Reports*, their association with 'madness' was hardly discussed beyond the structural demands of writing the *Reports*.

Life inside the asylum

Certain specific features need to be spelt out at this point. Going by the *Reports* over the period it does not seem that the system of the inmates sleeping with their excreta and urine changed over the years. There is no mention about this aspect in the *Reports*, excepting for a reference to the Cuttack Lunatic Asylum paying a 'latrine tax' to the Municipality, although the 'night soil' was 'trenched' in the Asylum. This was stopped in 1900 after which it was removed daily by the municipal staff.[107] If one were to speculate, the practice observed in 1864 – that was indeed exceptional insofar as the Asylums of Bengal were concerned – most probably stopped, with privies being built inside the compound that replaced the old system. Even then, as reported in 1876, the Asylum had the highest death rate among the Lunatic Asylums of Bengal, especially due to dysentery and diarrhoea that reflect on the health standards of the Asylum.[108] Alongside by 1881 the Asylum spent the lowest amount of money – viz. 36 rupees – per inmate.[109]

The sufferings of the inmates did have serious implications. Thus, an inmate described as a 'complete imbecile' committed suicide in his cell with the help of another inmate in 1872.[110] There were also attempts to escape from the Asylum. Thus whereas in 1888 an inmate escaped from the Asylum, the next year, another man got over the Asylum wall but did not succeed in his attempt.[111] The desire to run away – whether through suicide or escaping from the 'lunatic' asylum – reflects on the agonies and sufferings of the inmates, some of whom had been exposed to the brutalities in the district jails or the Cuttack Jail as 'criminal lunatics', or after their entry into the Asylum, where some of these practices continued.

The *Reports* mention how the inmates were entertained in several ways. Some of them were fond of and were encouraged to play *pachisi* – an indigenous game of cards. Books in Oriya were supplied by the Orissa Baptist Mission Press of Cuttack that had been established in 1855–56 but were read by very few of the inmates.[112] The idea of encouraging music (1865) and organizing *nautches* (by Dr. Stewart, 1867) to entertain the inmates in the Asylum was 'abandoned' since these excited some of the inmates.[113] Interestingly, Dr. Stewart's experiment drew the critical attention of the Oriya middle class. Thus, the *Utkala Dipika* published a short note 'Efforts to entertain the mad patients' (*Baya rogimanaka manoranjan prachesta*), criticizing Dr. Stewart for introducing prostitutes to dance in the mad 'haspatal' (hospital) for two hours every Saturday evening, for which the government hired them. As expressed, this was gradually transforming the 'haspatal' to resemble the Lucknow Nawab's palace.[114]

Case histories

In attempting to understand case histories in the *Reports* and the testimonies recorded by officials, one encounters serious difficulties, especially as many of these were written by people who did not have any understanding of an alien culture or its language, were directly associated with colonialism and suppressed, as we have already seen, many unpleasant truths.[115] In fact it was a 'triple' narrative since the testimonies were not directly recorded in the Cuttack Asylum by the officials who wrote them, but by an intermediary before they were 'fitted' into the narrative pattern and style of the *Reports*.[116]

Case 1

In 1864, there was the first instance of a woman committing suicide. Her son – most probably not an adult – had accompanied her to the Asylum. She was described as 'old' and had all the characteristic attributes of a 'mad woman', in the sense that she was 'excitable' and 'maniacal'. She was 'disturbed' due to the loss of her property and the 'supposed' death of her son, who had been taken away from the Asylum the previous day by 'his grandmother'. She ended her life by strangulating herself with her own sari in her ward, after it was cleaned at 4 P.M. The male guard who saw her attempting suicide ran to inform the 'native' doctor instead of preventing her strangulation that led to her death.[117]

Cases 2, 3 and 4 – 'religious' causes

Under the heading of 'Religious' causes, there were two 'helpless cases' who believed that they had been cursed by a debi (goddess) and had set out on a pilgrimage to 'appease her wrath'. The third concerned a Baptist whose study of the 'Revelations' had led him to hallucinate, and seeing and conversing with angels. He was cured.

Case 5 – Mussummut Rani

Then there was Mussummut Rani, who was described as a 'sad case'. She had quarrelled with her husband in 1861 who had 'abused her' after which she left her village (near Burdwan) for Puri. She was accompanied by her uncle and father-in-law and their wives. At Puri, her uncle sent her to the tank for water and told her that Gunesh Pundah would take care of her. Pundah flattered her and promised her gold ornaments and persuaded her to go to visit a sonar (goldsmith). After that he took Rani to his house and kept her for two and a half years, after which she escaped when he had gone to collect pilgrims, leaving his sister in charge of Rani. She was discovered making her way to Bengal near Balasore, where she was found 'naked, starving and quite mad' and sent to the Cuttack Asylum. On her recovery she was sent to Puri, where the magistrate took steps to initiate legal pro-ceedings against Pundah, who it was discovered, had died of cholera. After this, Rani was sent to her relatives in Burdwan.

Case 6

This was a 12-year-old girl who was found wandering in Cuttack by a 'baboo,', 'insane, naked and sick'. She was sent to the Asylum, where she suffered from choleric symptoms. She recovered from the latter but 'remained insane afterwards'. She had a fight with her family and left with two of her sisters for Puri. A pundah, whose name she could not remember, met them on the way and 'induced' her to leave her sisters, after which she lost contact with them. She did not remember her original place of residence or the places that she passed through, excepting that she spoke in Bengali and said that she lived at 'Lal Bazar', but her family could not be traced. After her recovery she was taken by a 'benevolent' lady at Cuttack who looked after her and edu-cated her.

Case 7

This was an orphan girl who was from Madras and was travelling by ship to Calcutta, en route to Assam. The captain of the ship ill-treated the 'coolies', but some officers who visited the ship 'ordered their release'. After reaching the shore the girl started to 'walk to Madras' and 'went mad' on the way. She was taken to the Asylum and after her recovery she was taken by a lady who employed her as a servant.[118]

Case 8

This relates to Kundree Singh, a 'very powerful man' (i.e. strong). Along with fellow inmates Kundree Singh worked in the garden on the morning (21 December, 1868). The two others included Sabar Naik ('a criminal [lunatic] who has been sane for a long period' and had been 'recommended for discharge') and Ram Naik ('a harmless patient' who had been 'recommended . . . to be sent to his friends'). Suddenly Singh struck 'violent blow[s]' on the 'head[s]' of both the other inmates with a 'gentee' (viz. an instrument for digging the earth). Both Sabar and Ram lost consciousness, and the latter died at night. Singh who had never been 'violent' before was 'shut up' (viz. locked up in isolation), though a 'detached ward for violent patients' did not exist.[119]

Discussion

How does one read these case histories? Although most things are not clear from the *Reports*, Case 1 seems to be a typical case of a woman being exposed to patriarchal violence and tortured within the domestic world, most probably after the death of her husband, over property. The reference to her son being taken away by 'his grandmother' was probably his paternal grandmother. The level of concern for human life in a space controlled by colonialism is clear. The non-existence of monetary inputs prevented trained, female staff in the female wards.

As far as Cases 2 and 3 are concerned, colonialism's fears and insecurities of those stereotyped as fakirs or mendicants who had to be confined is evident. It is rather unusual to expect two friends who had 'gone mad' to decide to set out on a pilgrimage (possibly to Puri) to counter the curses of a Hindu goddess. It is probable that these were extremely poor people who were trying to work out strategies of survival, and succeeded in subverting the colonial classification system in order to enter the Asylum – a phenomenon we have noted earlier. At the same time, even though we are not told anything about the progress of these two men, the recovery of the 'Baptist' (Case 4) possibly asserts sectors of supremacy associated with colonialism.

Mussammat Rani (Case 5) seems to be facing the problem of patriarchy working out the idea of getting rid of her. A typical feature seems to be the idea of abandoning women whose responsibilities were considered burdensome at pilgrimage sites, like Puri. It is not possible to go by the fact that a domestic squabble with her husband alone led to the subsequent development, and what seems to have been told by Rani after what she went through cannot be taken at face value. The reference to her uncle – who could well be a person related to her husband since words like *mausa* could be translated both as paternal and maternal uncles, and could be also used to address any senior male in a village – needs to be highlighted. If studied closely, Rani's case also reflects on the trafficking of women. Here one has to underscore the fact that perhaps Pundah who was supposed to look after Rani sent her to sexually gratify the sonar on the promise of gold ornaments, and that he kept her as a sex slave for over two years with his sister's assistance. One would of course never know if Rani's presence at her parent's place (in Burdawan) was considered burdensome by them, and what happened to her there.

The question of trafficking girls/women is also clear from Case 6. What needs emphasis is that the girl did not remember her place of origin, but talked in Bengali and only remembered 'Lal Bazar' – viz. red-light area – most probably of Calcutta. It is difficult to say anything about why the three sisters had decided to escape, and if one were to speculate this was perhaps occasioned by their resistance to the efforts made to sell them. Besides, the Pundah seems to have taken her back to where she had tried to escape from. This resulted in her effort to escape yet again, and explains her state at the time when she was discovered. What is striking is the way her relocation is described. This is indeed difficult to accept in a context where the Asylum authorities were more interested in getting her out of the Asylum after she recovered, unless there was some connection with the missionaries at Cuttack.

Regarding the orphan girl travelling from Madras to Assam (Case 7), it is again difficult to decipher anything clearly from the *Report*. The reference to the 'coolies' travelling in a ship from Madras to Calcutta, en route to Assam – probably to work in the plantations – is intriguing since it included a girl. Consequently, it seems that she had been despatched along with the 'coolies' who were heading to work in the Assam tea plantations or as indenture labourers in some other part of the colonial world, though she had been sold and was being 'trafficked' to someone in Lal Bazar, Calcutta. Whereas the 'civilising mission' of the colonial establishment wanted the girl to be out of the Asylum and relocated after her recovery, the 'charitable' lady who took her away actually recruited a domestic child labourer or 'slave', considering that she was an orphan and had nowhere to go, and nobody to look after her.

And finally Kundree Singh's action (Case 8) clearly demonstrates how, while criminalizing 'insanity,' colonialism had – through the Asylum (and perhaps also the Jail) – actually succeeded in brutalizing a man who had never before acted in a violent way. Colonialism's beastly organization of the Asylum insofar as the living conditions and the way in which this 'strong man' had been exposed to hard 'coolie labour' (in the name of 'gardening') had succeeded in transforming him into a man that matched the stereotype of a 'criminal lunatic.' Singh's 'isolation' after the incident would have most probably reinforced this brutalization.

Conclusion

The Cuttack Asylum closed down in the context of the Partition of Bengal. On 30 March 1906, 37 inmates (36 males and 1 female) of the Asylum were shifted to the Berhampore Asylum (Bengal) 'without any mishap'.[120] Predictably the Cuttack Asylum was merged with the Jail building, for which the decision had already been taken.[121] The most striking aspect related to the Asylum's existence demonstrates how colonialism itself was entrapped by the idea of the 'unchanging east' that it had invented. The virtually unchanging existence of the Cuttack Lunatic Asylum served to reinforce this myth.

This micro-study has great relevance. The story of the Cuttack Asylum highlights a host of complexities and interactions with the outside world contributed to this diversity. As has been emphasized, the idea behind establishing the Asylum was not to treat patients but to confine 'lunatics' and make life secure for those outside – a point that becomes clear from most of the scholarly engagements that have been mentioned. As for the Cuttack Lunatic Asylum, it is necessary to reiterate the role of caste, class, patriarchal practices, fears and insecurities of the internal order of exploitation and the Oriya middle class that stood behind and legitimized colonialism. As elaborated, many of the problems faced by those who were considered to be 'mad' were ironically conditioned by the presence and expansion of colonialism and its internal collaborators over the nineteenth century.

One should not generalize too much about conditions in the Cuttack Lunatic Asylum, though certain commonalities exist when it comes to most of the studies that have been mentioned. These include the logic of criminality associated with the insane and the manner in which the poor were located in the health programmes and agendas of a colonial government. What is of course striking is that nothing seems to have been learnt from these experiences, especially when it comes to the latter aspect. Today the Indian ruling classes are busy dismantling the public health system that developed in postcolonial India, even as they re-enact the moribund policies of the colonial ruling classes.

Notes

1 I would like to acknowledge a 'Research Award' from the University Grants Commission and an 'International Visiting Fellowship' from Oxford Brookes that enabled me to, among other things, collect the source materials that have been used here from the Orissa State Archives (Bhubaneshwar), the West Bengal State Archives (Bhowani Datta Lane, Calcutta) and the British Library (London). Thanks are also due to Dr. Shilpi Rajpal for being generous with her 'virtual library', providing me with a copy of the Report of James Clark's Enquiry and her incisive comments.

2 One still remembers Porter's essay, 'The Patient's View: Doing Medical History from Below', *Theory and Society*, 14, no. 2 (March 1985), 175–98. Significant contributions also include Elaine Showalter, *The Female Malady: Women, Madness and English Culture, 1830–1980*, London: Virago Press, 1987; Andrew Scull, *The Most Solitary of Afflictions: Madness and Society in Britain, 1700–1900*, New Haven: Yale University Press, 1993; Roy Porter, *Madness: A Brief History*, Oxford: Oxford University Press, 2002; and Joseph Melling and Bill Forsythe, *The Politics of Madness: The State, Insanity and Society in England, 1845–1914*, London: Routledge, 2006.

3 For details, see Fakirmohana Senapati, *Chamana Athaguntha*, Cuttack: Friends Publishers, 1902 (reprinted, 1990), chapter 27, 140–3. Fakirmohana was critical of 'traditional medicine'; for details *Chamana*, chapter 28, 143–46.

4 It is indeed difficult to outline the range of research done by Waltraud Ernst on the subject and what is cited here is directly connected to the present chapter; see for example, 'The Establishment of "Native Lunatic Asylums" in Early Nineteenth-Century British India', in G. Jan Meulenbeld and Dominik Wujastyk (eds.), *Studies in Indian Medical History*, New Delhi: Motilal Banarsidas, 2001, 169–204; and, 'Feminising Madness-Feminising the Orient: Gender, Madness and Colonialism, c. 1860–1940', in S. Kak and B. Pati (eds.), *Exploring Gender: Colonial and Post-Colonial India*, New Delhi: Nehru Memorial and Museum Library, 2005, 57–92; James H. Mills, *Madness, Cannabis and Colonialism: The 'Native-Only' Lunatic Asylums of British India, 1857–1900*, Basingstoke: Palgrave Macmillan, 2000; James Mills, 'Indians into Asylums: Community Use of the British Colonial Medical Institution', in Biswamoy Pati and Mark Harrison (eds.), *Disease, Medicine and Empire: Perspectives on Colonial India*, New Delhi: Orient Longman, 2001, 165–85; and *Cannabis Britannica: Empire, Trade and Prohibition*, Oxford: Oxford University Press, 2003.

5 Debjani Das, 'Houses of Madness: "Insane" Women and Asylums in Nineteenth Century Bengal', Ph.D. Thesis, Centre for Historical Studies, Jawaharlal Nehru University, New Delhi, 2012, which enabled me to get

an overall picture of the Bengal Asylums, and her very recently published book *Houses of Madness: Insanity and Asylums of Bengal in Nineteenth Century Bengal*, New Delhi: Oxford University Press, 2015; Anouska Bhattacharyya, 'Indian Insanes: Lunacy in the "Native" Asylums of Colonial India', Ph.D. Thesis, History of Science, Harvard University, 2013; Shilpi Rajpal, '"Madness" and "Delinquency" in Colonial North India, *c.* 1850–1947', Department of History, New Delhi University, 2014; and Pranjali Srivastav, ' "Lunatic Asylums" to Mental "Hospitals": Studying Madness in Colonial India, 1858–1930', M.Phil. Dissertation, Centre for Historical Studies, Jawaharlal Nehru University, New Delhi, 2014.

 6 Michel Foucault, *Madness and Civilization: A History of Insanity in the Age of Reason* (translated from the French original by Richard Howard), New York: Vintage Books, 1988; and the non-abridged edition, *History of Madness*, London: Routledge, 2006.

 7 I have in mind the process of India's colonization that poses serious complications, along with factors like caste, religion and race, to which I shall return later.

 8 For leprosy see Jane Buckingham, *Leprosy in Colonial South India: Medicine and Confinement*, Basingstoke: Palgrave Macmillan, 2002; Sanjiv Kakkar, 'Medical Developments and Patient Unrest in the Leprosy Asylum', in Biswamoy Pati and Mark Harrison (eds.), *Health, Medicine and Empire: Perspectives on Colonial India*, New Delhi: Orient Longman, 2001, 188–216; Biswamoy Pati and Chandi P. Nanda, 'The Leprosy Patient and Society: Colonial Orissa, 1870s–1940s', in Biswamoy Pati and Mark Harrison (eds.), *The Social History of Health and Medicine in Colonial India*, London: Routledge, 2009, 113–28.

 9 For details, see Sekhar Bandyopadhyay, *From Plassey to Partition: A History of Modern India*, New Delhi: Orient Longman, 2004, 45; 83–6.

10 For details, S.L. Maddox, *Final Report on the Survey and Settlement of the Province of Orissa (Temporarily Settled Areas) Vol. 1, 1890–1900*, Calcutta: Secretariat Press, 1900; and W.W. Dalziel, *Final Report on the Revision Settlement of Orissa 1922–32*, Patna: Superintendent Government Printing, 1934. Sanjeev Raut, 'Rural Stratification in Coastal Orissa 1866–1900', *Social Science Probings*, 3, 1 (1986), 136–50; Pradipta Chaudhury, 'Peasants and British Rule in Orissa', *Social Scientist*, 19, 7 (1991), 28–56; and S.P. Padhi, *Land Relations and Agrarian Development in India: A Comparative Historical Study of Regional Variations*, Thiruvananthapuram: Centre for Development Studies, 1999, analyze the details related to these settlements.

11 Ranchi Archives, 'A Collection of Archival Sources on the Agrarian Movements in Eastern India, 1757–1857'; B.P. Sahu, a historian friend, remembers his grandfather (located at Berhampur, Ganjam) mentioning about many Kandhas being hanged in the aftermath of this *meli*.

12 For details, see Biswamoy Pati, 'The Diversities of Tribal Resistance in Colonial Orissa, 1840s–1890s', *Economic and Political Weekly*, XLVIII, 37 (2013), 49–58.

13 These details are based on *Report of the State of Police in the Divisions of Chittagong and Cuttack, 1840*, Calcutta: Bengal Military Orphan Press, 1842, 24–32; 43; 46; 57; 63; 67; *Report on the Police of the Cuttack for 1852*, Calcutta: Bengal Secretariat Press, 1854, 1; 3; 10; *Report on the*

Police of the Province of Cuttack for 1853, Calcutta: Bengal Secretariat Press, 1854, 1–2; 4–5.

14 Andrew Stirling, *Orissa: Its Geography, Statistics, History, Religion and Antiquities*, London: John Snow, 1846, 15.

15 Fakirmohana Senapati, *Atma Jibana Charita* ('Autobiography'), Cuttack: Jagannath Ratha, 1927; reprint 1965, chapter 4.

16 For details, see Hermann Kulke, ' "Juggernaut" Under British Supremacy and the Resurgence of the Khurda Raja as "Rajas of Puri" ', in Anncharlott Eschmann et al. (eds.), *The Cult of Jagannath and the Regional Tradition of Orissa*, 346, 345–57.

17 Though Puri was described in missionary discourses as a 'valley of death' where 'vultures hovered over dead bodies', the early years hardly saw any serious effort to focus on health beyond the immediate concerns that has been delineated. In fact, the 'Pooree Pilgrim Hospital' was one of the few health establishments that had been set up, as late as 1836. However, although it admitted women, even in 1853 a critical remark was made about the absence of female attendants in this Hospital; see for example, H. Ricketts, *Selections from the Records of the Bengal Government – Reports on the Districts of Pooree and Balasore*, 1853, Calcutta, F. Carberry, Military Orphan Press, 1859, 21.

18 G. Toynbee, *A Sketch of the History of Orissa, from 1803 to 1828*, Calcutta: Bengal Secretariat Press, 1873, 78–9.

19 Michel Foucault, *Madness and Civilisation: A History of Insanity in the Age of Reason*, New York: Vintage Books, 1988, mentions how: 'John Howard, at the end of the eighteenth century . . . made pilgrimages to all the chief centres of confinement – "hospitals, prisons, jails" – and his philanthropy was outraged by the fact that the same walls could contain those condemned by common law, young men who disturbed their families' peace or who squandered their goods, people without profession and the insane'; 45–6. The details related to the Cuttack Jail are from *Report on the Jails of Bengal, Bihar and Orissa for the Year 1854–55*, Calcutta: Calcutta Gazette Office, 1956, Appendix, xxxi.

20 The 'profits' of the Cuttack Jail amounted to 1,236.6.9 rupees in 1853–54; 1,057.8.2 3/4 rupees in 1855–56; and 401.3.6 rupees in 1856–57, respectively; for details see *Report on the Jails of Bengal, Bihar and Orissa 1854–55*, Appendix, xxxi; xi, Table 8; F.J. Mouat, *Report on the Jails of the Lower Provinces of the Bengal Presidency for the Year 1856–57*, Calcutta: Military Orphan Press, 1857, 79. Needless to say, a sharp decline is visible in 1856–57, which was perhaps due to the 1857 Rebellion.

21 In 1792, Philippe Pinel was appointed chief physician and director of the Bicêtre asylum (Paris), where he was able to put into practice his ideas on treatment of the mentally ill, who were commonly kept chained in dungeons at the time. Pinel petitioned to the Revolutionary Committee for permission to remove the chains from some of the patients as an experiment and to allow them to exercise in the open air. When these steps proved to be effective, he was able to change conditions at the hospital and discontinue the customary methods of treatment, which included bloodletting, purging and physical abuse; for details see http://psychology.jrank. org/pages/494/Philippe-Pinel.html, accessed on 15 July 2015.

22 Waltraud Ernst, 'Madness and Colonial Spaces: British India, c. 1800–1947', in Leslie Topp, James E. Moran and Jonathan Andrews (eds.), *Madness, Architecture and the Built Environment: Psychiatric Spaces in Historical Context*, New York: Routledge, 2007, 229, 215–38.

23 According to the Old Poor Law, each parish had to look after its own poor and those who were unable to work were given some money to help them survive. However, the cost of the Poor Law stood at £7 million in 1830, and the upper classes were very keen to change it as they did not like the idea of providing for the poor through taxes. For details see E.P. Thompson, *The Making of the English Working Class*, Harmondsworth: Penguin, 1982, 247; 294–96.

24 For the Utilitarian position, see James Mill, *History of British India*, London: Baldwin, Cradock and Joy, first edition, 1817; for missionary discourses related to early colonial Orissa see Biswamoy Pati, ' "Ordering" "Disorder" in a Holy City: Colonial Health Interventions in Puri during the Nineteenth Century', in Biswamoy Pati and Mark Harrison (eds.), *Health, Medicine and Empire: Perspectives on Colonial India*, New Delhi, Orient Longman, 270–98.

25 As the Note of the Inspector of Jails to the Magistrate of Cuttack put it: 'Although in some respects a convenience, the prison is really a most unfit place for lunatics', 'Memorandum on Cuttack Jail', 30 January, 1859, Accession no. 338C Judicial Department, Orissa State Archives, Bhubaneshwar, was out of tune given the reality that has been discussed.

26 The term 'criminal lunatic' had a long life, and survived over the nineteenth century. Even some like Commissioner T.E. Ravenshaw – an icon of the colonial and postcolonial Oriya middle class for his reformative initiatives – referred to it in 1869; for details, T.E. Ravenshaw, *Annual Report on the Police of the Orissa Division for the Year 1869*, Calcutta: Bengal Secretariat Press, 1870, 4; T.H. Hendley, *The Annual Returns of the Lunatic Asylums in Bengal with Brief Notes for the Year 1901*, Calcutta: Bengal Secretariat Press, 1902, continued to refer to the 'criminal lunatics' in the Tables, 10–11.

27 Waltraud Ernst, *Colonialism and Transnational Psychiatry: The Development of an Indian Mental Hospital in British India, c. 1925–1940*, London: Anthem Press, 2013, 35.

28 James H. Mills, ' "More Important to Civilise than Subdue"? Lunatic Asylums, Psychiatric Practice and Fantasies of "The Civilising Mission" in British India 1858–1900', in Harald Fischer Tine and Michael Mann (eds.), *Colonialism as Civilising Mission: Cultural Ideology in British India*, London: Anthem Press, 2003, 171–82.

29 The position of colonial officials who focused on the three coastal districts (i.e. the three coastal districts of Orissa), along with a generation of postcolonial historians who sustained and reinforced it, is contradicted by the new research on this tract which sees this having far wider implications since it affected the western Orissan states and the Chotanagpur tract; see for example Biswamoy Pati, 'Beyond Geographical Boundaries: Chotanagpur and North-Western Orissa, 1850s–1930s and Vinita Damodaran', in Lata Singh and Biswamoy Pati (eds.), *Colonial and Contemporary Bihar and Jharkhand*, New Delhi, Primus Booksm 9–28; 59–90.

30 Slavery was formally abolished in 1834, but continued to flourish in the colonies in a reinvented form; here I am referring to the forcible recruitment of indenture labour for the tea gardens in Assam, or for areas like Natal, Mauritius and Fiji, conscious of the fact that there is no serious scholarly work on highland Orissa on this area.

31 With the type of research available today, it would be impossible to accept the 'old' or the 'new' positions of a variety of scholars ranging from M.D. Morris, 'Towards a Reinterpretation of Nineteenth-Century Indian Economic History', *The Journal of Economic History*, 23, 4 (1963), 606–18 to Tirthankar Roy, *The Economic History of India:1857–1947*, New Delhi: Oxford University Press, 2000, second edition, 2006 about the 'progress' and 'development' made under the aegis of colonialism in colonial India. Besides, no nationalist historian would be able to argue today that these problems can be traced singularly to the rise and growth of imperialism. The structure of growing rural indebtedness, famines and dispossessions/displacements are serious metaphors that illustrate the role of internal exploiters who were integrated to the colonial machine of exploitation that had been triggered by the Industrial Revolution.

32 J.M. Coates, M.D. Superintendent of the Cuttack Lunatic Asylum, 'Report on the Cuttack Lunatic Asylum', in J. Mc Clelland (ed.), *Annual Report on the Insane Asylums in Bengal for the Year 1864*, Calcutta: Military Orphan Press, 1865, 66–9. I am avoiding the other details that would be examined when I take up some typical themes later on, since my focus here is oncontinuities between the Jail and the Asylum.

33 W.A. Green, *Annual Report on the Insane Asylums in Bengal for the Year 1865*, Calcutta: Military Orphan Press, 1866, 2; Medical Department Proceedings, 1–6, April 1865 (hereafter, MDP), West Bengal State Archives Calcutta (hereafter WBSA).

34 Green, *Annual Report Insane Asylums 1865*, 91–2.

35 W.A. Green, *Annual Report on the Insane Asylums in Bengal for the Year 1866*, Calcutta: Office of the Superintendent of Government Printing, 1867, 7; 72; 75; 81.

36 W.A. Green, *Annual Report on the Insane Asylums in Bengal for the Year 1867*, Calcutta: Office of the Superintendent of Government Printing, 1868, 94.

37 J. Murray, *Annual Report of the Insane Asylums in Bengal for the Year 1868*, Calcutta: Office of the Superintendent of Government Printing, 1869, 54.

38 Here, I am invoking Marx's well-known writing, 'The Eighteenth Brummaire of Louis Bonaparte'; for details, www.marxists.org/archive/marx/works/1852/18th-brumaire/ch01.htm, chapter 1, second paragraph.

39 For details, see Waltraud Ernst, ' "Useful Both to the Patients as Well as to the State": Patient Work in Colonial Mental Hospitals in South Asia, *c*. 1818–1948', in Waltraud Ernst (ed.), *Work, Psychiatry and Society, c.1750–2015*, Manchester: Manchester University Press, 2016, chapter 5.

40 James Irving, *Annual Report on the Insane Asylums in Bengal for the Year 1877*, Calcutta: Bengal Secretariat Press, 1878, 9; 23.

41 MDP 72, 4 January 1868, WBSA; using waterways was a point that was repeated later on as well.

42 In fact, Rajpal, ' "Madness" and "Delinquency" in Colonial North India', refers to the Indian Lunacy Act No. IV of 1912, Chapter IV, Section 87, that legitimized this idea of extracting any money or valuables in the possession of the lunatics for their maintenance; 78.

43 Waltraud Ernst, *Mad Tales from the Raj: The European Insane in British India, 1800–1858*, London: Routledge, 1991, highlights this aspect very well; emphasis added.

44 The part on the Cuttack Lunatic Asylum was written by W.D. Stewart, Officiating Civil Assistant Surgeon. Bhattacharyya, 'Indian Insanes', discusses this Enquiry in chapter 3; see Shilpi Rajpal, 'Colonial psychiatry in mid-nineteenth century India: The James Clark Enquiry', *South Asia Research*, 35, 1 (2015), 61–80; The 14 asylums that were covered by Clark include Nagpore, Jubbulpore, Benaras, Bareilly, Lucknow, Delhi, Lahore, Patna, Dacca, Bhowanipore, Dullunda, Moydapore, Cuttack and Rangoon.

45 While responding to Clark, James Wise, the Superintendent at the Dacca Asylum remarked that the criminal in a jail got 54 'superficial' feet a man that was in any case insufficient for the 'lunatics'; cited by Rajpal, 'Colonial psychiatry', 73.

46 'Memorandum from W.D. Stewart, Officiating Assistant Civil Surgeon, Cuttack, no. 44, dated 19 June 1868' to the Deputy Inspector General of Hospitals, Presidency Circle, in Hospitals of the Bengal Presidency, *Bengal James Clark Committee Report, 1868*, 37 (37–40); emphasis added.

47 'Memorandum from W.D. Stewart', 37.

48 J. Murray, *Insane Asylums in Bengal for the Year 1869*, Calcutta: Bengal Secretariat Office, 1870, 42.

49 'Memorandum from W.D. Stewart', 37; 39.

50 'Memorandum from W.D. Stewart', referred to the inmates as 'patients', 37. Ernst, *Colonialism and Transnational Psychiatry*, mentions that any person charged with a crime and considered mentally ill had to be produced before a magistrate and jail officials for admission to the region's general mental hospital; 35. What perhaps needs to be added here is this part could also work in a different way with the suspected 'insane' being picked up and transferred to the lunatic asylum.

51 Waltraud Ernst, 'Madness and Colonial Spaces', correctly mentions the spatial expression of madness in British India being defined by race, social class, caste and communal background, which illustrates how the colonial context determined these characteristic features, 232; however, what she ignores is the associated criminalization/penal components that have been stressed in this chapter.

52 What I say about the Cuttack Lunatic Asylum broadly matches Rajpal's, 'Colonial psychiatry', which is a macro exploration of some the asylums based on Clark's Enquiry.

53 MDP 30, April 1869, Cuttack, dated 12 February, 1869 WBSA.

54 MDP 31, April 1869, WBSA.

55 MDP 16–20, August 1871; letter to the Officiating Secretary, Government of Bengal, 4 August 1871, WBSA.

56 A. Fleming, *Annual Report on the Insane Asylums of Bengal for the Year 1871*, Calcutta: Bengal Secretariat Press, 62.

57 Report of W.D. Stewart in R. Cockburn, *Annual Report on the Insane Asylums in Bengal for the Year 1874*, Calcutta: Bengal Sect Press, 1875, 16.
58 Green, *Annual Report Insane Asylums 1865*, 94.
59 J. Campbell Brown, *Annual Report on the Insane Asylums in Bengal for the Year 1872*, Calcutta: Calcutta Central Press Co., 1873, 99.
60 Report of W.D. Stewart in R. Cockburn, *Annual Report Insane Asylums 1874*, 16.
61 A.J. Payne, *Annual Report on the Insane Asylums in Bengal for the Year 1880*, Calcutta: Bengal Secretariat Press, 1881, 4.
62 MDP 59, 16 June 1873, WBSA. While discussing the 'native' troops stationed at Cuttack, the 'Report of the Royal Commission on the State of the Indian Army' 1860 observed that 3 per cent of the hospital inmates had venereal diseases, and considered it to be 'highly advantageous' to have a 'lock hospital at every military station' (obviously for the white troops), 575. As it appears, Cuttack did not have a 'lock hospital' and it is possible that it was not considered to be a favourable site to shift of the Asylum in order to keep this entire area *secure* for implementing such a plan in the future; I owe this reference to Ms. Divya Iyer, who is presently completing her M.Phil. Dissertation (at the Department of History, Delhi University) on the lock hospitals in colonial India; emphasis mine.
63 Murray, *Insane Asylums in Bengal 1869*, 44.
64 MDP 59, 16 June 1873, WBSA.
65 MDP 59, 27 August 1873, WBSA.
66 Home Department, Medical Branch, File no. 44–6 & KW, January 1876, National Archives of India, New Delhi.
67 J. Fullerton Beatson, *Annual Report on the Insane Asylum in Bengal for the Year 1876*, Calcutta: Bengal Secretariat Press, 1877, 28; 5; emphasis added. The idea of using waterways – viz. the river Mahanadi as mentioned earlier, and the sea – was rather irresponsible and perhaps echoed memories of the 'ship of fools'.
68 W.W. Hunter, *Statistical Account of Bengal: Cuttack and Balasore, Vol. XVIII*, London: Trubner and Co., 1877, 64, and 266–67; and W.W. Hunter, *Statistical Account of Bengal: Puri and the Orissa States, Vol. XIX*, London: Trubner and Co., 1877, 27, 30; and 208, respectively. Henry Waterfield, *Memorandum on the Census of British India 1871–72*, London: Eyre and Spottiswoode, 1875, mentions that the distinction between insane persons and idiots were not understood by the enumerators; that the inmates of lunatic asylums were in many cases returned as idiots; and that the number of afflicted males were in most instances largely in excess of the females, probably since the information about the latter was withheld; 37.
69 Beatson, *Annual Report Insane Asylums, 1876*, 25.
70 J. Campbell Brown, *Annual Report on the Insane Asylums in Bengal for the Year 1871*, Calcutta: Calcutta Central Press Co., 1872, 63; the *Report on the Cuttack Lunatic Asylum* was drafted by Surgeon Major A. Fleming, who regretted the decision.
71 Green, *Annual Report Insane Asylums, 1865*, 89; this was a part of an ongoing process that finally criminalized the tribes (1871).
72 J.M. Coates, 'Report on the Cuttack Lunatic Asylum', in J. McClelland (ed.), *Report on the Asylums in Bengal for the Year 1864*, Calcutta, Bengal Secretariat Office, 1864, 73.
73 Green, *Annual Report Insane Asylums, 1865*, 95.

74 Murray, *Annual Report Insane Asylums, 1868, 53.*

75 Beatson, *Annual Report Insane Asylums, 1876,* 43; 3; 27.

76 Irving, *Annual Report Insane Asylums, 1877,* 23.

77 James Irving, *Annual Report on the Insane Asylums in Bengal for the Year 1878,* Calcutta: Bengal Secretariat Press, 1879, 23; 37; 24. Once again we are not told anything about where the zamindar was housed inside the Asylum.

78 A.J. Cowie, *Annual Report on the Insane Asylums in Bengal for the Year 1884,* Calcutta: Bengal Secretariat Press, 1885, 28.

79 A. Hilson, *Annual Report on the Lunatic Asylums of Bengal for the Year 1890,* Calcutta: Bengal Secretariat Press, 1891, 24.

80 Coates, *Annual Report Lunatic Asylum 1864,* 67.

81 Ibid., 67; Green, *Annual Report Insane Asylums, 1865,* 94; and Green, *Annual Report Insane Asylums 1866,* 79.

82 A.J. Payne, *Annual Report on the Insane Asylums in Bengal for the Year 1881,* Calcutta: Bengal Secretariat Press, 1882, 27.

83 Ernst, 'Madness and Colonial Spaces', 225; 232, mentions most of these points, and stresses the class component.

84 L.S.S. O'Malley, *Census of India, 1911, Vol. V, Bengal, Bihar and Orissa and Sikkim,* Part 1, Calcutta: Bengal Secretariat Book Depot, 1913, 414.

85 S.C. Roy, *Mundas and Their Country,* Bombay: Asia Publishing House, 1970, 279.

86 *Census 1911,* 414.

87 Ibid., 416.

88 For details, 'Tracing the Social History of a Famine: Kalahandi (1800–1992)', in Biswamoy Pati (ed.), *Situating Social History: Orissa (1800–1997),* New Delhi: Orient Longman, 2001, 99–139.

89 James Clark Enquiry; in fact Stewart puts these points at the very end of the Report.

90 Coates, *Annual Report Insane Asylum 1864,* 72.

91 Green, *Annual Report Insane Asylums, 1865,* 3; Table – 'Annual Register of Insane Patients treated in Cuttack Asylum in 1865'; I have not put in all the details cited in the *Report.*

92 Green, *Annual Report Insane Asylums, 1866,* 3; 82–3; I have not put in all the details cited in the *Report.* Murray, *Annual Report Insane Asylums, 1869,* refers to the 'miserably starved condition' of a large number of inmates, who on admission to the Asylum required 'more nourishing food'; 42.

93 G. Toynbee, *A Sketch of the History of Orissa from 1803 to 1828,* Calcutta: Bengal Secretariat Press, 1873, mentions the available options for procuring opium in the 1815–17 phase, which included the illicit opium and government opium, and also illicit ganja, which was grown widely in Orissa; 68. Henry Rickets, *Selections from the Records of the Bengal Government: Reports on the Districts of Pooree and Balasore,* Calcutta: Bengal Hurkaru Press, 1859; 8; 44. Gorachand Patnaik, *The Famine and Some Aspects of the British Economic Policy in Orissa, 1866–1905,* Cuttack: Vidyapuri, 1980, 211; nevertheless, as a true empiricist he sees this as an indicator of the cultivators getting a better price for their produce.

94 Mills, *Cannabis and Colonialism* and *Cannabis Britannica* provide valuable insights to explain this dimension; about medical journals I have in mind journals like *The Lancet* from the period 1880s; *The Report of the Indian Hemp Drugs Commission, 1894–95,* Simla: Government Central Printing Office, 1894.

95 Thomas S. Szasz, *The Medicalization of Everyday Life: Selected Essays*, Syracuse, NY: Syracuse University Press, 2007, 84.

96 Thomas S. Szasz, *The Manufacture of Madness: A Comparative Study of the Inquisition and the Mental Health Movement*, Syracuse, NY: Syracuse University Press, 1997, 185.

97 Amit Ranjan Basu, 'Emergence of a Marginal Science in a Colonial City: Reading Psychiatry in Bengali Periodicals', *Indian Economic and Social History Review*, 41, 2 (2004), 119–20.

98 Coates, *Annual Report Insane Asylums 1864*, 70–1.

99 Green, *Annual Report Insane Asylums 1865*, Table – 'Annual Register of Insane Patients treated in Cuttack Asylum in 1865'.

100 Green, *Annual Report Insane Asylums 1866*, 82–3; Green, *Annual Report Insane Asylums 1867*, 99.

101 Coates, *Annual Report Insane Asylums 1864*, 67; MDP 34–6 April 1865.

102 J.G. Pilcher, *Annual Report on the Lunatic Asylums of Bengal for the Year 1892*, Calcutta: Bengal Secretariat Press, 1893, 12.

103 Hilson, *Annual Report Lunatic Asylums of Bengal 1890*, 12; Hendley, *The Annual Returns Lunatic Asylums 1901*, 18–19.

104 Murray, *Annual Report Insane Asylums, 1868*, 50.

105 Irving, *Annual Report Lunatic Asylums 1878*, 23.

106 Coates, *Annual Report Insane Asylums 1864*, 72; Green, *Annual Report Insane Asylums 1867*, 90; *Annual Report Insane Asylums 1865*, 3; Green, Murray, *Annual Report Insane Asylums 1868*, 52.

107 Hendley, *Annual Returns Lunatic Asylums 1900*, 16.

108 J. Fullerton Beatson, *Annual Report Insane Asylums 1876*, 11.

109 A.J. Payne, *Annual Report on the Insane Asylums in Bengal for the Year 1881*, Calcutta: Bengal Secretariat Press, 5; this was based on a comparison of the figures of Cuttack with Dullunda, Dacca, Patna and Berhampore.

110 Brown, *Annual Report Insane Asylums 1872*, 101.

111 A. Hilson, *Annual Report on the Lunatic Asylums of Bengal for the Year 1888*, Calcutta: Bengal Secretariat Press, 1889, 4; A. Hilson, *Annual Report on the Lunatic Asylums of Bengal for the Year 1889*, Calcutta: Bengal Secretariat Press, 1890, 10. One needs to refer to 'Drapetomania', a term from the slave days that was used to describe a type of mental illness in which the symptoms made slaves addicted to attempting escape, or escaping slavery; the suggested cure was to cut off their toes.

112 Green, *Annual Report Insane Asylums 1867*, 91; the indigenous Oriya Press was established in 1866.

113 MDP 34–46, April 1865; Green, *Annual Report Insane Asylums 1867*, 8.

114 *Utkala Dipika*, 28 December 1867.

115 Most of the existing scholarship has engaged with 'case histories' of the inmates in some of the Asylums. See Mills, 'Indians into Asylums'; Ernst, 'Feminising Madness – Feminising the Orient', and Debjani Das, *Houses of Madness*, focus on the Indian women in the Asylums; Rajpal, ' "Madness" and "Delinquency" in Colonial North India', chapter 5, and Srivastav, ' "Lunatic Asylums" to Mental "Hospitals" ', chapter 3 do refer to case histories.

116 Carol Berkenkotter, *Patients' Tales: Case Histories and the Uses of Narrative in Psychiatry*, Columbia: University of South Carolina Press, 2008,

9, makes an interesting point; as she puts it: '[F]rom a discursive perspective the clinical case history is actually a *double narrative*. The patient's "story", his or her narrative of personal experience, is subsumed into the narrative pattern and thought style of clinical psychiatry'; 2 (emphasis in original); I have merely extended this idea to Asylum *Reports* written in a colonial context.

117 Coates, *Annual Report Lunatic Asylum 1864*, 68; we have already mentioned a case of suicide in 1872, where details are not provided. It is indeed unfortunate that the details of the Asylums in the *Reports* get shorter, and this is more so when it comes to the inmates, as one proceeds over years 1864 and 1906.

118 Cases 2 to 7 are from Green, *Annual Report Insane Asylums 1865*, 88–9.

119 MDP 62, 21 December, 1868; and 63.

120 R. Macrae, *Annual Returns of the Lunatic Asylums in Bengal with Brief Notes for the Years 1906*, Calcutta: Bengal Secretariat Book Depot, 1907, 1. For details related to the factors that determined the closing down of several Asylums and the move to have centralized asylums by the end of the nineteenth century, see Rajpal, ' "Madness" and "Delinquency" in Colonial North India', chapter 2, 65–9.

121 R. Macrae, *Triennial Report on the Lunatic Asylums in Bengal for the Years 1903, 1904 and 1905*, Calcutta: Bengal Secretariat Book Depot, 1906, 1.

10 What did the 'wise men' say?

Gender, sexuality and women's health in nineteenth-century Bengal

Sujata Mukherjee

In nineteenth-century Bengal numerous writings of reform-minded Bengali authors – including home manuals, medical and quasi-medical literature – produced a normative discourse on the family, which included guidelines for proper home management, scientific nurturing of children, regulation of dietary habits, creation of hygienic environment and so forth. This corpus of writing included advice books addressed simultaneously to men and women and also included books and writings in journals where the audience intended were unclear. By far the largest number of writings included in this collection was manuals written specifically for women. Between 1860 and 1900 more than forty advice-for-women manuals were written in Bengali (most in the 1880s) and thirty-seven women's magazines and journals came into existence between 1860 and 1910.[1] Advice contained in these writings were part of an attempt to reshape and redefine Hindu domestic life and household organization. Whether published as separate books or within the pages of contemporary women's magazines, these works sought to disseminate, among other things, knowledge about health, hygiene, scientific nurturing of children, proper diet and treatment of sick family members. They formed part and parcel of a transnational discourse on domesticity.[2] This chapter focuses on some of these issues and concerns.

Domesticity, social reforms and the 'new woman'

During the nineteenth century, a set of ideas about the proper ordering of home and family relations became integral to bourgeois ideology and self-identity in Europe which are linked by most contemporary scholarship with the beginnings of industrialization, industrial capitalism and the new modes of production of the late eighteenth and early nineteenth centuries.[3] As a secular discourse, domesticity – a product of nineteenth-century bourgeois ideology – was deeply imprinted with enlightenment themes of order, reason and science. System, discipline and efficiency were considered to be essential components of daily domestic life, elements that must of necessity inform all the practices to which that life gave rise. The hegemonic ambitions of nineteenth-century European bourgeois classes led them to promote domesticity (as well as reason, citizenship and market economics) as a natural and universal category of human life.[4] In the colonies, bourgeois domestic discourse and the practices to which it gave rise were incorporated into the civilizing mission of colonialism itself.[5] It has been argued that nineteenth-century domestic literature produced in India is indigenous, local and authentic; it is also hybrid in that it brings a transnational domestic discourse to bear on local concerns.[6] They profoundly highlight the significant contestations of late nineteenth-century Bengali and Indian society. In the nineteenth century, the dominance of British power in India imposed an alien culture on the indigenous life worlds of that region. From the point of view of the colonized, the presence of colonial modernity as an alternative cultural system problematized all areas of indigenous life. The Hindu woman and her domestic world were at the centre of a debate over colonial modernity and indigenous home and family life. Colonial modernity had many meanings within late nineteenth-century India. Several scholars have explored its relationship to emerging nationalist discourses, its connections with the revitalizations of the Hindu Renaissance, its role in transforming traditions of music and art and its incompatibilities with indigenous aesthetics.[7] It can also be added that new notions of health and hygiene and diseases became part of a new ideal of restructuring of indigenous society through which the indigenous reformers sought to negotiate and reformulate the received notion of colonial modernity.

In India, colonial administrators, to buttress their own legitimacy, disparaged the miserable conditions of women. Indian ideas of domestic life were described as 'barbaric' and demeaning for women when compared to Europe's 'civilized' notions about domesticity in general and women's freedom and equality in particular. In *The History of British India* (1826), James Mill stated: 'nothing can exceed the habitual contempt which the Hindus entertain for their women. [They] . . . are held . . . in extreme degradation'.[8]

To the colonial critique of Indian domestic practices (including women's supposed inferior position) and to changing demands of life under British rule, English-educated and Western-influenced Indian men responded by focusing on the need of reforming women's conditions, most particularly women's literacy and education – which they saw as the key to both India's progress and their own. It has been argued that by 1860 social conditions became more favourable to the implementation of social reforms than before.[9] Apart from individual reformers' (Radhakanta Deb, Vidyasagar and others) attempts for upgrading women's conditions, it was the Brahmo Samaj (founded as a religious organization by Rammohun Roy in1828) as a group which provided support for reform of women's conditions in Bengal. Issues like child marriage, widow remarriage, the breaking of Purdah and the education of women all were associated with one or another sect of the Brahmo Samaj.[10] After the first schism in the Brahmo Samaj in 1866, the Brahmo Samaj of India led by reformer and religious leader Keshab Chandra Sen (the other sect led by Debendranath Tagore was known as Adi Brahmo Samaj) became staunch supporters of social reform more than ever. The 1870s witnessed serious debates and discussions amongst the Brahmo reformers regarding patterns of female education to be adopted. While the mainstream Brahmos like Keshab Sen and Umesh Chandra Dutt advocated limited educational reforms, radical Brahmos like Dwarkanath Ganguly, Manmohan Ghosh, Durga Mohan Das and Sivnath Shastri felt that both men and women should have equal opportunities in life. They became vocal about giving the same opportunity to women in the field of education as was available to the male members of the society.

In the colonial situation, most of the English-educated bhadralok were subjected to humiliation in their working lives. It has been suggested by scholars that new British ideas of time, office work, the harshness and humiliation of office work, or *chakri*, impacted the consciousness and identities of the Bengali educated middle classes.[11] The educated Indians required the type of wife who could provide sympathetic care and create the atmosphere of a 'peaceful haven in their own homes'.[12] The Western-educated elite section of the society imbued with liberal ideas sought educated wives as companions or 'helpmates'.[13] Newly educated women were expected to develop as companions to men, as scientific nurturers and as members of civil society, and they were to remain a socially distanced class from the common or lower-class women, inhabiting a world of unrefined, coarse, popular culture.[14] It has been pointed out that the nationalist reformers of this period offered women participation in a 'new patriarchy' in place of older indigenous patriarchal traditions which had demanded that women remain illiterate and uneducated, confined to the home's inner quarters, the *antahpur*.[15] Colonially modern Indian men imagined a new order which would facilitate women's literacy and education but also maintained that women would remain in a dependent and subordinate status within Indian society. It has been asserted that the Hindu nationalists who were excluded from the political power structure of the British Raj came to define the domestic world as their own – outside the purview of colonial intervention. This was to be the private domain of the nation over which they could achieve some measure of mastery and autonomous self-identification. Thus, long before the nationalists began their political struggle with British imperialism, Partha Chatterjee has argued, they had produced a domain of sovereignty within colonial society itself, a domain that included the domestic world of women and the family.[16]

The 'new woman' of nationalist construction was to inculcate in her

> the virtues – the typically bourgeois virtues characteristic of the new social norms of 'disciplining' – of orderliness, thrift, cleanliness, and a personal sense of responsibility, the practical skills of literacy, accounting, hygiene, and the ability to run the household according to the new physical and economic conditions set by the outside world.[17]

In colonial India, many of the Western-educated citizens argued that colonial modernity – as symbolized by the habits of daily domestic life – was both superior and preferable to indigenous practice. Punctuality, cleanliness, order and discipline were seen as the inherent characteristics of European homes; dirt, disorder and disease characterized the indigenous household.[18]

The reading woman and health advice

It has been argued by Benedict Anderson that print literature (along with the print capitalists who produced it) was of particular importance to the nineteenth-century bourgeoisies, the middle classes of Europe and Americas. It is through print, Anderson argues, that these middle classes came to imagine their mutual existence.[19]

In colonial India, too, nineteenth-century discourse on domesticity was produced in the world of print and was consumed naturally by literate members of the society. Growth of a class of educated girls also created demand for books in print. By the mid-nineteenth century, a substantial publishing industry had grown up in urban centres of the British Raj. In Bengal the publication of Bengali-language books had become an income-producing activity for many. Growth of a class of educated girls also created demand for books in print. Over the nineteenth century, the number of girls attending schools continued to rise. In 1862–63, the government's *Report on Public Instruction* published its first statistics on women's educational institutions in Bengal. It recorded the existence of 15 schools for girls and 530 attending students.[20]

By 1881 government reports for Bengal listed the number of women's schools at 1,042 and of girl students at 44,096. By 1891 the number of schools had doubled to 2,239 and the number of students had risen to 78,865.[21]

Newly literate women needed new reading materials. The first manuals appeared in the 1860s just as schools for girls became statistically visible. Over the rest of the century, the number of manuals increased along with (and as a result of) the growth of girls' literacy and of women's schools throughout the province.

Bengali writers initially produced advice literature for girls to use at home – for home education (the zenana system) and for home tutoring, both of which were popular in the 1860s and 1870s. Zenana education was promoted by European female missionaries who were employed by educated families to give private tuition to the female members. Home education or instruction provided by male members of the family to the female members was a scheme which was adopted more frequently than school education. Home education and zenana education were accepted by those who did not desire to break purdah restrictions by sending girls to schools. Despite some disadvantages, homeschooling remained popular at least until the end of the nineteenth century.[22]

Between 1880 and 1900, the publication of domestic manuals surged. A number of medical and quasi-medical manuals were published on birth management, childcare and other topics, many of which were adaptations or translations of English-language guidebooks. In 1857, the first of a continuing stream of mother and childcare manuals, an adaptation of Andrew Combe's *Treatise on the Physiological and Moral Management of Infancy*, appeared under the title of *Sisupalan*, and subtitled *Infant Treatment* authored by Shib Chunder Deb.[23]

Childcare manuals aimed at modernizing child-rearing practices in Bengali families mostly emphasized the need of following a regular routine in matters of the infant's breast-feeding and also spacing of the diet to be delivered to a child.[24] *The Duties of Women* [*Ramanir Kartavya*], composed by two authors Giribala Mitra and Jayakrishna Mitra (1890), contained sections on 'Child Rearing' where readers would learn what to feed a baby from infancy up to 2 years of age. It included general advice on which food items were nutritious and also pointed out that every room of a house should be regularly and thoroughly cleaned since cleanliness was necessary to improve everyone's health.[25] Different women's magazines also published health advice to impart knowledge to women. In a number of writings emphasis was put on the necessity of a sense of cleanliness, hygienic environment and fresh air for protection of health and prevention of diseases. It was even pointed out that an indispensable part of *garhyasthya dharma* and compulsory domestic duty to be performed by a Hindu female consisted in cleaning and washing bed linen and dusting twice daily and purifying drinking water.[26]

One way of improving health conditions was for mothers themselves to know something of different hygienic, dietary and medical principles and apply those to deliver healthcare. Women had to play a crucial and far more important role than before in the standardized, reformulated style of domesticity. With the emergence of family as a site where nationalist restructuring was to be carried out, women were awarded a special, augmented status in remodelling the private domain of the nation. *Bhadramohila* was expected to master the technique of becoming a *sugrihini* by acquiring elementary knowledge of all sorts of medical remedies – allopathy, homeopathy, kabiraji as well as Unani or *hakimi* for treating at least common ailments which would save the family a lot of expenses in doctors' fees.[27]

Allopathic treatment was criticized by some for its harmful side effects, and too much dependence on this kind of treatment was assumed to be an outcome of women's loss of knowledge regarding local herbal remedies. Women were often criticized for having lost the expertise in 'native' folk medicine held by women of previous generations and for harming children by giving them Western medicine. Rajnarain Bose, for example, pointed out that children of recent generations were weaker than in the past because their mothers treated them with Western rather than 'native' medicines.[28]

It may be pointed out that the heterogeneous nature of health advice contained in domestic manuals as well as in articles published in different periodicals addressed to women helps us understand the contested medical world which influenced the new world of domesticity. The educated middle class or *bhadraloka* as well as *bhadramahila* in colonial India tried to blend indigenous tradition with modern or Western medicine in a reformulation of the Western ideal of domesticity of which the formation of hygienic and healthy habits was an indispensable part.

As pointed out by researchers, biographical evidence shows that some women did try to follow the advice given in the manuals. However, there is no direct evidence that would prove conclusively that the kind of knowledge disseminated here actually filtered down to the majority of the *bhadramahila*. The value of these manuals and other writings lies in the fact that they reflect the attitudes of the writers.

With the institutionalization of medicine in the nineteenth century and the emergence and spread of the knowledge of a group of professional doctors, more and more families were becoming exposed to various kinds of expertise on medical matters, child rearing and other topics. In this new situation, parents, especially mothers, were expected to educate themselves to be able to understand and execute the medical experts' instructions to which the family had become exposed.

Instructions like the following, for instance, directed towards women were quite common: 'For the proper rearing of children, for proper knowledge about the child's nutrition and health, you should read appropriate books, you should take advice from expert physicians'.[29] Home manuals and other didactic writings thus imparted a dual responsibility to women for their families' health: a woman should be competent enough to provide care herself, yet at the same time should entrust the care of her family's health to a physician. In their capacity as mothers, they were to play a central role in national health regeneration. It was even pointed out that women who were ignorant of the rules of the body would not only harm themselves, but by producing weak and deficient children would also destroy the nation.[30] Pratapchandra Majumdar, one of the early authors on the new role of women, remarked: 'Because of the flaws of the mother, the child is ruined; when the child is ruined, the family is ruined; when family life crumbles, society decays; and when society is polluted, no nation can advance.'[31]

Degeneration of national health, Indian women and sexuality

This linking of individual and national body can be placed against the context of the growth of a medico-social rhetoric of degeneration. British colonial stereotypes that depicted Indians as 'decadent', 'weak' and 'effeminate' were not unknown to the English-educated Indians in the city of Calcutta (mostly high-caste Hindus), or in other parts of India.[32] A large number of publications on the subject of health and diseases which included discussions on – among other topics – the physical condition of Bengalis reflected the middle-class Bengali Hindus' concern and anxiety about the supposed continuous deterioration of the health of the nation, and of the Bengali community in particular. The starting point of the discussion in many writings on national health was the physical weakness and lack of strength of Indians, especially Bengalis, even though there was a complementary view that the Bengali was second to none in intelligence. The causes of this supposed deterioration of the health of Bengalis and the measures to be adopted to improve health conditions formed the subject matter of intense debate and discussion in a number of essays.[33] Out of these writings there emerged a medico-social rhetoric of degeneration, emphasizing that the question of how best to preserve or restore health should be regarded as a matter of urgent national security, requiring immediate attention. One author pointed out in an essay titled 'The Revival of National Health' published in a periodical called *Chikitsa Sammilani*: 'Most foreigners and some thinking Indians strongly believe that the people of our country have a frail body and a short lifespan, and that is certainly not far from truth.'[34] According to some observers the reasons behind such declining status of health could be grouped under two broad headings, namely (a) natural or local and (b) gradual pollution induced.[35]

It was also argued that natural or local factors like environment, climate and so forth were hard to eliminate. Many middle-class Bengalis of the time in fact were influenced by an environmental determinism promoted by the miasmatic theories and the medico-topographical surveys carried out by the Europeans since the early nineteenth century.[36] Different medical investigations of climate and topography contributed towards fashioning the idea of a pathogenic Bengal. Uncongenial environments of Bengal seemed to encourage diseases like malaria. Malaria was described as an 'emasculating disease' that threatened reproduction, rendered individuals weak and sickly, and thus seemed to accentuate the division (already entrenched in colonial ideology and practice) between the 'manly' and 'martial' races of the north and northwest and the 'effeminate' Bengalis.[37]

Medical topographer and surgeon in the Native Hospital in Calcutta James Ranald Martin pointed out that climate imparted to the Bengalis a constitution that 'partakes more of the lymphatic and phlegmatic temperaments than the sanguineous, predisposing them more to corpulence from laxity of cellular tissue and deposition of fat, than robustness from growth of muscular fibre'.[38] Martin published his *Notes on the Medical Topography of Calcutta* in 1837.[39] One important aspect of Martin's view is an emphasis on the interconnectedness of the effects of topography, culture and government – which reinforced each other's effects. Thus he writes, 'When we reflect on the habits and customs of the "natives", their long misgovernment, their religions and morals, their diet, clothing, etc., and above all their *climate*, we can be at no loss to perceive *why* they should be what they are.'[40] He also expressed the belief that influence of good government and English culture could bring in change and reform. This optimistic outlook regarding the power of reform was also embedded in the views of Dr. John Roberton – Manchester surgeon – who articulated these in a liberal-racialist manner. Roberton published a few articles in the 1840s in the *Edinburgh Medical and Surgical Journal* on the subject of menstruation among 'Hindus', 'Negroes', 'Esquimaux', which were later published in the form of a book.[41] According to him not climate, but social customs and cultural practices such as early marriages, precocity, men refusing to eat with women, polygamy, the treatment of widows, lack of education and other factors were responsible for creating divergence among races which had bearing on women's bodies. Roberton even argued that women's menstrual cycles in different parts of the globe could give an indication of racial difference.

He concluded:

> The difference between the European and the Hindu . . . must be sought in race, for if the early menstruation of tropical women was found to be a natural fact, then their inferiority is determined; and it will be in vain, by means of the missionary, of education, or of enlightened legislation, to attempt the reversal of laws based on physiological difference.[42]

Roberton based his observations on sources like Monstuart Elphinstone's *History of India*, W. Adam's *Reports on Education in Calcutta*, N.B. Halhed's A *Code of Gentoo Laws* and Allan Webb's *Pathologica Indica*. Dr. Gooddeve, professor of midwifery at the Calcutta Medical College, helped him with statistics on puberty. Dr. Gooddeve cited 90 cases of Hindu women and the average age of menarche was established as 12 years, whereas the average age for English women was established as 14 years, based on the evidence collected from 2,169 cases.[43]

Allan Webb, the curator of the Museum of the Calcutta Medical College, presented discussions on the female body based on pathological specimens in the Museum of the Calcutta Medical College. He noted the morbid state of the sexual and reproductive organs of 'native' women in his book *Pathologica Indica* published in 1848. According to Webb, Indian women did not menstruate earlier than 12 years unless 'unnaturally forced' by mechanical or mental stimulation.[44] He tried to explain the cause of abortion among the Hindu population and pointed out that attractive young wives of polygamous, aging kulin Brahmin grooms who became widows soon after marriage were lured into illegitimate sexual liaisons. In their attempts to get rid of the unwanted pregnancies, the Hindus, 'more than any other race', indulged in feticide. It was perceived to be a cultural phenomenon without a natural, biological or climatic basis, which could be reformed as well. Thus evidently by the mid-nineteenth century the conjugal and sexual practices were accepted in imperial discourses as ethnological indicators and were also accepted as an area with potential for reform. Female body was also perceived to be a symptom of culture and palpable to reform.

No doubt the 'native' experts and reformers turned the colonizer's liberal-racist discursive formulation of otherizing the Bengali into a tactic of self-criticism and reform.[45] In discussions on national health, the nature of social customs (like child marriage), sexual relations and habits of the indigenous people and the means of controlling sexual acts became subjects of open analysis. Social customs as well as harmful habits were blamed for the deterioration of physical strength and the decline of the health of Bengalis. The hope was expressed that changes which resulted from pollution or harmful practices and made the physique weak and fragile could be controlled through individual will or reform of damaging social norms. Some major factors identified as harmful for health were listed as (a) child marriage, (b) multiple marriages, (c) improper food habits, (d) lack of physical exercise, (e) alcoholism, (f) masturbation and nocturnal pollution, and (g) indiscriminate coital indulgence.[46]

With the progress and institutionalization of medical knowledge, a vernacular discourse on sexuality (and body) was formulated in the shadow of race, pathology and degeneration. This medicalized concept of sexuality became closely linked with the nature and goal of sexual relations, on the one hand, and national health, on the other. Sexual discipline was considered an important element of reform which would function as a corrective mechanism of health degeneration.[47]

In different writings on conjugal life and sexual activities published in the nineteenth century, it was pointed out emphatically that in the private domain of family the production of children was the sole aim of sexual union of husband and wife. In *Baigyanik Dampatya Pranali*, the writer stated

> the sexual union which produces children is described as the true satiation of sensual proclivities. The satiation of the senses affects every part of the body, physical and mental well-being is greatly decreased, and as a result the basic material of which the body is

composed is lost and destroyed. The satiation of the senses is in itself harmful, whether in excess or in a balanced manner, whether at the proper or the improper time, whether out of necessity or out of desire, the satiation of the senses will definitely lead to a loss of physical health. In the act of sensual satiation, many disgusting materials are lost from the body.[48]

Controlled sexual intercourse between men and women was proclaimed as divine rule. It was argued:

> Since the organs meant for procreation do not help the body in any way, the functions related to those organs, including coitus between men and women, also do not help the body in any way; but if such activities including coitus cross the sanctified limits and become perverted, then they harm the body, and that is why it is necessary to abide by God's rules.[49]

Sometimes opinions of European doctors were also cited in this and other matters relating to sexual practices. It was pointed out that Dr. Trall, a noted physician and author of the late nineteenth century (also considered to be the one of the founders of the natural hygiene movement),

> says in his book entitled *Sexual Pathology* that generating children is the main purpose of sexual intercourse between men and women, so that you should avoid periods of pregnancy and breast feeding and also avoid the first four days of menstruation; if coitus happens within the next 12 days and if both the young partners are free from diseases, then the woman would conceive.[50]

It was pointed out that 'the ovaries in women and the testicles in men are needed just for producing children and they do not help the body in any other way.'[51]

Proper ways of eating, bathing, drinking, sleeping and non-indulgence in aimless sex-related behaviour were interpreted as part of divine-ordained rules. It was also pointed out that a married couple could indulge in sexual union at an interval of 20 months.

One major cause of concern was the ill effects of child marriage on the health of young husbands and wives as well as their offspring. It was stated:

> Some Hindus and many Muslims of this country get married at a very young age. Among the Hindus, girls eight/nine years old get

married to boys 11/12 years old. Marriage at such a young and immature age results in the girls having their first issues around the age of 11/12; being as feeble and fragile as their parents, these babies either do not live long, or grow up to be weak and sickly. Second, the girl-mothers face a lot of problems during pregnancy and difficulties and pain at the time of delivery often leading to maternal mortality. Third, even if these girls are spared their lives during childbirth, they become subject to a lifetime of ill health.[52]

In the beginning of the twentieth century also a great deal of emphasis was put on the intimate relation between marriage and health. It was pointed out in an essay published in *Swasthya*: 'when entering into matrimony one must always remember one's responsibilities for the nation's health and the fact that health and marriage are inextricably linked.'[53] Polygamy and debauchery were criticized on health grounds. It was pointed out that multiple sexual intercourse which could be an outcome of polygamy or debauchery 'makes the bodies of men and women so weak that they can never be healthy and virile again.'[54]

Another issue highlighted as a cause of serious concern in the discussion on sexuality was the practice of masturbation. Masturbation and nocturnal pollution were identified as two vices which not only weakened the body, but also 'lead to a number of serious diseases such as impotence, epilepsy, sex mania, mental imbalance, loss of intelligence, etc.'[55] In a letter written in 1885 to the editor of the *Chikitsa Sammilani*, a medical journal published in Bengali from Calcutta, a reader described how he suffered because of his habit of masturbation and even after he was cured of this habit after being taught about its ill effects in 'English School', how he was haunted by wet dreams which enfeebled him. His appearance became skeletal; his face and body appeared to be bloodless and his eyes were blank. His penis became twisted and diminished. He lost his appetite as well as his courage.[56] According to the editor, the journal received hundreds of such letters each month. The anxiety was expressed that masturbation was a disease that affected not only individuals but afflicted the community and the race as a whole. The masturbator was the symptom as well as the cause of a degenerate, enfeebled, effeminate nation.

A great deal of concern was expressed in different writings regarding the adverse impact of masturbation on the health of adolescent boys and girls. One of the main objections raised against masturbation was that it was aimless; there was no relation between this habit and reproduction, so this habit only led to a deterioration of health. Further, masturbation, through individual physical deterioration, was seen to lead to the social decline of the country and identified as one of the main causes of India's backwardness. It was observed: 'In any case, boys through bad company, natural inclination or through other reasons ruin their body by masturbation, but girls aged 9, 10, 11 or 12 years do not ruin themselves in exactly this manner.'[57] Even so, books written at this time also discussed the masturbation of girls.[58] It was pointed out that women who indulged in masturbation become reluctant to face social gatherings. Moreover,

> They have thin bodies, pale faces and sunken eyes with dark circles around them, their heartbeat and their pulse run slow and their bodies emit a kind of bad odour. The sweetness of their voice and behaviour and the beauty of their bodies are gradually lost, and they feel ashamed to look at men.[59]

Dr. Annada Charan Khastagir observed in *A Treatise on the Science and Practice of Midwifery with Diseases of Children and Women*, a textbook written for the students of the Bengali class at the medical school, that

> masturbation by young girls was a cause of hypertrophy of the clitoris. Apparently the practice was common in many schools, and was believed to be addictive and damaging to the brain . . . To stop masturbation; the remedy prescribed was a grain of opium and three grains of camphor made into a paste and taken three times daily, as well as the application of ice on the clitoris. The clitoris was medically recognized as the central organ of arousal. To increase desire, an electric current through the clitoris was recommended, and to decrease it, the clitodorectomy operation; less drastically, a strong caustic lotion or ice could be placed on the clitoris.[60]

One important aspect of public discussions regarding sexual disciplining was the anxious preoccupation of 'native' experts and reformers with the question of reformulating sexual norms and practices within the household by targeting women. Sometimes it was pointed out that in the *andarmahal* (inner quarters), a lot of female conversation was centred on *adiras* or sexual matters. Women were often criticized for unrefined tastes revealed through crude conversations of a sexual nature. Apparently one of the ways of passing leisure time by women was listening to stories related to sex. According to S.C. Bose, women's amusements included needlework, cards and listening to puerile stories. He even observed, 'Their social tone is neither so pure nor as elevated as becomes a polished, refined community.'[61] Complaints were made about the fact that in such an environment where sex-related matters were openly discussed little girls became exposed to discussions of sexual matters from such an early stage that they were corrupted.[62] One alleged source of ill health of women was uncontrolled sexual desire. It was stated:

> Excessive sexual intercourse with one's own husband also breaks a woman's health and changes her behaviour considerably. A wife who used to be gentle in her attitudes and tender in her speech becomes quarrelsome, irate, and short-tempered. Such women stay healthy if they live away from their husbands for a long stretch, but suffer from over bleeding or under-bleeding during menstruation and other diseases when they live with their husbands. This is why men and women are all going to have broken health and short life spans unless they get rid of such unhealthy and harmful habits, and they will never be able to generate healthy and strong children to help the development of the country.[63]

Abinashchandra Kaviratna, the editor of *Chikitsa Sammilani*, wrote:

> Everybody seems to be aware, by virtue of subtle perception or natural intelligence that till the first appearance of menses it is not at all appropriate for girls to have sex with their husbands. Scriptures enjoin this and everyone, wise and foolish alike, is aware of this fact. As it happens, owing to the arousal of sexual desire from close proximity to their husbands, girls begin to menstruate and become pregnant at a premature age which causes irreparable damage to the health of the children born of them.[64]

Many popular marriage manuals published during the close of the nineteenth century put emphasis on the regulation of sexuality and the danger and disorder which would result if sexuality was not controlled. In fact a great deal of emphasis was put on the need to control female sexuality. Some of the popular manuals, including *Yuvak-yuvati* by Bipradas Mukhopadhyaya (first published in 1891), Yogindranath Mukhopadhyaya's *Jiban Raksa* (1887) and Baradakanta Majumdar's *Naritattva* (1889), went into great detail regarding sexual matters. *Yuvak-yuvati* dealt with subjects like development of the female body, sexual intercourse, pregnancy, birth and child rearing. It also contained many traditional Hindu rules regarding the times suitable for intercourse and the code of conduct for menstruating women.[65] The widely accepted notion in Bengali society that girls in the company of their husbands were sexually stimulated and thus reached puberty at an early age is mentioned here.[66] Baradakanta Majumdar's book *Naritattva* expounded reformist views on medical questions regarding consummation of marriage and prescribed that a prolonged period of gaona or the bride's residence at her father's house during the period between marriage and sexual maturity should be observed so as to delay the onset of the first menses.[67]

Conclusion

Thus, the family was made a medium of vigilance and policing in matters related to sexuality. In fact, by restructuring the private domain of the nation a great deal of emphasis was put on making women aware of different health-related problems, reforming and controlling their habits and practices including precocious sexuality. In discussions on early marriage, forced puberty and sexual aberrations (including masturbation), women were portrayed both as victims as well as the source of degeneration of the health of the nation. Aberrant sexuality was sought to be disciplined and controlled through dissemination of medical knowledge in 'Advice literature'. As modern medicine established the object reality of the physical body, prescriptive literature on new forms of vigilance, discipline and control were produced which linked the individual body to the social body. Some writers argued that it was essential that women should be made aware of their future responsibilities as housewives and mothers through ethical, religious and practical education since they could not concentrate and think logically like men.[68] Women's main role as biological reproducers tended to be highlighted. Curiously enough, women's voices would become less and less important in the growing medical discourse on degeneration of national health. Didactic writings of 'native' experts and reformers encoded women's bodies more and more predominantly as a potent site of reform – whose main function and utility consisted in becoming biological reproducers of a healthy race.

Notes

1 Usha Chakraborty, *Conditions of Bengali Women Around the 2nd Half of the 19thCentury*, Calcutta: Self-Published, 1963, 184–85; 190–1.
2 Outside Bengal, too, throughout British India in this period, an equally large domestic literature for Indian women came into existence in a wide range of formats (manuals, journals and novels).

3 See Carmen Luke, *Pedagogy, Printing and Protestantism*, Albany, NY: State University of New York Press, 1989; Leonore Davidoff and Catherine Hall, *Family Fortunes: Men and Women of the English Middle Class, 1780–1850*, Chicago: University of Chicago Press, 1987; Jean Comaroff and John L. Comaroff, 'Home-Made Hegemony', in K. Hansen (ed.), *African Encounters with Domesticity*, New Brunswick, NJ: Rutgers University Press, 1992. Central to this domestic discourse was a conviction that the 'natural' order of human relations involved a patriarchal family system with a gendered separation of spheres of activity and the husband at the head of the family unit. See Davidoff and Hall, *Family Fortunes*.

4 The Comaroffs argue that far from being a universal standard for human family life, nineteenth-century European middle-class domesticity is a discourse and argument marshalled by particular European classes at a particular historical moment who aimed to advance their own claims to cultural hegemony. See Jean Comaroff and Comaroff, 'Home-Made Hegemony', 39.

5 Comaroff and Comaroff, 'Home-Made Hegemony', 39.

6 See Judith E. Walsh, *How to be the Goddess of Your Home: An Anthology of Bengali Domestic Manuals*, New Delhi: Yoda Press, 2005.

7 See for example, works like Partha Chatterjee, *Nationalist Thought and the Colonial World*, Minneapolis: University of Minnesota Press, 1986; 'The Nationalist Resolution of the Women's Question', in K. Sangari and S. Vaid (eds.), *Recasting Women*, New Brunswick, NJ: Rutgers University Press, 1990; *The Nation and Its Fragments*, Princeton, NJ: Princeton University Press, 1993; Sumit Sarkar, *Writing Social History*, New Delhi & New York: Oxford University Press, 1997, Tanika Sarkar, *Words to Win*, New Delhi: Kali for Women, 1999, and her *Hindu Wife, Hindu Nation*, Bloomington: Indiana University Press, 2001; Lakshmi Subramaniam, 'The Master, Muse, and the Nation', *South Asia*, 23, 2 (2000), 1–32; Brian Hatcher, *Idioms of Improvement*, New Delhi: Oxford University Press, 1996; Dipesh Chakrabarty, *Provincializing Europe: Postcolonial Thought and Historical Difference*, Princeton, NJ: Princeton University Press, 2000.

8 Quoted in Geraldine Forbes, 'Negotiating Modernities: The Public and Private Worlds of Dr.Haimabati Sen', in Avril A. Powell and Siobhan Lambert-Hurley (eds.), *Rhetoric and Reality: Gender and the Colonial Experience in South Asia*, New Delhi: Oxford University Press, 2006, 225.

9 Meredith Borthwick, *The Changing Role of Women in Bengal, 1849–1905*, Princeton, NJ: Princeton University Press, 1984, 47.

10 Some of the important historical works on Brahmo Samaj are David Kopf, *The Brahmo Samaj and the Shaping of the Modern Indian Mind*, Princeton, NJ: Princeton University Press, 1979; Meredith Borthwick, *Keshub Chunder Sen: A Search for Cultural Synthesis*, Calcutta: Minerva Associates, 1977; Sivnath Sastri, *History of the Brahmo Samaj*, Calcutta: Brahmo Mission Press, 1974 (2nd edition).

11 See for example, Sumit Sarkar, *Writing Social History*, New Delhi & New York: Oxford University Press, 1997.

12 Borthwick, *The Changing Role of Women in Bengal*, 116.

13 Ibid., 114–24.

14 Geraldine Forbes, *The New Cambridge History of India, IV.2, Women in Modern India*, Cambridge University Press, First South Asian Paperback Edition, 1998, 41. Also see Sumanta Banerjee, 'Marginalization of Women's Popular Culture in Nineteenth Century Bengal', in Kumkum Sangari and Sudesh Vaid (eds.), *Recasting Women: Essays in Colonial History*, New Delhi: Kali for Women, 1989.

15 Partha Chatterjee, *Nationalist Thought and the Colonial World*, Minneapolis: University of Minnesota Press,1986; *The Nation and Its Fragments*, Princeton, NJ: Princeton University Press, 1993.

16 Chatterjee, *The Nation and Its Fragments*, 6.

17 Ibid., 129–30.

18 Dipesh Chakrabarty, 'Postcoloniality and the Artifice of History', in R. Guha (ed.), *A Subaltern Studies Reader1986–1995*, Minneapolis: University of Minnesota Press, 1997, 277.

19 See Benedict Anderson, *Imagined Communities: Reflections on the Origin and Spread of Nationalism* (Revised and extended ed.), London: Verso, 1991.

20 Jogesh C. Bagal, 'History of Bethune School and College 1849–1949', in K. Nag (ed.), *Bethune Centenary Volume*, Saraswati Press: Calcutta, 1949, 25; Chakraborty, *Conditions of Bengali Women Around the 2nd Half of the 19th Century*, 47.

21 Ghulum Murshid, *Reluctant Debutant*, Rajshahi: Rajshahi University Press, 1983, 43.

22 Ibid., 43.

23 ShibChunder Deb, *Sisupalan, Part I*, Serampore, 1857; part 2, Calcutta: 1862.

24 Borthwick, *The Changing Role of Women in Bengal*, 170–8.

25 Judith E. Walsh, *How to be the Goddess of Your Home: An Anthology of Bengali Domestic Manuals*, New Delhi: Yoda Press, 2005.

26 'Narirkartabya', *BP*, 2, 3,196 (May 1881), Kumudini Ray, 'Hindu narir garhasthya dharma', *BP*, 5, 3, 359 (December 1894); 'Swasthyaraksa', *BP*, 2, 2, 188 (September 1880). Also cited in Borthwick, *The Changing Role of Women in Bengal*, 207.

27 In 1878, a 'native' doctor's fee varied from 3 to 10 rupees; a European doctor charged 16. Lady doctors charged 10 rupees per visit. Borthwick, *The Changing Role of Women in Bengal*, 217.

28 Rajnarain Bose, *Se kal r e kal*, Calcutta, 1976 (1874), 87. Also cited in Borthwick, *The Changing Role of Women in Bengal*, 220.

29 Pradip Kumar Bose, 'Sons of the Nation: Child Rearing in the New Family', in Partha Chatterjee (ed.), *Texts of Power: Emerging Disciplines in Colonial Bengal*, Calcutta: Samya, 1996, 123.

30 *Prasannatara Gupta-Paribarikjiban*, Calcutta: Kuntaleen Press, 1903, 82. Also cited in Pradip Kumar Bose, 'Sons of the Nation: Child Rearing in the New Family', in Partha Chatterjee (ed.), *Texts of Power: Emerging Disciplines,* Calcutta: Samya, 1996.

31 Pratapchandra Majumdar, *Stricharitra*, Calcutta: Nababidhan, 1891,1. Also cited in Bose, 'Sons of the Nation: Child Rearing in the New Family'.

32 See Indira Chowdhury, *The Fragile Hero and Virile History: Gender and Politics of Culture in Colonial Bengal*, New Delhi: Oxford University Press, 2001; Mrinalini Sinha, *Colonial Masculinity: The Manly Englishman and*

the *Effeminate Bengali in the Late Nineteenth Century*, Manchester: Manchester University Press, 1995.

33 See articles like 'Indigenous Health Science' published in *Swasthya*, Magh (January–February), B.S.1307 (1901) in Pradip Kumar Bose (ed.), *Health and Society in Bengal: A Selection from Late 19th-Century Bengali Periodicals*, New Delhi, Thousand Oaks &London: Sage, 2006, 126–38. 'Precepts for Good Health' published in *Vigyan Darpan, Bhadra* (August–September), B.S. 1289 (1882), in Pradip Kumar Bose (ed.), *Health and Society in Bengal*,120–2, 'The Revival of National Physical Health', published in *Chikitsa Sammilani*, Baisakh (April–May), B.S. 1292 (1885).

34 *Chikitsa Sammilani*.

35 'The Revival of National Physical Health', in *Chikitsa Sammilani*, Baisakh (April–May), B.S.1292 (1885).

36 See David Arnold, *The New Cambridge History of India III: Science, Technology and Medicine in Colonial India*, Cambridge: Cambridge University Press, 2008, 75–81.

37 For discussions on malaria see Arabinda Samanta, *Malarial Fever in Colonial Bengal 1820–1939 Social History of An Epidemic*, Kolkata: Firma KLM Private Limited, 2002; David Arnold, *Colonizing the Body: State Medicine and Epidemic Disease in Nineteenth Century India*, New Delhi: Oxford University Press, 1993; D. Arnold, *The New Cambridge History of India 111·5, Science, Technology and Medicine in Colonial India*, Cambridge: Cambridge University Press, 2000; Kabita Ray, *History of Public Health: Colonial Bengal 1921–1947*, Calcutta: K P Bagchi & Company, 1998; Mark Harrison, *Public Health in British India: Anglo-Indian Preventive Medicine 1859–1914*, Cambridge: Cambridge University Press, 1994; Ihtesham Kazi, 'Environmental Factors Contributing to Malaria in Colonial Bengal', in Deepak Kumar (ed.), *Disease and Medicine in India: A Historical Overview*, New Delhi: Tulika, 2001; Ira Klein, 'Malaria and Mortality in Bengal, 1840–1921', *The Indian Economic and Social History Review*, IX, 2 (June 1972). Sujata Mukherjee,'Environmental Thoughts and Malaria in Colonial Bengal: A Study in Social Response',*Economic and Political Weekly*, XLIII, 12 and 13 (March 22–April 4, 2008), 54–61, Rohan Deb Roy, ' "An Awful, Unseen Visitant": The Return of Burdwan Fever', *EPW*, XLIII, 12 and 13 (March 22–April 4, 2008), 62–70.

38 Fever Hospital Committee, *Abridgement of the Report of the Committee Appointed by the Right Honorable the Governor of Bengal for the Establishment of a Fever Hospital and for Inquiring into Local Management and Taxation in Calcutta*, Calcutta: Bishop's College Press, 1840, 153.

39 For a detailed discussion see Mark Harrison,*Climates and Constitutions: Health, Race, Environment and British Imperialism in India, 1600–1850*, New Delhi: Oxford University Press, 1999, 43; Partha Datta, 'Ranald Martin's *Medical Topography* (1837): the Emergence of Public Health in Calcutta', in Mark Harrison and Biswamoy Pati (eds.), *The Social History of Health and Medicine in Colonial India*, London & New York: Routledge, 2009, 15–30.

40 James Ranald Martin, *Notes. . . 52*.

41 John Roberton, *Essays and Notes on the Physiology and Diseases of Women, and on Practical Midwifery*, London: John Churchill, 1851.

42 Ibid., 22.
43 Ibid., 22.
44 Allan Webb, *Pathologica Indica, or, the Anatomy of Indian Diseases, Medical and Surgical: Based Upon Morbid Specimens from All Parts of India in the Museum of the Calcutta Medical College: Illustrated by Detailed Cases, with the Prescriptions and Treatment Employed, and Comments, Physiological, Practical and Historical*, 2nd edn, London: W. H. Allen and Co., 1848, 254–60. Also cited in Ishita Pande, *Medicine, Race and Liberalism in British Bengal: Symptoms of Empire*, London & New York: Routledge, 2010, 155.
45 See Pande, *Medicine, Race and Liberalism in British Bengal Symptoms of Empire*.
46 'The Revival of National Physical Health', in *Chikitsa Sammilani*, Baisakh (April–May), B.S.1292 (1885).
47 Widespread prevalence of literature on sexuality predated the emergence of the practice of linking of national health to sexual practices in Bengal. Rev. James Long's list mentioned several books on the subject of sex and sexuality including *Adirasa* (Eroticism), *Veshyarahasya* (A treatise on Prostitutes), *Ratibilash* (Erotic Pleasures), *Sambhogratnakar* (A Treasury of Erotic Love, with 16 illustrations), *Ramaniranjan* (A book on Pleasing Women), *Sringar Tilak* (Jewels of Coition), *Ratibilap* (Lament of Eros), *Ratimanjari* (A Compendium of Coition), *Ratishastra* (Art of Coitus). Rev. James Long, *A Descriptive Catalogue of Bengali Works, Containing a Classified List of Fourteen Hundred Bengali Books and Pamphlets Which Have Issued from the Press During the Last Sixty Years with Occasional Notices of the Subjects, Prices and Where Printed*, Calcutta: Sandars, Cones and Company, 1855.
48 Suryanarayan Ghosh, *Baigyanik Dampatya Pranali*, Dacca, 1884, 32.
49 *ChikitsaSammilani*, Baisakh (April–May), B.S.1292 (1885).
50 'The Revival of National Physical Health', published in *Chikitsa Sammilani*, Baisakh (April–May), B.S. 1292 (1885).Also cited in Bose,*Health and Society in Bengal*, 113.
51 *Chikitsa Sammilani*, Baisakh (April–May), B.S. 1292 (1885).
52 'The Revival of National Physical Health', in *Chikitsa Sammilani*, Baisakh (April–May), B.S. 1292 (1885).
53 'National Health – How Marriage Affects It', in *Swarthy*, Math (January–February), B.S.1307 (1901).Also cited in Bose, *Health and Society in Bengal*, 138.
54 'The Revival of National Physical Health', published in *Chikitsa Sammilani*, Baisakh (April–May), B.S. 1292 (1885).
55 'Having an ejaculation while sleeping is known as nocturnal pollution.' See 'The Revival of National Physical Health', published in *ChikitsaSammilani*, Baisakh (April–May), B.S. 1292 (1885). Also cited in Bose, *Health and Society in Bengal*, 109.
56 Editor, 'Deshiya swasthya bigyan: *Abhigaman o stri purusha sangsara*' (Indigenous medical science: Sex or the union of men and women) in *Chikitsa Sammilani*, 1885. Reproduced in Pradip Basu, Samayiki. *Purono Samayikpatrer Prabandha Sankalan*, Vol.1, Calcutta: Ananda, 1998, 194.
57 *Chikitsa Sammilani*, Baisakh (April–May), B.S. 1292 (1885).

58 Annada Charan Khastagir, *A Treatise on the Science and Practice of Midwifery with Diseases of Children and Women: Manabjanmatattwa, dhatri bidya, nabaprasuta sisu o strijatir byadhisangraha*, 2nd ed. Calcutta, 1878 (1868).

59 *Chikitsa Sammilani*, Baisakh (April–May), B.S. 1292 (1885).

60 Khastagir, *A Treatise on the Science and Practice of Midwifery with Diseases of Children and Women*, 624–5. Also cited in Meredith Borthwick, *The Changing Role of Women in Bengal 1849–1905*, Princeton, NJ: Princeton University Press, 1984, 135–6.

61 S.C. Bose, *The Hindoos as They Are: A Description of the Manners, Customs and Inner Life of Hindu Society in Bengal*, Calcutta, 1881, 8. Also cited in Borthwick, *The Changing Role of Women in Bengal*, 19.

62 See Borthwick, *The Changing Role of Women*, 18–19.

63 'The Revival of National Physical Health', published in *Chikitsa Sammilani*, Baisakh (April–May), B.S. 1292 (1885).

64 Bose, *Health and Society in Bengal*, 152.

65 Bipradas Mukhopadhyaya, *Yuvak-yuvati*, Calcutta, 1922, 1st ed., 1891, 42–51.Also cited in Dagmar Engels, *Beyond Purdah? Women in Bengal 1890–1939*, New Delhi: Oxford University Press, 1996, 82.

66 Mukhopadhyaya, *Yuvak-yuvati*, 42.

67 Baradakanta Majumdar, *Naritattva*, Calcutta, 1889, 40–1. Also cited in Engels, *Beyond Purdah?*, 83.

68 Majumdar, *Naritattva*, 30–5.

11 Feminizing empire

The Association of Medical Women in India and the campaign for a Women's Medical Service

Samiksha Sehrawat

The 'medical needs' of Indian women were championed by the Association of Medical Women in India (AMWI) at the beginning of the twentieth century, twenty years after the establishment of the Dufferin Fund. This Association, representing the professional interests of British women doctors in India, campaigned for a Women's Medical Service that would parallel the Indian Medical Service (IMS) but would have an entirely female cadre. Its agitation demonstrated the rising prominence of female experts in India, and involved reconfiguring the colonial gender order and racial hierarchies. The AMWI's campaign marked the beginning of the 'feminization' of empire as British women doctors called for a reconceptualization of colonial development to include medical care for Indian women.

Medical care for Indian women

The Kittredge Fund (established in 1882) and the Dufferin Fund (established in 1885) were both meant to provide zenana medical care for Indian women. These organizations were founded because it was believed that Indian women had been prevented from seeking medical care by rules of female seclusion that severely limited contact with male medical staff. Zenana medical care sought to provide female medical staff and restructure hospitals and dispensaries as spaces that facilitated female segregation. The Dufferin Fund received considerable support from colonial administrators, was successful in raising funds in Britain and was popular among conservative elites in India. The interests of British medical women, who were employed in large numbers in India by the beginning of the twentieth century, were also linked closely with the trope of the zenana patient who was widely described as suffering from lack of medical attention due to 'barbaric' practices of female seclusion. Scholarships from the Dufferin Fund for training medical women in Britain were an integral aspect of the early history of the London School for Medical Women, and employment opportunities in Indian zenana hospitals were crucial in the early years of the professionalization of British medical women.[1]

The trope of the zenana patient signified all Indian women and disregarded the many Indian women who did not observe female seclusion. It elided the differences in practices of female seclusion and variation in the extent to which these were observed.[2] Given the variety in practices of female seclusion among different social, economic and cultural groups, debates about how to provide zenana medical care had arisen since the formation of the Dufferin Fund.[3] Those constructing and maintaining women's hospitals were faced with a range of choices regarding staffing, which patients were admitted and the physical organization of medical spaces. Since practices of female seclusion prescribed who women could interact with, arrangements had to be made to ensure that zenana patients did not come into contact with men from beyond their immediate kin group whom they were meant to avoid.[4] While male patients could clearly not be allowed in a zenana hospital, objections were even raised to the admittance of male children as patients at the Victoria Dufferin Hospital, Calcutta.[5] Some hospital committees also objected to the presence of low-caste and working-class female patients. Since female seclusion was meant to maintain social distance and uphold moral standards, intermixing of upper-caste and lower-caste women in zenana hospitals was perceived by some elites as violating purdah practices. This was especially the case in Calcutta, where the temporary building of the zenana hospital had been located close to the red-light district of Bow Bazaar between 1886 and 1898.[6]

Publications and speeches about zenana medical care also acknowledged the need for enclosing the hospital – which was a public space – to ensure that zenana women could move within it without compromising their seclusion. Saleni Armstrong-Hopkins describes the use of chick curtains and screens on windows to prevent the zenana hospital compound in Hyderabad, Sind, from being overlooked.[7] Similar arrangements were also made at the Victoria Dufferin Hospital at Calcutta.[8] These arrangements prioritized the needs of those Indian women who observed female seclusion and disregarded a large number of women from lower castes who had to work outside the house and who did not observe seclusion or only observed it to a very limited extent. The latter could use public spaces such as hospitals more freely and did not require the considerable elaboration of detail and expense necessary for zenana hospitals. The Punjab government, recognizing this, chose to fund wards and branch dispensaries for women, which cost less than a zenana hospital to construct and to run. This strategy was in contrast to the emphasis of the United Provinces government on subsidizing zenana hospitals. In both provinces the average annual increase in hospital beds for women (Punjab: 21.78 per cent, UP: 10.30 per cent) was higher than the average annual percentage increase in beds for male patients (Punjab: 10.77 per cent, UP: 6.13 per cent) between 1905 and 1925. However, in the United Provinces, the number of female hospital beds did not increase as rapidly as in Punjab during this period – by 1925 the gap between the provision of male and female beds in Punjab had been narrowed, while it had expanded in UP.[9]

Shaping medical institutions to accommodate practices of female seclusion often resulted in a preference for an entirely female staff. For instance, objections to the presence of male janitorial staff at the Victoria Dufferin Hospital, Calcutta, had led to their dismissal.[10] Decisions regarding medical staff were more convoluted. Many local bodies keen to open dispensaries, hospitals or wards for women did not have sufficient resources to employ women doctors, especially as special living arrangements had to be made for British or American women doctors and because they expected higher salaries and regular furloughs.[11] Questions about the medical staff of women's hospitals were at the heart of the AMWI's campaign in the first decade of its formation.

British women doctors, racial difference and reworking the colonial gender order

The AMWI, founded in 1907, brought together women doctors employed in zenana hospitals in criticism of the Dufferin Fund. Though the group was primarily interested in campaigning for better work conditions and improved pay, its demands were couched in a rhetoric that evoked the trope of the suffering zenana patient. The AMWI's criticism drew upon existing debates about how zenana medical care was to be delivered and employed a language of medical reform which had been used by nineteenth-century British medical periodicals arguing for the reform of Poor Law hospitals in the late nineteenth century.

Articles about zenana medical care published by the Association's *Journal* criticized the Dufferin Fund for failing to provide appropriate facilities for zenana patients. Members of the Association presented evidence of medical buildings that did not screen zenana patients from public view and criticized the admission of 'disreputable' women in zenana hospitals.[12] In this they were echoing criticism of the Fund by sections of the Indian press, with one article declaring: 'We should be very glad if some Indians would express their views'.[13] By urging greater fastidiousness in adapting hospitals for 'proper' observation of female seclusion, these women doctors were launching a potent criticism of the Dufferin Fund and appropriating to themselves the authority to speak for the zenana patient. Discussions about who would form the appropriate medical staff for zenana hospitals were also appropriated by the AMWI to advance the claims of British women doctors. Formally named the National Association for Supplying Female Medical Aid, one of the aims of the Dufferin Fund had been to provide female medical staff for women's hospitals in India. The Fund's reports referred to medical staff of zenana hospitals as 'lady doctors'.[14] The AMWI argued that this category lumped together women doctors, women sub-assistant surgeons, and in some cases, even unqualified women. One letter to the Association's *Journal* claimed, 'women's hospitals . . . in most cases are provided with the class of "lady doctor" who in England would be debarred from practice.'[15] By being placed in the same category as unqualified women and women with lower qualifications, women doctors were liable to receive a lower pay and often had to put up with living conditions and conditions of work that they considered unsuitable to their position. While the employment of unqualified women was easily condemned, the AMWI was keen to distance women doctors from female sub-assistant surgeons, especially because the latter were more ubiquitous and because hospital committees who made decisions about staffing often failed to distinguish between the two, categorizing both as 'lady doctors'.

This was not the first time that professionalizing women doctors had sought to distance themselves from other women practising medicine. Burton shows that in late nineteenth-century Britain, women doctors had been motivated by similar concerns of shoring up professional status when they sought to distance professionally trained women doctors from unskilled missionary medical practice.[16] Asserting the superiority of women doctors' training over that of female sub-assistant surgeons was one of the strategies employed by the AMWI. In a typical tirade, an AMWI member decried 'the evil of the partly qualified (often wholly unfit) woman Hospital Assistant [later sub-assistant surgeon], who is so large and septic a factor in India'.[17] Women holding the position of sub-assistant surgeon held a Licentiate of Medicine and Surgery (L.M.S.) – a lower medical qualification offered by several medical colleges in India. Women doctors held medical degrees which could be registered in Britain and were considered superior to the licentiates. This distinction had created a well-recognized professional hierarchy among male medical staff of civil hospitals and dispensaries. Civil surgeons (with medical degrees) belonged to the IMS (which was dominated by British doctors) and supervised Indian male sub-assistant surgeons who held licentiates.[18] Indeed, the licentiates had been instituted to train a body of Indian practitioners who would provide subordinate medical employees for the colonial state's military and civil establishment. While the professional hierarchy of the colonial medical establishment overlapped neatly with a racial hierarchy, British women doctors felt frustrated by the lack of such clear distinctions in zenana hospitals.

The AMWI, ostensibly representing all women doctors in India, was dominated by British women doctors, especially in its first decade of existence. Committee members and contributors to the *Journal* were overwhelmingly white and British despite the existence of a significant number of Indian women holding medical degrees.[19] A few Indian women doctors presented papers and were active in the Bombay branch, but did not hold positions in the Association's Council.[20] The demands of the AMWI mirrored closely the interests and concerns of British women doctors, despite its claims of representing all women doctors.[21] Indian women, when they were discussed in the pages of the *Journal*, denoted the hapless zenana patient who needed rescuing.[22] In this, British women doctors writing in the *Journal of the Association of Medical Women in India (JAMWI)* were drawing on a tradition of British feminists using the trope of the helpless and suffering colonized woman to establish British women's fitness for citizenship in the British imperial-nation state.[23] Antoinette Burton shows that articles about Indian women in Victorian feminist periodicals were used to imagine and exercise the authority of British feminists over colonial womanhood and were accompanied by the increasing activism of British women on behalf of Indian women.[24] Mirroring these strategies, articles published in the *JAMWI* assumed that Indian women did not 'have a voice in their own concerns'.[25] The 'dumb needs' of Indian women were evoked by Dr. Annette Benson, the president of the AMWI, in her evidence to the Royal Commission on Public Services and by those presenting the AMWI's demands to the secretary of state for India.[26] In the protracted battle to win the right to a medical education waged by British women, Indian zenana hospitals had provided an important source of employment at a time when there were few opportunities for practising their professional skill in Britain.[27] By 1910 they had come to the realization that their professional status was under threat from Indian female sub-assistant surgeons who could be used to staff women's medical institutions in India more economically, the sexist attitudes of male IMS officers who had been placed in a position of authority above them and the memsahib who played an important role in hospital committees and at various levels in the Dufferin Fund hierarchy.[28] British women doctors' criticism of the Dufferin Fund therefore set out arguments to improve the position of British women doctors in racial hierarchies by showing them to be superior to Indian female sub-assistant surgeons and to improve their position in the colonial gender order by showing them to be equal to white male civil surgeons.

The AMWI advanced the claims of white women doctors by asserting that they understood the 'medical needs of Indian women' best and were best placed to serve them. Which medical practitioners could perform surgery on zenana patients was crucial to these claims. Members of the AMWI argued that since Indian female sub-assistant surgeons were not sufficiently qualified to hold sole charge of a medical institution, they required the supervision of senior doctors. This implied that unless female sub-assistant surgeons were under the charge of women doctors with British qualifications, their zenana patients would receive surgical treat-ment from male civil surgeons under whose supervision they worked.[29] For members of the AMWI, this clearly established that women doctors were to be preferred over Indian female sub-assistant surgeons due to the latter's inability to preserve the female seclusion of patients during sur-gery.[30] Equally problematic for the AMWI were the Dufferin Fund's rules requiring (male) government medical officers to appoint and supervise its female medical employees, which members believed did not sufficiently acknowledge the superiority of women doctors over female sub-assistant surgeons.[31] The possibility of being subjected to the same level of pro-fessional supervision as the female sub-assistant surgeon eroded women doctors' professional status. Though contributors acknowledged that IMS officers often accorded women doctors professional courtesies appropriate to an equal, they found the possibility that some civil sur-geons may not do so disquieting. As one member argued:

> The lady doctor in charge of a Pardah hospital ought herself to be in a position to decide whether or not a man is to be called in, and then only do it with the patient's and her friends' permission. She will have to decide whether the Civil Surgeon is a better man than herself and whether if he is, the fact of calling in outside assistance will tend to loosen confidence in the Women's Hospital. It prob-ably will, unless the Civil Surgeon is courteous enough to invite the lady on occasions to assist at his operations.[32]

The zenana patient was therefore used as an argument against the control of women doctors by civil surgeons, since this control allowed them to enter a zenana hospital for inspection and claim the right to perform surgery on zenana patients. Arguing that the Dufferin Fund's rules ought to be modified to prevent the violation of female seclusion by a male medical officer's interference, the AMWI asserted the primacy of women doctors over all other medical professionals in treating zenana patients.

Hospital committees were also criticized for the arbitrary exercise of their power to employ and dismiss women doctors. Wives of colonial officials (memsahibs) often served on zenana hospital committees and on Dufferin Fund branch committees along with colonial officials and Indian men who had donated substantially to the local hospital. These incorporated wives were especially criticized for their lack of interest in such welfare work and for their lack of professional knowledge which left them ignorant of the requirements of a medical institution.[33] Arguing that women doctors possessed authentic professional knowledge of the needs of women patients, the AMWI urged the necessity of greater professional control of zenana hospitals by women doctors, especially in decisions relating to equipment and subordinate staff. The AMWI thus asserted the equality of women doctors with IMS civil surgeons and memsahibs – two groups it located as having a favourable social position. By claiming equality with these groups, it could improve the social position and influence of British women doctors. The AMWI simultaneously distanced British women doctors from Indian female sub-assistant surgeons, who were tainted by low social status, on grounds of professional superiority.

Arguing for Indian women's 'medical needs': female medical experts and colonial development

The criticism of the Dufferin Fund by the AMWI in 1909 and 1910 increasingly cast it as a voluntary organization that had failed in its raison d'etre – providing medical care for the zenana patient. Its *Journal* recounted its various shortcomings – its failure to provide adequately equipped women's hospitals, to inspect hospitals included in its report, the uneven distribution of these hospitals, its 'capricious and inefficient' branches and the ways in which the Fund misrepresented its achievements to its subscribers.[34] The Fund was dismissed as a skeletal and 'un-business'-like organization – one which was badly organized for the work it sought to do.[35] These criticisms of the Dufferin Fund were remarkably similar in tone to earlier criticism of Poor Law hospitals in the British medical press of the 1880s and even harked back to tropes from earlier campaigns for reform in the medical periodical press.[36] By invoking these campaigns of medical reform, women doctors sought to identify themselves with earlier medical experts who had called the attention of the public to abuses in the medical system, leading to greater medical regulation and a more prominent position for medical professionals.[37]

The AMWI's attempts to establish the importance of female medical experts in colonial administration foregrounded medical women's professional knowledge that they believed gave them a unique insight not merely into Indian women's 'medical needs' but even the needs of the 'people of India'.[38] Arguing that this knowledge placed the Association under an obligation to represent the Indian people, the AMWI claimed that it needed to be 'regarded as a body to be referred to for expert opinion'.[39] Women doctors' claims of expertise centred especially on the zenana patient, women's hospitals and were extended during the 1920s to include maternal and infant welfare and all matters related to the health and medical training of women in India.[40] The 'medical needs' of Indian women were evoked repeatedly by members of the AMWI in articles and letters published in the *JAMWI* in 1911 and 1914 and a *JAMWI* editorial claimed that '[o]ur object is to further the cause of medical work amongst women in India'.[41] The AMWI argued that by sharing their expertise, women doctors could 'do much for the benefit of the country'.[42] These claims were accepted widely – for instance, *The Times* acknowledged that 'the development of India cannot be carried on without the co-operation of the medical woman'.[43] The failure of the Indian government and the Dufferin Fund to recognize 'the advisability of consulting women experts in matters pertaining to women' was attributed by Benson to the backwardness of India.[44] Women doctors claiming expert status in India were demanding a role in colonial development by claiming that they could improve the 'health of the race' in India and advance the claims of empire in the face of rising anti-colonial protests.[45] They were making these claims at a time when the role of experts in grappling with the challenges of improving national efficiency was widely accepted in Britain.[46]

Oliver MacDonagh's articulation of the revolution in government in nineteenth-century Britain that gave rise to experts outlined five stages. Of these the first two were the exposure of a social evil leading to legislation and the employment of experts in executive capacities to implement this legislation.[47] These steps were rehearsed by women doctors who were staking their claims to expertise in early twentieth-century

India. They projected the Dufferin Fund's failure to provide for the zenana patient as a social evil to be remedied. They also linked the fulfilment of the 'medical needs' of Indian women with improving the work conditions of women doctors, arguing that the government ought to employ female medical experts in a state-run medical service. In a general meeting of the AMWI, the president, Benson, declared:

> Looking at the Medical Profession in India. . . [w]e see [that] women [are] a nondescript, scattered number of isolated units, at the mercy of chance employment and still more chance conditions of service, and almost all in subordinate positions. Yet the majority of better class women of India have no one to look to for help in sickness and childbirth but these same isolated units. For the good of this large factor of the population and therefore in the name of the Public Weal, we aim . . . to improve the conditions under which Medical Women work.[48]

Discussion of Indian women's 'medical needs' routinely dovetailed into pointing to the poor work conditions of medical women, with articles in the *JAMWI* arguing that women doctors in 'Dufferin' hospitals were overworked.[49] The AMWI claimed that the pay and conditions of service offered to medical women were too low to attract good professionals, leading to the appointment of medical staff with lower qualifications or incompetent medical women.[50] So disenchanted were women doctors employed by the Dufferin Fund with their work conditions that one of them quipped: 'Dufferin Service and Suffering Service are terms somewhat identical'.[51] Poor pay, overwork, poor living arrangements, lack of furlough opportunities and unfair interference by hospital committees and civil surgeons were among the conditions highlighted for amelioration in the name of 'helping the women of India by the development of an official class of medical women with ethical standards worthy of their calling'.[52]

In early 1909, the *JAMWI* proposed a scheme for organizing a Women's Medical Service to redress this dissatisfaction with poor conditions of work.[53] This proved popular with members of the AMWI with initial proposals stressing the need to have a uniform set of rules for pay, appointments and conditions of work across India. Several respondents called on the government to organize a service for medical women employed in zenana hospitals and the IMS was increasingly mentioned as the model on which the proposed Women's Medical Service would be based.[54] By the end of 1910, the AMWI's campaign had come to focus on demanding a state medical service of women doctors independent of the Dufferin Fund.[55] The Fund was perceived as obstructing reform of women doctors' work conditions, despite its attempts to address the grievances of the AMWI.[56] In June 1908, the Dufferin Fund applied for an annual government grant of 50,000 rupees to allow it to raise the salaries of female doctors in its employ.[57] The Fund's request for a grant, though supported by the Indian government, was rejected by Secretary of State for India Lord John Morley in 1908.[58] For the next two years, the Indian government worked behind the scenes with the Dufferin Fund to develop proposals for funding that would meet the approval of the India Office.[59] Utterly disenchanted with the lack of concrete action and with the Dufferin Fund, the Association increasingly demanded state intervention. The AMWI interpreted the Dufferin Fund's failure as signifying the failure of the colonial state's policy of leaving medical care provision for Indian women to the private and voluntary sectors. Benson argued that 'voluntary work . . . could not touch the enormous number of women and their great needs'.[60] Another letter to *The Times* echoed this argument – 'two-thirds of the women [of India] have been practically ignored by the State and left to three nonofficial agencies . . . The Lady Dufferin Fund has done work worthy of the honoured name it bears, but is not equal to meeting a great Imperial demand.'[61] The government's neglect was seen as an indication of the low priority given to Indian women's medical needs by the state – 'of so little consequence. . . [that provision] is left to charitable contributions'.[62] The AMWI argued that funding for zenana medical care could not be left to Indian philanthropy as Indians were incapable of 'independent' effort.[63] Through such claims, the AMWI yoked utilitarian ideals of government intervention in India to a duty to provide medical care for Indian women. It outlined the colonial state's duty given that

> the country is not sufficiently advanced to be willing to pay for well qualified practitioners apart from Government aid; that the people as yet cannot distinguish the qualified from the unqualified, and if left to itself [sic] would certainly not spend large sums on medical research work and on hospitals for the poor. Government therefore steps in.[64]

The duty of the state to intervene also reiterated older tropes of rescuing the indigenous woman from the poor treatment she received from her society.[65] The press campaign launched by the AMWI in Britain especially attracted attention to the need to allay the suffering of the zenana patient and the Indian government's failure to do so.[66]

While these attempts to gain public support relied on earlier ideological justifications of empire, the AMWI's arguments also marked a shift towards newer conceptions of imperial duty towards indigenous subjects and a foregrounding of service to colonial women in justifications of imperial rule. Kate Vaughan argued in an early editorial 'Surely they [Indian women] are subjects of the Empire as well as men, and proper provision for them in sickness should be provided by public funds.'[67] The AMWI advocated healthcare as a welfare measure, seeking to highlight the state's duty to reduce the 'immense mortality and suffering among women and children' in India.[68] The expansion of medical care through state provision was seen as a natural extension of the state's role given the rising political opposition from the nationalist movement. Supporters claimed that such welfare measures could 'evolve a remarkable response of good will in every home' counteracting the nationalist 'political agitation' against the Raj.[69] Such ideas clearly found support in British public opinion, especially among the middle classes, with *The Times* locating medical care provision for Indian women among other 'developmental' activities advocated by the colonial state, such as irrigation, sanitation, education and encouragement of industries.[70] In a potent counter-argument to the government's protestations that it did not have the financial resources to extend the remit of development to provision of medical care, the AMWI argued: 'the plea of financial inability [is not] at all convincing; for surely the preservation of the lives of women and children should be the first duty of every civilized State, and should therefore be the last to be starved for want of funds.'[71]

The AMWI not only conducted a strong press campaign in India and Britain, it also energetically lobbied for support amongst the highest echelons of policy making, including in its ambit Viceroy Hardinge, and three vicereines – Lady Minto, Lady Hardinge and the founder of the Dufferin Fund, Lady Dufferin.[72] In November 1910, some members of the AMWI and other British medical women presented a memorial to Secretary of State Morley demanding a state service for medical women in India.[73] Given the tardy response of the Indian government to these demands, in 1912 the AMWI presented the case for the formation of a Women's Medical Service again to the new secretary of state, Lord Crewe, reiterating arguments made by its earlier deputation. The two intervening years saw an intensification of the AMWI's campaign, with questions in the Parliament meant to embarrass the government into admitting that it had made insufficient provision for the needs of the zenana patient.[74] Although demi-officially both the Indian government and the India Office continued to argue that the colonial state had 'never accepted the responsibility [for providing government funded medical attendance] either for men or women',[75] this campaign proved sufficiently embarrassing for the India Office to lead to a more conciliatory attitude. Crewe pressed the Indian government to respond to claims made by the AMWI and to take into account its suggestions for a service.[76] Most importantly, Crewe marked a break from his predecessor's opposition to a government grant to the Dufferin Fund, signalling strong support for a government grant to the Dufferin Fund to enable it to improve the pay of women doctors.[77] The inauguration of the Women's Medical Service in India (WMSI) in September 1913[78] represented an acknowledgement from the government of its 'responsibility' to provide treatment for Indian women by 'doctors of their own sex'.[79] By insisting on the role of the Dufferin Fund in the formation of the WMSI, however, the colonial state continued to assert the importance of the voluntary and private sectors in medical provision, shying away from any state-run service that could potentially be used to argue for greater state funding for medical care. State aid for the WMSI was conceived as assistance towards

> the creation of an independent profession of female medical practitioners [rather] than to create a service of medical women employed by the State. . . [T]o secure this end, it is essential that there should be a limited number of European medical women of high professional qualifications both to take charge of exemplar hospitals in the larger towns and to assist in the medical education of indigenous female practitioners.[80]

This amounted to only a very partial acknowledgement of the AMWI's claims that as part of its imperial obligations the Indian colonial state was responsible for providing medical care for Indian women. It nevertheless amounted to a greater acceptance of the role of the female medical expert in the colonies. The Dufferin Fund's rules were amended to concede the AMWI's demand for greater representation of women doctors on the Fund's central and provincial committees and on hospital committees. The need for inspection of women's hospitals by women doctors was also accepted, though no formal provision was made for this.[81] Finally, members of the WMSI in independent charge of a hospital were given full professional control, deciding the thorny issue of a civil surgeon's control over Dufferin employees in favour of medical women.[82] The scheme made a clear distinction between women doctors with qualifications that could be registered in Britain and female sub-assistant surgeons with lower qualifications, with suggestions that the latter be organized in provincial subordinate medical services for women.[83] These proposals were welcomed by the AMWI, but with reservations that the pay had not been sufficiently increased and about the continuing prominence of the Dufferin Fund.[84] Over time, prominent members of the AMWI came to play a greater role in the running of the Dufferin Fund and the WMSI, leading to greater identification of the goals of all three.[85]

Conclusion

The activities of the AMWI represented a transition from an older politics of 'maternal imperialism' associated with British women to a later 'feminization' of empire. Barbara Bush and Helen Callaway have shown that the inter-war years associated with this feminization witnessed an increase in the number of women professionals in the colonies, and a reconceptualization of empire involving a 'move from (masculine) power to (feminine) service'.[86] This is believed to be distinct from the politics of an earlier era. Burton has argued that Victorian feminists' campaigns in the name of the colonial woman did not amount as much to a feminization of empire as 'a refiguration of imperial power'.[87] The AMWI adopted many of the strategies of these Victorian feminists, with members appropriating colonial women to argue for a greater role in the empire for British women doctors and for improving the position of the latter within the gender order and racial hierarchies of colonial India. However, what set the AMWI apart was its demands for a more prominent imperial role for women professionals, and for greater emphasis on the 'medical needs' of Indian women in colonial development. In this, it anticipated later changes associated with the feminization of empire. Yet, the Indian colonial state did not embrace the AMWI's vision of imperial service in its entirety. The emphasis on colonial development and 'welfare' in justifications of empire came after the First World War in response to rising anti-colonial movements and a changed geopolitical context.[88]

Notes

1 Antoinette Burton, 'Contesting the Zenana: The Mission to Make "Lady Doctors for India", 1874–85', *Journal of British Studies*, 35, 3 (1996).
2 Especially troublesome for colonial tropes of purdah were peasant women who followed codes of female modesty but also worked outside their homes in the fields, see for example, Prem Chowdhry, *The Veiled Women:*

Shifting Gender Equations in Rural Haryana, 1880–1990, New Delhi: Oxford University Press, 1994.

3 For criticism of the Dufferin Fund in the Bengali press, see Dagmar Engels, *Beyond Purdah? Women in Bengal 1890–1939*, Oxford: Oxford University Press, 1996, 138–9 and Chandrika Paul, ' "The Uneasy Alliance": The Work of British and Bengali Women Medical Professionals in Bengal, 1870–1935', Unpublished Ph.D. Thesis, University of Cincinnati, 1997, 270–1, 282.

4 Generalizing about practices of female seclusion is problematic as these are best studied in relation to the cultural context in which they are found. Nevertheless, some broad similarities were observed by Papanek, who felt that generally Muslim women are expected to avoid contact with men from outside the kin group and Hindu women tend to show respect to affines by avoiding them through practices of female seclusion, Hannah Papanek, 'Purdah: Separate Worlds and Symbolic Shelter', in Hanna Papanek and Gail Minault (eds.), *Separate Worlds: Studies of Purdah in South Asia*, New Delhi: Chanakya, 1998, 19–26.

5 Paul, 'The Uneasy Alliance', 287.

6 Ibid., 275.

7 Saleni Armstrong-Hopkins, *Within the Zenana*, New York: Eaton and Mains, 1898, 27, 32.

8 Paul, 'The Uneasy Alliance', 278.

9 There were 1,175 more hospital beds for men than for women in UP hospitals in 1900 – this number had grown to 1,652 in 1925. In Punjab the gap had stood at 1,194 in 1900 and was narrowed to 1,095 by 1925. Statistics from *Punjab Hospital Reports, 1900–25* and *United Provinces Hospital Reports, 1900–25*. This could be partly explained by the higher per capita expenditure on medical care by Punjab. According to Chand, Punjab spent 112.80 rupees per 1,000 of population in 1897 and UP spent 32.76 rupees. This trend continued in 1907 (Punjab: 58.42 rupees; UP: 46.14 rupees), in 1912 (Punjab: 132.56 rupees; UP: 61.80 rupees) and in 1921 (Punjab: 206.45 rupees; UP: 114.63 rupees). Gyan Chand, *The Essentials of Federal Finance*, Madras: Oxford University Press, 1930, 384, 388, 391, 395.

10 Paul, 'The Uneasy Alliance', 282, 297.

11 *Dufferin Fund Report [DFR] 1890*, 10. Also see *DFR 1911*, 10.

12 'Editorial', *Journal of the Association of Medical Women in India [JAMWI]*, 1, 4 (November 1908), 3; 'Provisional Report on the working of the Countess of Dufferin's Fund', *JAMWI*, 1, 4 (November 1908), 8–13. Also see 'Editorial', *JAMWI*, 1, 5 (February 1909), 2.

13 'Report by a Member of the Association on a "Dufferin Ward" marked as Dispensary on the Map', *JAMWI*, 1, 4 (November 1908), 22.

14 A distinction between first-, second- and third-class 'lady doctors' had been made by Harriot Dufferin, the founder of the Dufferin Fund (DF), in Harriot Dufferin, *A Record of Three Years' Work of the National Association for Supplying Female Medical Aid to the Women of India*, Calcutta: Thacker Spink and Co, 1888, 15–16.

15 'Extracts from the *Pioneer*', letter by 'Commonsense', *JAMWI*, 1, 12 (November 1910), 27. Also see Editorial, *JAMWI*, 1, 3 (May 1908), 4. Another member related an imaginary inspection of a Dufferin hospital

in which the 'lady doctor' was none other than an illiterate indigenous midwife. Galena, 'A Christmas Dream', *JAMWI*, 1, 10 (May 1910), 25.

16 Burton, 'Contesting the Zenana', 368–97.

17 'Comment by Other Members of the Association', *JAMWI*, 1, 4 (November 1908), 17. Also see M. Balfour, 'The Training of Hospital Assistants in Obstetrics', *JAMWI*, 1, 11 (August 1910), 14–17.

18 Those holding licentiates complained about the 'casteism' of this hierarchy. Roger Jeffery, 'Recognizing India's Doctors: The Institutionalization of a Medical Dependency, 1918–39', *Modern Asian Studies*, 13, 2 (1979), 317–19.

19 For the careers of some pioneering Indian women doctors, see Geraldine Forbes, *Women in Colonial India: Essays on Politics, Medicine and Historiography*, New Delhi: Chronicle Books, 2005, 89–90, 109–14; Paul, 'The Uneasy Alliance', 94–148.

20 For instance, Dr. Avanbai Mehta was Honorary Treasurer and Dr. Hilla Banajee-Batliboi was Honorary Secretary for the Bombay Branch in 1910, 'Report of the Bombay Branch', *JAMWI*, 1, 10 (May 1910), 3; Hilla Banajee-Batliboi, 'Report of the Bombay Branch', *JAMWI*, 1, 5 (February 1909), 11. It was not until the 1920s and 1930s that Indian women became more prominent in the AMWI. For the latter, see Mridula Ramanna, *Health Care in Bombay Presidency 1896–1930*, New Delhi: Primus, 2012, 138–42.

21 The AMWI's argument that women doctors' health suffered during long periods of service in India and that furlough arrangements were essential indicate the preponderance of British women within the AMWI. See for instance, arguments by Elizabeth Garrett Anderson, Burton, 'Contesting the Zenana', 387. In Bengal the DF was associated with Western cultural imperialism and the continued dominance of white women within the AMWI rendered it suspect, see Engels, *Beyond Purdah*, 138–41. Forbes and Paul point to the marginalization of Indian women doctors in appointments by the Dufferin Fund, Forbes, *Women in Colonial India*, 112–13; Paul, 'The Uneasy Alliance', 290–3.

22 This has parallels with the Victorian feminist periodical press examined by Burton, which also discussed the activities of English women in articles about India, while neglecting those contemporary Indian women who destabilized the trope of the passive Indian woman, Antoinette Burton, *Burdens of History: British Feminists, Indian Women, and Imperial Culture, 1865–1915*, Chapel Hill & London: University of North Carolina Press, 1994, 116–17.

23 Ibid.

24 Ibid., 97–125.

25 Letter by 'Commonsense', *JAMWI*, 1, 12 (November 1910), 32.

26 Evidence of A.M. Benson to the Royal Commission on Public Services, reprinted in *JAMWI*, 5, 2 (May 1914), [hereafter, 'Benson's Evidence to Royal Commission on Public Services'], 2; 'Report of a Deputation to the Marquess of Crewe', printed in enclosure to *JAMWI*, 4, 8 (November 1912), [henceforth, 'Deputation to Crewe, 1912'], 9.

27 For a classic account of the struggle of women to be allowed to study and acquire a medical degree, see Edith Bell, *Storming the Citadel: The Rise of the Woman Doctor*, London: Constable, 1953. Also see Mary Elston,

'Women Doctors in the British Health Services: A Sociological Study of their Careers and Opportunities', Unpublished Ph.D. Thesis, University of Leeds, 1986.

28 Colonial officials' wives were referred to as *memsahibs*. For their involvement in the DF, see Mary Procida, *Married to the Empire: Gender, Politics and Imperialism in India, 1883–1947*, Manchester: Manchester University Press, 2002, 43–5, 165, 168, 171.

29 Letter to the Editor by 'Commonsense', *JAMWI*, 1, 12 (November 1910), 31.

30 Such arguments ignored the popularity of female hospital assistants such as Haimabati Sen, Sen and Geraldine Forbes (eds.), *The Memoirs of Dr. Haimabati Sen: From Child Widow to Lady Doctor*, trans. Tapan Raychaudhuri, New Delhi: Roli Books, 2000. Paul points to the credibility of Bengali newspapers' claims that female sub-assistant surgeons could better understand the needs of Indian patients due to their cultural proximity and linguistic proficiency, Paul, 'The Uneasy Alliance', 292–3, 297.

31 In March 1912, a special meeting of the DF was held in Calcutta to amend the rules of the Fund to ensure that women doctors were not considered subordinate to civil surgeons, which K.O. Vaughan (editor of the *JAMWI*) and K.O. Platt (first principal of the Lady Hardinge Medical College who later became a member of the AMWI) attended. See Vaughan's objections to the Fund's rule, *Proceedings of the Special Meeting Held at Government House, Calcutta, 6 March 1912*, Calcutta: Superintendent Government Printing, 1912.

32 Letter to the Editor, 3 June 1909, *JAMWI*, 1, 7 (August 1909), 37.

33 'Government Service versus Charitable Effort', *JAMWI*, 1, 9 (February 1910), 26.

34 See Samiksha Sehrawat, *Colonial Medical Care in North India, c. 1830–1920: Gender, State and Society*, New Delhi: Oxford University Press, 2013, chap. 4.

35 Vaughan, 'The Dufferin Fund', *JAMWI*, 1, 11 (August 1910), 8–9. Also see, 'Memorial from the United Kingdom Branch of the Association of Medical Women in India', *JAMWI*, 2, 1 (February 1911), 7.

36 Criticism of the abuses of the Poor Law infirmaries from the 1860s by the British Medical Association had emphasized the need to increase the salaries and conditions of work of Poor Law medical officers to improve conditions for patients of Poor Law medical services. See Steven Cherry, *Medical Services and the Hospitals in Britain 1860–1939*, Cambridge: Cambridge University Press, 1996, 30; P.W.J. Bartrip, *Mirror of Medicine: A History of the British Medical Journal*, Oxford: Clarendon Press, 1990, 51–5. The medical reform campaign had characterized lay governance of medical institutions as 'irrational', Michael Brown, 'Medicine, Reform and the "End" of Charity in Early Nineteenth-Century England', *English Historical Review*, 124, 511 (2009), 1353–88.

37 For medical reform in the mid-nineteenth century, see Ivan Waddington, 'General Practitioners and Consultants in Early Nineteenth-Century England: the Sociology of an Intra-Professional Conflict', in J. Woodward and D. Richards (eds.), *Health Care and Popular Medicine in Nineteenth-Century England: Essays in the Social History of Medicine*, London: Croom Helm, 1977, 164–88. For the rise of the medical expert, see Roy McLeod, 'The Anatomy of State Medicine: Concept and Application', in F. Poynter

(ed.), *Medicine and Science in the 1860s*, London: Wellcome Institute of the History of Medicine, 1968, 199–227.

38 Benson to Lord Hardinge, 26 December 1911, published in *JAMWI*, 3, 5 (February 1912), 15.

39 Council Meeting of the AMWI, Bombay, 24 January 1914, *JAMWI*, 5, 1 (February 1914), 16.

40 See, for instance, Margaret Balfour and Ruth Young, *The Work of Medical Women in India*, Bombay: Humphrey Milford, 1929, 162–3.

41 Editorial, *JAMWI*, 1, 5 (February 1909), 2; 'Medical Work Among Women in India', reprinted from the *BMJ*, *JAMWI*, 2, 2 (February 1911), 28; Mervyn Smith, 'The Medical Needs of India: Lady Doctors', *JAMWI*, 5, 1 (February 1914), 1; 'Benson's Evidence to Royal Commission on Public Services', 2–3, 6, 8; 'Work Done by the Association', *JAMWI*, 2, 1 (February 1911), 19. Margaret Balfour, Letters to the Editor, 7 June 1912, *JAMWI*, 3, 7 (August 1912), 35.

42 'Secretarial', *JAMWI*, 5, 8 (November 1915), 17.

43 'Indian Women and Their Needs: The Dufferin Fund', *The Times* (27 March 1913), 5.

44 Letter to the President, Association of Registered Medical Women from the Council of the AMWI, 24 January 1914, *JAMWI*, 5, 1 (February 1914), 21. Benson to Lord Hardinge, 26 December 1911, published in *JAMWI*, 3, 5 (February 1912), 15. See also, 'General Notes', *JAMWI*, 3, 7 (August 1912), 36.

45 'Extracts' from the *Pioneer*, *JAMWI*, 1, 12 (November 1910), 32. Also see arguments about the importance of state intervention to safeguard the 'future of the race' in India, 'Indian Women and Their Needs: The Dufferin Fund', 5.

46 Roy MacLeod points out that despite the British bureaucracy's success in curbing the power of experts by relegating them to specific functions within departments, they were perceived as playing an important role in government and society in the run-up to the First World War, MacLeod, 'Introduction', in Roy MacLeod (ed.), *Government and Expertise: Specialists, Administrators and Professionals, 1860–1919*, Cambridge: Cambridge University Press, 1988, 1–24.

47 For a restatement of this revolution in government, see Oliver MacDonagh, 'The Nineteenth-Century Revolution in Government: A Reappraisal', *Historical Journal*, 1, 1 (1958), 52–67. For a later overview see, Valerie Cromwell, 'Interpretations of Nineteenth-Century Administration: An Analysis', *Victorian Studies*, 9, 3 (1966), 245–55.

48 Equating the interest of 'better class [Indian] women' to the 'Public Weal' ignored the many Indian women from lower social strata who could and did use dispensaries not supervised by women doctors. Such elisions were essential for the success of the AMWI's demands. 'General Meeting', *JAMWI*, 1, 6 (May 1909), 6.

49 'Editorial', *JAMWI*, 1, 5 (February 1909), 4.

50 Letter by R.N. Cohen, 'Letters to the Editor', *JAMWI*, 1, 6 (May 1909), 10; 'The Countess of Dufferin Fund', *JAMWI*, 1, 11 (August 1910), 5.

51 'Reform', 'Services under the Dufferin Fund', *JAMWI*, 1, 4 (November 1908), 22.

52 'The Address from the A.M.W.I. to H.M. the Queen Empress', *JAMWI*, 3, 4 (November 1911), 4. For a more detailed account of women doctor's grievances, see Sehrawat, *Colonial Medical Care*, esp. chap. 4.

53 'General Meeting', *JAMWI*, 1, 6 (May 1909), 7.

54 Ibid., 10; *JAMWI*, 1, 5 (February 1909), 39.

55 O'Brien, 'Proposals for a Medical Women's Service', *JAMWI*, 1, 12 (November 1910), 4–9.

56 In 1909, Benson, Mildred Staley and Kate Vaughan were invited to represent the AMWI on a DF sub-committee considering reforms, 'The Meeting of the Sub-committee of the DF at Simla', *JAMWI*, 1, 7 (August 1909), 2–4; 'General Notes', *JAMWI*, 1, 9 (February 1910), 33; *DFR 1910*, 2. Vaughan, an outspoken critic of the DF, also acted as one of the inspectors of Dufferin hospitals appointed by Lady Minto, 'Editorial', *JAMWI*, 1, 8 (November 1909), 2.

57 Joint-Secretary, DF to Home Dept., GOI, 25 June 1908, Government of India (GOI), Home Department (H), Medical Branch (M), September 1908, 54–6A, National Archives of India (NAI), Delhi, 7–8.

58 For details of the Fund's proposals and the Indian government's response, see Sehrawat, *Colonial Medical Care*, chap. 5.

59 GOI, H, Med., February 1909, 16–20A, NAI; GOI, H, Med., August 1909, 195A, NAI; GOI, H, Med., February 1911, 1–26A, NAI.

60 'Indigenous Midwives and Victoria Memorial Scholarships', *JAMWI*, 1, 6 (May 1909), 33. Also see letter by 'M.B. Lond', *The Times* (14 May 1913), 5; 'Benson's Evidence to Royal Commission on Public Services', 6.

61 Letter by 'Retired Administrator', *The Times* (2 January 1912), 8. Lely claimed that 'more than 80 millions – women and children – stand outside the pale of medical relief provided by Government', 'Deputation to Crewe, 1912', 8.

62 'Editorial', *JAMWI*, 1, 4 (November 1908), 2.

63 'Government Service versus Charitable Effort', *JAMWI*, 1, 9 (February 1910), 25.

64 'Work Done by the Association', *JAMWI*, 2, 1 (February 1911), 17.

65 'Government Service versus Charitable Effort', *JAMWI*, 1, 9 (February 1910), 25–6.

66 See for instance, 'Indian Women and their Needs: The Dufferin Fund', 5; 'Medical Women for India', *The Times* (20 January 1912), 9; Letters to the Editor, by May Thorne, *The Times* (22 December 1911), 10; by Meroy Ashworth, *The Times* (23 December 1911), 10 and by R. Pitt, *The Times* (20 January 1912), 6.

67 'Editorial', *JAMWI*, 1, 4 (November 1908), 2. Also see, G.E. O'Brien, 'Proposals for a Medical Women's Service', *JAMWI*, 1, 12 (November 1910), 4.

68 'Benson's Evidence to Royal Commission on Public Services', 2.

69 Lely in 'Deputation to Crewe, 1912', 8.

70 For a discussion of Indian and British conceptions of development during a later period, see Benjamin Zachariah, *Developing India: An Intellectual and Social History, c. 1930–50*, New Delhi: Oxford University Press, 2005.

71 O'Brien, 'Proposals for a Medical Women's Service', *JAMWI*, 1, 12 (November 1910), 5.

72 For details see Sehrawat, *Colonial Medical Care*, chaps. 5 and 6.

73 The account of the meeting, the text of the memorial and the scheme for a Women's Medical Service were published in the *Journal, JAMWI*, 2, 1 (February 1911), 4–11.

74 House of Commons Question no. 82, 10 June 1912, Public and Judicial Departmental Papers, Annual Files, File 1228, India Office Records, Asia Pacific and Africa Collections, British Library, London.

75 Note by T. Holderness, Revenue Secretary, India Office, 19 June 1912, ibid.

76 Secretary of State (SoS) Revenue Despatch no. 87 of 1912, 6 September 1912, GOI, H, M, April 1913, 32A, NAI.

77 Telegram from SoS, 4 July 1913, GOI, H, M, September 1913, 87–96A, NAI.

78 Note issued by the DF Committee, Simla, 10 September 1913, GOI, H, M, September 1913, 87–96A, NAI, 17. Also see coverage in *Tribune*, 17 October 1913, *Selections from Indian Newspapers Published in the Punjab*, 26, 42, 917–18.

79 Finance Despatch no. 259 of 1912 from GOI to SoS Crewe, 12 September 1912, Simla, GOI, H, M, Sep. 1912, 54–6A, NAI, 15–16.

80 Ibid., 16.

81 Honorary Secretary, DF, to Home Secretary, GOI, 6 October 1913, GOI, H, M, November 1913, 63A, NAI. Indeed, the Punjab government's proposals to appoint Margaret Balfour as a female inspector of hospitals were initially rejected because it was believed that it could give renewed impetus to calls for the creation of a state service of medical women, GOI, H, M, August 1913, 32–4A, NAI.

82 'Women's Medical Service: Rules and Regulations', *JAMWI*, 4, 12 (November 1913), 14.

83 Ibid., 14–15.

84 Ibid., 11–19. Also see 'Editorial: Women's Medical Service for India', *JAMWI*, 4, 12 (November 1913), 20–1; *JAMWI*, 5, 1 (February 1914), 17.

85 For instance, Margaret Balfour, who had been an active member of the AMWI from its beginning in 1908, was joint-secretary to the DF from 1916 until 1924, and was appointed chief medical officer of the WMSI in 1920. Balfour subsequently became the president of the AMWI (1928–32). 'List of Members', *JAMWI*, 1, 3 (May 1908), 8; *JAMWI*, 20, 2 (May 1932), 5; 'Obituary Dr Margaret Balfour', *The Times* (3 December 1945).

86 The phrase is from Margery Perham, 'African Facts and American Criticisms', cited in Barbara Bush, 'Gender and Empire: The Twentieth Century', in Philippa Levine (ed.), *Gender and Empire*, Oxford: Oxford University Press, 2004, 80; for a succinct appraisal of the feminization of empire, see ibid., 86–90. Also see Helen Callaway, *Gender, Culture and Empire: European Women in Colonial Nigeria*, London: Macmillan Press, 1987, 83–162.

87 Burton, *Burdens of History*, 17.

88 Zachariah, *Developing India*; Marc Matera, 'An Empire of Development: Africa and the Caribbean in God's Chillun', *Twentieth Century British History*, 23, 1 (2012), 12–37; and Penelope Hetherington, *British Paternalism and Africa, 1920–1940*, London & Totowa, NJ: F. Cass, 1978.

12 Indian physicians and public health challenges

Bombay Presidency, 1896–1920

Mridula Ramanna

Indian doctors were vital intermediaries in the promotion of Western medicine in colonial Bombay. While their role in the formulation of sanitary or medical policy was negligible in the nineteenth century, they tended to subscribe to the then current contagionist or miasmic theories about the causation of cholera and smallpox, which struck the city regularly in epidemic proportions. Being trained in Western medicine, at the Grant Medical College (established in 1845), they were convinced of its efficacy, and actively endorsed sanitary reforms as a means of combating cholera and enthusiastically carried out smallpox vaccination. They were familiar with the local languages and with Indian cultural practices, and hence were in a better position to tackle the opposition and reservations that these measures encountered than their British counterparts. Their presence in hospitals made possible the acceptance of the very idea of hospitalization, which was unfamiliar to many. During the plague epidemic of 1896–97, when drastic controls were introduced to contain its spread and public protests were brushed aside, it was Indian doctors who played a significant role, not only in identifying it as plague but also in assuaging the fears of the terrified public. The outrage over the unparalleled medical interventionism turned to vehement opposition, which led to the abandonment of this policy by the colonial government. Now, public support was sought in promoting plague control measures, even as plague continued to appear in the first decade of the twentieth century.

Indian doctors were in the forefront in propagating and dispensing the plague prophylactic, which had been developed by Waldemar Mordecai Haffkine in 1897. Other public health concerns were malaria outbreaks and increased incidence of tuberculosis, and it was the Bombay medics who were vital participants in the anti-malaria and anti-tuberculosis campaigns. They propagated the preventive measures through local forums like the Bombay Medical Union (BMU established in 1884) and promoted sanitary consciousness through the Bombay Sanitary Association (BSA started in 1904). The aim of this chapter is to showcase the contributions of individual doctors to coping with health challenges in these two and half decades. The public response to epidemic controls, in relation to cholera, smallpox and plague outbreaks, between 1900 and 1919, by drawing on evidences from different parts of the Bombay Presidency, has been studied by this author.[1]

In order to understand the role of these doctors, it is worth briefly looking at their views and experiences in combating the killer diseases of cholera and smallpox, scourges of the nineteenth century. Cowasjee Nowrojee wrote a treatise entitled *Notes on Cholera and How to Avoid It* (1877) in what he described as 'an easy and popular style'. He wanted to convince his readers that cholera was preventable by the timely adoption of suitable precautionary means, which included sanitary measures. Consumption of pure water and properly cooked food, the avoidance of unwholesome drinks and indigestible 'food', of crowded and damp localities, of purgatives and fasting and the cultivation of 'an equable state of mind' were prescribed by Nowrojee. He further stated that, like his teacher, Dr. Charles Morehead, Principal of Grant Medical College (GMC), he did not accept the contagion theory, which, he argued, had 'done vast mischief by bringing our fears into conflict with our duties to the sick'.[2]

K.R. Kirtikar, another eminent graduate of the GMC who served in the Indian Medical Service, suggested in a paper read at the Bombay Medical and Physical Society that cholera spread not only through contaminated water but also through clothes, food and air.[3] These doctors thus tended to subscribe to the then current miasmatic and contagionist theories regarding causation of diseases and were convinced of the efficacy of Western medicine to treat them. The peak of cholera deaths in Bombay city, however, had been reached by the last quarter of the nineteenth century.[4] The contributory stimuli for their containment by the early 1900s were civic improvements, like the completed water supply and the slowly progressing drainage schemes. It will be shown later in this chapter that some of their colleagues made valuable observations about the city's water supply at the Bombay Medical Congress held in 1909.

The involvement of Bombay's medical fraternity in the promotion of smallpox vaccination has been detailed by this author.[5] It was due to the propagation of Jenner's vaccine by the brothers Bhau Daji and Narayan Daji Lad and Atmaram Pandurang Tarkhadkar, graduates of GMC, that smallpox vaccination gradually came to be accepted in *urbs prima in Indis*. Ananta Chandroba Dukhle was appointed vaccination superintendent in 1858, and for over two decades, laboured on, supervising six vaccination 'stations', including one located on the veranda of the house of his classmate, J.C. Lisboa. But it was no easy task, as he recounted in the annual vaccination reports that he filed. Dukhle described the difficulties he encountered: superstition, apathy, the belief that vaccination offered slight immunity and led to syphilis and leprosy, the 'procrastination', with mothers concealing their infants or giving false addresses, or not bringing their children for inspection. The fear of *Shitala Devi*'s wrath led to abstention from vaccination. There were propitiatory ceremonies to be performed after vaccination and hence some would forgo or postpone it, if they could not afford the expenditure. Doubts and fears were magnified when some vaccinated cases succumbed to smallpox. There were, at times, abuse and assaults on Dukhle's assistants. He recorded his own initial diffidence, in view of the lack of success of the previous fifty years, but at the end of his career, in the 1880s, he asserted that his faith in the efficacy of vaccination remained unshaken. The government recorded its gratitude for his zealous and unremitting labours during smallpox epidemics, which regularly appeared in the 1870s and 1880s. Sakharam Arjun, Dukhle's colleague, contended that no better evidence of its efficacy, 'is needed than the fact that in spite of gross ignorance and rank superstition of the masses, which attribute a divine character to smallpox, the remedy of vaccination is sought year after year'.[6] Shantaram Kantak, who also served as superintendent of vaccination, made important observations on the state of the campaign in his paper presented at the Indian Medical Congress, 1884. He pointed out that vaccination was done throughout the year in Bombay and Madras, and not seasonally as in other provinces, local funds were used to a larger extent than elsewhere and princely states in western India also spent much more on vaccination than their counterparts in other provinces.[7]

By the time of the plague epidemic of 1896 these Indian physicians had established themselves and gained the confidence of some of the population of colonial Bombay. When the plague outbreak of 1896–7, occurred, the authorities neither knew where it came from nor how to treat it. Drastic controls were introduced to contain the outbreak, including mass disinfection, inspection, destruction of the clothing and bedding of the afflicted, segregation and isolation of plague victims, and hospitalization. These measures met with vigorous resistance from Indians, as has been shown in various studies.[8]

Dr. Accacio G. Viegas, then a member of the Bombay Municipal Standing Committee (later president of the BMC), was the first to diagnose the plague, on 23 September 1896. A number of persons were later interviewed by the Indian Plague Commission, set up in 1898, to determine its source. Of importance in view of the later discovery of the rat flea as the carrier was the evidence of Ismail Jan Mahomed. He had examined two cases with pneumonic complications and diagnosed them as plague, and reported that one of his patients lived in a house adjacent to the warehouse where rats had died.[9]

The very idea of segregation and isolation was opposed to the local traditions of family members tending to the sick and, besides, there were the issues of pollution attached to bodily discharges, or of ritual rules being broken by the caste of the attendant and of the cook. In order to overcome reservations about hospitalization and fears of possible pollution, twenty-nine caste and community hospitals were set up during the epidemic.[10] These were manned by doctors of the respective castes or communities. Kaikhosru Nasarwanji Bahadurji was the first to set up a hospital exclusively for Parsis, where he worked night and day until his premature death in 1898. Various contemporary newspapers paid tribute to him on his demise; thus *Kesari* commended his great learning, fearless independence of character and the work he did in the BMC.[11] The Pathare Prabhu Fever Hospital was maintained through 1898, with funds collected from the community members, including women. The committee, which managed this voluntary effort, included medical members A.V. Velkar, V.S. Trilokekar, S.B. Nayak and A.P. Kothare. The committee also ran health and segregation camps for families removed from plague-stricken homes where doctors, led by G.B. Prabhakar, conducted daily medical inspections free of charge. Members of the government's inspection team were impressed by the management of both the hospital and camps.[12] Mention is also made of Vajeram Shaketram Diwan, who manned a hospital for Jains.[13]

The work of doctors was commended in the local press. Viegas, Jan Mohamed, N.F. Surveyor and the popular Thomas Blaney were lauded by *Hindu Punch*, 'the bubonic mahatma is not very well pleased with the prying curiosity' of these doctors.[14] *Rast Goftar* mentioned the names of two doctors, Nanabhai Kunvarji Modi and Sorbaji Gandhi, as having worked for the enforcement of plague measures.[15] R.N. Ranina was commended for running the municipal dispensary at Mandvi, where he secured the confidence of many patients, 'through the influence of success in treatment'.[16] Another doctor who worked during this period was Annie Walke, who graduated from GMC in

1888 and was working at the Cama Hospital for women and children and succumbed to plague in 1898.[17]

Nasserwanji Hormusji Choksy was designated extra assistant health officer and placed in charge of the Arthur Road infectious diseases hospital (AR, today the Kasturba Hospital) during the peak of the epidemic and left a candid report of his experiences. While members of the various plague commissions who visited the AR hospital may have envied Bombay for possessing such a well-situated institution, Choksy maintained that he had insurmountable problems in running the institution.[18] The hospital was short staffed and there were difficulties in finding recruits, since few had ever been inside a hospital. Those who were induced to join 'ran' away within hours or days and did not even come back to claim their wages. They had never seen so many persons die as they did in plague, for the largest number died at the hospital, both because of the numerous admissions and because so many cases were brought in a moribund condition, the percentage of mortality being 73.26 per cent. Most cases were sent there under compulsion when they were beyond all help, and Choksy had to contend with their ignorance and prejudice. There were rumours that the authorities took people to hospitals to make a speedy end of them, so that their hearts could be taken out to be sent to the Queen in England to appease her wrath on account of the disfigurement of her statue, which had occurred in the beginning of the epidemic. The means used to resuscitate patients, through subcutaneous injections, were misconstrued.[19]

The hostility culminated in a raid on the hospital on 29 October 1896, when an estimated 800–1,000 mill hands rushed in, broke open the gates and scaled the walls in order to wreak vengeance on the staff for allegedly killing patients. Some of them reached the wards and even injured the patients, but no one was seriously hurt. They were dispersed by the police, who continued to be stationed on the premises for some time. As for relatives and friends, Choksy said they were welcomed with the hope that they would supplement the efforts of the nursing staff, but they were so terror stricken that they would not venture beyond the gates once the patient had been admitted. He had to counter what he termed a host of 'pseudo-specialists', who pretended to know all about plague, and, for a time, forgot their regular avocations as tram conductors, railway guards, engineers, postal inspectors or clerks and suddenly blossomed into specialists, 'vaunting their nostrums' day after day.[20] Children were brought to hospital by their parents who gave incorrect addresses and could not be traced afterwards. These children were later either adopted or cared for by the All Saints Sisters who managed the nursing. He also paid tribute to his colleagues who volunteered during the peak of the epidemic: P.N. Davda, who succumbed to the disease; Pilgaokar and Maneck Tarkhad Bahadurji (daughter of Dr. Atmaram Pandurang, among the early graduates of GMC).

Choksy remained in charge of the AR hospital until 1922, and of the Maratha plague hospital from 1902 until 1921. Begun as a plague hospital for Maratha, the latter institution later provided treatment to plague patients of all communities. He collated statistics of patients, gender- and occupation-wise, and noted that, as with cholera, lower social status coupled with want, poverty, over-crowding, unsanitary conditions and intemperance were vital factors in lowering the power of resistance. Even though the incidence of plague declined by 1920, case mortality was not affected because plague did not alter its virulence nor abate its toll of life. Many patients were brought in when it was too late and enforcement never worked.[21] Nevertheless, doctors did not always accept adoption of controls. Thus, the forcible segregation of smallpox patients at the AR hospital in 1905 was condemned by doctor municipal councillors, and it was felt that a repetition of the 'foolish measures' attempted during the plague epidemic of 1896–7 was being tried again because Europeans had a dread of smallpox. The solution was to popularize vaccination, to vaccinate all persons in areas where the infected stayed and to provide comfortable hospital accommodation at convenient locations.[22] Choksy showed that the efficacy of even one primary vaccination reduced case mortality. It was not only cholera, smallpox and plague from other regions of India, but also jigger and sleeping sickness from East Africa that were treated at the AR hospital, as were mumps, erysipelas and cerebro-spinal meningitis.[23] John Andrew Turner, Bombay's Health Officer (1901–19), lauded the hospital, 'which has done valuable work and saved lives'.[24] By 1922, there were 6 wards for Indians with 132 beds and 4 wards for Europeans, with 56 beds. An infectious diseases hospital was also started in Poona, while separate wards for such cases were set aside in civil hospitals in other cities.

Choksy, whose name became synonymous with the treatment of infectious diseases, was honoured both by the government, with the Companion of the Order of the Indian Empire, and the Bombay Medical Union, for his devotion to duty, particularly during epidemics.[25]

Plague prophylactic

Haffkine informed the Government of India on January 1, 1897, that he had developed a prophylactic in Bombay, which he had tried on himself with a dosage four times stronger than that which was later accepted as standard. The details of the preparation were published both in the *British Medical Journal* and the *Indian Medical Gazette*, in May and June, 1897. Haffkine's Indian assistant was R.M. Kalapesi, and others on the staff of the Plague Research Laboratory at the time were R.J. Kapadia, J.B. Quadros and A.S. Paymaster.[26] The medical establishment hoped that Indians would accept inoculation, since they were familiar with smallpox vaccination. This is where the role of Indian doctors was vital. The BMU declared the conviction of its members in its effectiveness, as did the Pathare Prabhu Medical Committee, which observed that of the deaths in their hospital, very few occurred among those inoculated and none among those who had been inoculated twice. By October of that year, 8,142 persons had been inoculated, including 77 'leading citizens'. The Khojas, under the leadership of the Aga Khan, had been the first to accept inoculation in Bombay, and in Karachi. S.M. Kaka, the city's health officer, recorded that he had inoculated 3,756 men and 2,063 women, in 1898.[27] Burjorji Sorabsha was employed by the Parsi Panchayat to perform inoculations in Bharuch. Vishram Ghole, assistant surgeon in Poona, advocated its use in the *Kesari*, in 1899.[28] Not everywhere did doctors meet with success; even though a medical graduate, who had worked with Haffkine, was employed by the state of Porbandar to perform inoculations, the plan had to be given up when the plague showed signs of abating and Brahmins there were most reluctant to get themselves inoculated.

Shortly after the introduction of the prophylactic, Bhalchandra Krishna Bhatvadekar shared his observations with his colleagues at a meeting of the Grant College Medical Society. Four cases of an 'analogous nature', all of whom had suffered from fever, had been placed at his disposal by Haffkine, but he had cured them with the inoculation. Two of the cases were themselves doctors. As to the question often raised, whether the health of a person suffered after inoculation, he cited the case of the Khojas who had lower mortality from general causes among those who had been inoculated. He clarified that neither the inoculated person nor the plague sufferer acted as a source of infection to the un-inoculated, the source of immediate danger being the 'locality', which had the 'poison'. He asserted that he was convinced of its efficacy and had personally undergone inoculation. Bhatvadekar hailed Haffkine as the 'benefactor of mankind'.[29] In answer to Lokamanya Tilak's queries about the probable ill effects of the inoculation, he clarified that it was unsuitable only in cases of phthisis (pulmonary tuberculosis), rheumatism, kidney diseases and general debility.[30] Bhatvadekar as Chairman, Standing Committee, Bombay Municipal Corporation, had an impact on its acceptance.

The 1908 successful propagation of the prophylactic in Poona was particularly significant since that city had been in the forefront of agitation against it in the previous decade. *Maratha* had maintained that the interventionist measures enforced by the plague administration, in the first epidemic, had fully justified the popular demand made that local bodies should be entrusted with the task of carrying out all plague measures, under the guidance of the government.[31] Under the leadership of Gopal Krishna Gokhale and his team of volunteers, led by Gopal Krishna Devadhar, the Poona committee coordinated with the municipal authorities not only in propagating inoculation (persuading 15,250 persons to get inoculated) but also in rat destruction, evacuation and the disposal of the dead.[32] They compiled statistics showing 1,250 deaths among the un-inoculated and only 4 deaths among the inoculated, and concluded that there had not been a single instance in which 'evil effects' had resulted from inoculation.[33] The success of its promotion in Wai was attributed to the efforts by Dr. D.A. Turkhud.[34] At Ranebennur, it was popularized with the aid of magic lantern demonstrations, and under the aegis of the Dharwar District Sanitary Association, Dr. N.V. Dhavale gave plague inoculations. In 1915, the Sanitary Commissioner reported that 29,925 persons had been inoculated at civil hospitals and dispensaries.[35] Rakhmabai, one of the noted women physicians of these years, worked selflessly during the plague and influenza epidemics in the early 1900s during her service at Surat and Rajkot and was subsequently awarded the Kaiser-I Hind Medal in recognition of these efforts.

Sanitary consciousness

The Bombay Sanitary Association was founded in 1904 at the initiative of Turner and Choksy and was supported by civic leaders, philanthropists and the Bombay governor, Lord Lamington (1903–7). The creation of public awareness about hygiene and disease was one of the main objectives of the BSA, hence the very first lecture was delivered by Choksy on an issue of immediate urgency, 'Some common sense views on plague'. The lecture by K.B. Shroff (special assistant to Turner) on malaria and dengue drew large crowds because of the prevalence of dengue at the time. Other topics included 'Household and personal cleanliness', 'Rearing of children', 'Caring for the new born and lying-in woman' and 'Practical hints regarding nursing'. Both the English-language and the vernacular newspapers gave free publicity to these efforts. A health exhibition was mounted by the BSA in connection with the Industrial and Agricultural Exhibition of 1904. Magic lantern slides and a gramophone were used to attract audiences to lectures on temperance, sanitation, hygiene and first aid. A.L. Nair, A.V. Velkar, A.P. Cama, D.A. Turkhad, S.N. Ranina, N.N. Katrak and N.M. Kalapesi were among the physician members of the BSA.[36]

Pilgrimages had long been regarded as breeding grounds of epidemics. The BSA therefore regularly organized lectures at Pandharpur, explaining the causes of diseases and distributing pamphlets on plague and cholera. There were important contributions from men on the spot, like Da Gama, whose work during festivals at Pandharpur was particularly mentioned in the *Report of the Sanitary Commissioner* (1916) for improving conservancy in that pilgrim town.[37] Three years later, another Indian health official, Anthony D'Mello, Deputy Sanitary Commissioner, was credited with the elaborate arrangements that had been made for the smooth conduct of the fair. Sub-assistant surgeons, with their other duties being suspended, were attached to the different *palkhis* (palanquins commemorating the Bhakti saints of Maharashtra) on their inward and outward marches to Pandharpur and inspected them, weeding out all infectious cases, even before they reached their destination. Step wells were converted into draw wells for the protection of the existing water supply, trenches were dug, dustbins provided, extra sweepers employed, food stuffs inspected and sheets of muslin provided to sweet meat dealers to cover exposed sweets.[38] By the mid-1920s, it was stated that no fair or festival in Bombay Presidency was responsible for epidemics, and this gratifying achievement was attributed to the preventive work done under the direction of Jamshyd Munsiff, Acting Director of Public Health.[39]

It is noteworthy that some of the papers presented by Indian doctors at the Bombay Medical Congress, 1909, were based on their experiences during epidemics. Choksy reported on the results of serum treatment in plague cases, having treated 275 cases with the subcutaneous method of administration. He had found that meat eaters suffered more than vegetarians from the after-effects of this treatment, with rashes, oedema, joint and muscle pains. Bhatvadekar endorsed this finding of the efficacy of the serum treatment, which he too had tried in his medical practice. In another paper, Choksy showed the baneful effects of alcohol, internal antiseptics, anti-pyretics and the use of carbolic acid in the symptomatic treatment of plague. Choksy also presented his observations about 'relapsing fever', the so-called Indian variety then being regarded as the most fatal form. It was Henry Vandyke Carter, Principal of GMC, who had first identified the spirillum of the relapsing fever under the microscope, though the then governor, Richard Temple, seems to have alleged that he was observing his own eyelashes. This fever was associated with scarcity and poverty and claimed the largest number of victims during famines.[40] These doctors also criticized superstitions. Raghunath Row referred to the popular belief in Cambay that only after a person had an attack of 'the Delhi boil', also called *ashrafi*, was he regarded as having good health.[41]

Kavasji Dadachanji, President of the Bombay Medical Union, emphasized the importance to the individual of pure water, in view of the recognition that both cholera and typhoid were water-borne diseases. He advocated a constant supply to the city, for, otherwise, people resorted to storing water and there would be the possibility of pollution. To ensure purity of the water supply, he recommended the following measures: (a) location of villages or cities, 10 miles from water sources; (b) in cities, located close to the sea, the intake of water to be where the tide had no effect; and (c) no fishing or cattle to be allowed near pump houses, and no wells to be dug near manured ground. The water supplied in Bombay had been compared with that of London to see how potable it was. Dadachanji questioned why better results had not been secured, despite getting water from the lakes, fed by the annual monsoons. N.N. Katrak pointed out, however, that cholera deaths had been reduced since the introduction of water supply from the Vihar lake.[42] Sorab C. Hormusji discussed agents of disinfection, like pesterine, which had been used in homes where there had been plague cases. B.S Shroff, Medical Officer with the British India Steam Navigation Company, recommended the fumigation of shore godowns with sulphur cakes and the scrubbing of dock walls with caustic alkaline soda.

Malaria

An example of the part played by the man on the spot is to be seen in the anti-malaria campaign in Bombay. The disease topped the list of causes of deaths, and Charles Bentley, IMS, was appointed to carry out an investigation into the causes of malaria. He held that the obstinacy of the 'upper classes' was a greater obstacle in the prevention of malaria than 'the ignorance of the masses', though this had not prevented the adoption of a pure water supply, once the 'educated had decided that it was necessary'.[43] His conclusion that there was a higher rate of malaria among Parsis was strongly objected to by this community, which had been in the forefront of the acceptance of Western medicine. The municipal commissioner issued a directive to close wells or cover them. Three hundred and fifty Parsi priests submitted a petition, contending that they could not use water for religious purposes if it was pumped from covered-up wells, since they believed that it had to be exposed to the sun, which was considered a great purifier.[44] Bentley referred to a particular house owner who had threatened to take legal proceedings for trespass if any of his properties were visited by the inspection staff, and regretted that many Indian doctors practising in Bombay had little influence on their wealthy clients. In fact, some Parsi doctors made a vigorous onslaught on Bentley for holding their private wells responsible for the prevalence of infection.[45] But, subsequently, a committee of medical men appointed by the Bombay Zoroastrian Association supported Bentley's conclusions.[46] K.B. Shroff, himself a Parsi, referred to these as 'sentimental objections', including beliefs about the presence of 'saintly beings' resident in wells. Stocking of wells with fish, which had been recommended as a means of reducing mosquito larvae, was also objected to by the Jain community.[47]

Yet, while inspecting, Shroff saw that, in 90 per cent of cases, the trap doors were left open and larvae was found even in closed wells, indicating that they had been left open at nights. To bolster support for the campaign, public lectures were given at different venues by Shroff, Constancio Coutinho and Hirji Gini. The magnate Jamsetjee Jejeebhoy exhorted his co-religionists to cooperate with the authorities. To oppose the closure of wells, he said, 'was as much against the spirit and teaching of religion as against the laws of health'.[48] Pherozeshah Mehta maintained that the objections were more due to an inordinate attachment to custom than to 'a proper appreciation of the spirit which runs through religion'.[49] A weekly report of wells with larvae was even sent to local newspapers like the *Times of India*, *Jame-Jamshed*, *Bombay Gazette* and *Bombay Samachar*, so that it would have a salutary effect in convincing the recalcitrant. Finally, it seems the campaign worked.

Anti-Tuberculosis League

Another disease, which was recognized as having reached epidemic proportions, was tuberculosis. The local-level initiative taken to launch an anti-tuberculosis campaign resulted in the establishment in 1912 of the King George V Anti-Tuberculosis League (ATL). It was so named to commemorate the durbar and visit of King George V and Queen Mary. The ATL was founded consequent to the promise of an annual donation of 15,000 rupees for ten years by the industrialist philanthropist Ratan J. Tata. The executive committee of the ATL included other philanthropists like Sassoon, Jamsetji Jejeebhoy, Dinshaw Petit, Vithaldas Thackersey, Fazulbhoy Currimbhoy Ibrahim; and doctors Bhatvadekar, T.B Nariman, N.F. Surveyor, D.A. D'Monte; and British officials, the Municipal Commissioner P.R. Cadell, the Surgeon General R.W.S. Lyons and Glen Liston of the Bombay Bacteriological Laboratory. The speeches delivered at the inaugural give an idea of the proposed objectives. Governor Lord George Sydenham Clarke (1908–13) referred to the methods being applied in different countries to combat the disease, a decrease in mortality in England, Scotland, Wales and the Netherlands having been achieved not only due to advances in medical sciences, but also to methods adopted to give effect to these advances. For any campaign to succeed, the cooperation of the medical fraternity was necessary, hence he had sounded out Bhatvadekar, who had co-opted his colleagues. Government could assist by insisting on the teaching of elementary principles of sanitation in schools, the compulsory notification of phthisis already being in place since 1902. He pointed out that it was a fine opportunity for medical graduates to give lectures on the preventive measures.

Turner, in his speech, made an impassioned plea for more attention to tuberculosis. He pointed out that the health department was constantly fighting plague, cholera, smallpox and malaria and that these diseases were under control. Emphasizing the danger from tuberculosis, he said it was now known that plague and malaria were not spread from person to person, smallpox did not attack persons protected by vaccination and that sanitary reform kept cholera at bay, but tuberculosis caused more misery and illness with its slow and insidious progress, fatal termination and mode of spread. Turner's suggestions were comprehensive: education of the general public, of school children and their teachers; establishment of dispensaries, sanatoria and hospitals for advanced cases; home training; extermination of tuberculosis from cattle; rigorous supervision of milk and food supply; assistance to the family in case of the death of the bread winner and provision of employment to the cured cases. While he had often come against the argument that rules and regulations enforced elsewhere could not be applied in India, he believed that persuasion and sympathy must take their place. Bhatavadekar assured the support of the medical profession and of the Social Service League in the effort. He ascribed the disease to 'over crowding, insufficient ventilation, insanitary conditions and unwholesome food'.[50] T.B. Nariman contended that the preventive measures were more effective in tuberculosis. It is significant that a female physician, Kashibai Nowrange, attended and spoke at the inaugural. In her speech, she pointed out that, of late, tuberculosis was wreaking havoc among the poorer classes, especially women, who had to pass most of their time in seclusion. Women were more susceptible than men because of their 'habits' and the subject was vitally connected with sanitation and hygiene, and it was therefore necessary to educate the ignorant masses.[51] Rakhamabai had found, in her practice at Rajkot, that the fast-spreading custom of purdah, which was regarded a mark of social status, was responsible for the increased incidence of tuberculosis and stunted growth in girls.[52]

The methods of the ATL were to spread information about tuberculosis through lectures and pamphlets in English, Gujarati, Marathi and Urdu; with lantern slides; to conduct visits and medical inspections at schools, mills, docks and factories; and supervise milk and food supplies; and to create 'a special fund, to relieve distress'.[53] The *British Medical Journal*, commending this effort, had hoped that the public would respond amply, and it did, with a collection of 135,000 rupees.[54] Since its work was to be mainly preventive, the ATL started with a central dispensary and information bureau run by Constancio Coutinho and N.V. Dhavale, assisted by three nurses. Patients came to the dispensary on recommendations from charitable, religious and public institutions and medical practitioners, while district registrars in charge of free municipal dispensaries also sent cases. The patients received instructions regarding mode of life and habits and received treatment by drug inhalations and tuberculin.

The latter, introduced by Robert Koch in 1890, had not satisfied the expectations that it had raised but was brought back into extensive use in the twentieth century as a diagnostic aid in the detection of early pre-symptomatic tuberculosis.[55] It was noticed, however, that some patients gave up on their treatments when their immediate symptoms were relieved. Coutinho found that young adults from the ages of 16 to 20 were most prone to the disease; they constituted 22.9 per cent of all cases in 1914, and most of them were students or clerks. Of the 541 patients he treated in 1914, 199 were female, 18 were infants and the rest male.[56] Since Turner was health officer and an initiator of the ATL, the dispensary worked in close cooperation with the municipal health department. He claimed, with justifiable pride, that just as the Royal Victoria Dispensary, Edinburgh, founded by Sir Robert Philip, was the first of its kind in the world, the ATL was the first of its kind in India.[57] A museum was set up with exhibits, models and diagrams purchased from England.

A branch dispensary was started in 1915 in the crowded locality of Kamatipura when the Municipality placed the Bai Lingoobai dispensary at the disposal of the ATL, which was meant for the very poor.

By 1916, the number of patients treated rose to 2,461; the varieties of tuberculosis treated were thus classified: enlarged glands, pulmonary tuberculosis, bone tuberculosis, peritonitis, abscesses, ankle joints, tubercular diarrhoea, caries of the spine and pleurisy.[58] A small bacteriological dispensary was opened for pathological examination and for the preparation of vaccines. Turner and Choksy despaired of the conditions in the unsanitary *chawls* constructed by the City Improvement Trust (CIT), with their damp, dark and dirty appearances.[59] Coupled with insufficient food, children in these places had poor resistance and consequently succumbed to infection. Between 1916 and 1920, 2,567 house visits were made by doctors, and 5,914 visits by nurses.

The subject also engaged the doctors' attention in their forums. Sorab Engineer, in a paper presented at a meeting of the BMU, pointed out that statistics had shown that half of all death rates were attributable to tuberculosis. He outlined what the medical fraternity could do for the people of Bombay: educating lay people in such a way as to be useful to both themselves and to their neighbours. He cautioned that not by high-handedness or force, as was done during the plague, but by gentle persuasion could this be accomplished. In fact, he alleged that though the BSA existed, few people took interest in its proceedings. One lecture that the BSA had arranged on the disease was attended by only fifty persons, and lectures before collegians and mill hands, just once a year, were as good as 'not to have said a word'; and for the latter, it served as a 'picnic'.[60] He called upon the government, the municipality and the CIT to improve housing and recommended regulations against spitting, inspection of dairies and the establishment of dispensaries. R.B. Billimoria in his lecture entitled, 'Specific Treatment of Pulmonary Tuberculosis' chastised his colleagues for rushing to lay newspapers discussing tuberculin, sera and so forth, and for giving false certificates, so that patients gained access to convalescent homes not meant for consumptives. He stressed the importance of early diagnosis and of impressing upon the patient and the relatives the danger from sputa. Delineating his method of treatment, which included pyramidon with chloroform, and then an iodine compound, rest, gradual exercise and nourishing food, he emphasized that it was imperative to teach medics how to distinguish between hopeless and hopeful cases.[61]

Glen Liston and M.B. Soparkar, on the basis of their experiments at the Bombay Bacteriological Laboratory, explained in the *Indian Journal of Medical Research* that the human infection caused by tubercle bacilli of the bovine type was rare in Bombay Presidency, despite the use of cow dung in houses.[62] At the All India Social Service Conference, Bombay, 1923, B.S. Kanga, who was in charge of one of the dispensaries, maintained that it was the duty of the municipality to provide more parks and open spaces. This view was endorsed by his colleague, F.N. Moos, who called for more active participation by the municipality, the corporators having been 'dulled' by questions of public health. He contended that 'education and effective nutrition rather than disinfection and treatment would reclaim the veil so deeply ingrained in the habits, customs and lives of our people.'[63]

Conclusion

While a number of Indian doctors of Bombay pursued private practice, the fact remained that, during these years, they did not occupy the top positions in the medical administration, which remained the monopoly of the British and the Indian Medical Service.[64] The contemporary newspapers often voiced protests against what was perceived as injustice towards qualified Indians, Dr. Surveyor's appointment as professor of bacteriology in GMC, in 1907, being an exception.[65] Dr. Gilder pointed out in the Bombay Legislative Council, that even into the 1920s, the 'indigenous' profession was perceived to be 'hewers of wood and drawers of water', and beyond that they did not need to look for anything. He cited the example of a European doctor appointed to a professorship in preference to a locally qualified candidate.[66]

Thus, Indian physicians were by no means the policy makers, yet, serving in intermediate positions in government service and as private practitioners, they were the vital executors of that policy, as this regional focus has attempted to show. Their presence made the regulations imposed during epidemics and at pilgrim centres, requiring immediate compliance, acceptable to the public. In the promotion of preventive medicine, their role was to inform, persuade and cajole. They were initiators of the voluntary organizations, like the BSA & ATL, set up to push forward these measures. The BMU offered its services to the government during the First World War. Its members were powerful voices in Bombay's civic affairs and would invariably 'dissect' the reports of the health officer. Katrak and Blaney had indicted the health department just before the onset of the plague epidemic of 1896. Members of the municipal committee, Viegas, Jan Mahomed and Blaney, had 'hunted down the demon of culpable negligence, disgraceful carelessness and inexplicable dilatoriness, who had taken possession of the Bombay civic fathers and health department'.[67] Dadachanji asked the municipal commissioner whether he was aware that since necessary steps had not been taken to drain storm-water drains, they had become breeding grounds for mosquitoes.[68] During the influenza epidemic, 1918–19, the BMC formed a medical subcommittee under the chairmanship of Rahimtulla Currimbhoy, with Dadachanji, Sir Cowasji Jehangir and Dr. M.C. Javle as members. They visited dispensaries and brought to the attention of the Controller of Prices the need to reduce the high prices of medicines. D'Monte served in the governor's legislative council.[69]

Their growing confidence is reflected in the important suggestions that they made, based on their hands-on experience regarding combating public health challenges. Kantak made a case for more pay for vaccinators and interestingly for the employment of women vaccinators. This would be advantageous because the operations were usually endangered by the 'dirty condition of the children', and the extreme haste with which 'the vesicles were covered up with rags'.[70] Choksy, in articles on public health (*Times of India*, May and June, 1923), urged the creation of a special sanitary preventive and curative service under the ministry of health. The masses were not ready for an intensive campaign of sanitary education, what they needed was actual and concrete demonstration of the benefits promised. The *British Medical Journal* commended this article as being of great value in the effort to arouse public opinion. It had the merits of propounding a constructive policy and of being advocated by 'one whose medical education has been indigenous and who is intimately connected with the political and medical history of the country, its possibilities and aspirations and the social and sanitary conditions, which form such an obstacle to comprehensive and effective means of public health'.[71]

Notes

1 Mridula Ramanna, 'Coping with Epidemic: Indian Responses, Bombay Presidency, 1900–1919', in Arun Bandhophyay (ed.), *Science and Society in India, 1750–2000*, New Delhi: Manohar, 2010, 145–67.

2 Cowasjee Nowrojee, *Notes on Cholera and How to Prevent It*, Bombay, Bombay, 1877, 19, 54–7.

3 *Transactions of the Medical and Physical Society of Bombay*, Bombay: Bombay Education Society Press, new series, 7 (1884), v.

4 The names, Bombay and Poona, as they were then known, have been used here. They have since been changed to Mumbai and Pune.

5 Mridula Ramanna, *Western Medicine and Public Health in Colonial Bombay, 1845–1895*, New Delhi: Orient Longman, 2002, 137–43.

6 Sakharam Arjun, 'Vaccination A Scientific Remedy', *Transactions of the Medical and Physical Society of Bombay*, n. s, 7 (1884), 37.

7 Shantaram Kantak, 'Vaccination Systems in India', *Indian Medical Congress*, Calcutta: 1894, 252–7.

8 See Raj Chandavarkar, *Imperial Power and Popular Politics*, Cambridge: Cambridge University Press, 1998; Ian Catanach, 'Plague and the Tensions

of Empire: India, 1896–1918', in David Arnold (ed.), *Imperial Medicine and Indigenous Societies*, Manchester: Manchester University Press, 1988, 149–71; David Arnold, 'Touching the Body: Perspectives on the Indian Plague, 1896–1900', in Ranajit Guha (ed.), *Subaltern Studies*, V, New Delhi: Oxford University Press, 1987, 55–90; Kavita Sivaramakrishnan, *Old Potions, New Bottles: Recasting Indigenous Medicine in Colonial Punjab, 1850–1945*, New Delhi: Orient Longman, 2005; Mridula Ramanna, *Health Care in Bombay Presidency, 1896–1930*, New Delhi: Primus, 2012, 10–38.

9 *Report of the Indian Plague Commission*, 5 vols., London: Eyre and Spotiswode, 5, 1901, 453.

10 R. Nathan, *The Plague in India*, 3 vols., Simla: Government Central Press, 1898, I, 162–3.

11 *Report of Native Papers, Bombay Presidency* (hereafter *RN*) *East Indian*, 19 August, 1898, *Kesari*, 16 August 1898.

12 General Department volumes, Maharashtra State Archives, Mumbai (hereafter GD), 770 1898, Report of the Pathare Prabhu Fever Hospital.

13 *RN, Gujarati*, 25 July, 1897.

14 *Pickings from the Hindi Punch* (hereafter *HP*), November, 1896, 168.

15 *RN, Rast Goftar*, 25 July, 1897.

16 *Record of the Proceedings of the Standing Committee of the Municipal Corporation of Bombay*, Part II, XXII, 1898–99, 250, 450.

17 See Mridula Ramanna, 'Women Physicians as Vital Intermediaries in Colonial Bombay', *Economic & Political Weekly*, XLII, 12 &13 (2008), 71–8.

18 N.H. Choksy, *Report on Bubonic Plague*, Bombay: Times of India Press, 1897, 4.

19 Ibid., 5.

20 Ibid., 5.

21 *Administrative Report for the Municipal Commissioner for the City of Bombay*, (hereafter *ARMCB*), 1918, Bombay: The Times of India Press, 1919, Arthur Road Hospital Report, 1918, 88–9.

22 *RN, Gujarati*, 25 June, 1905. *RN, Sanj Vartaman*, 9 March, 1904. Mridula Ramanna, 'Gauging Indian Responses to Western Medicine: Hospitals and Dispensaries, Bombay Presidency, 1900–20' in Deepak Kumar (ed.), *Disease and Medicine in India: A Historical Overview*, New Delhi: Tulika, 2001, 233–48.

23 Since there was movement of people to and from this region to Bombay, the authorities wanted to keep out diseases like jigger and sleeping sickness which could be brought in by these people. The anxiety was to protect the city from any kind of infectious disease.

24 *ARMCB*, 1912–13, 53.

25 *British Medical Journal* (hereafter *BMJ*), 23 September, 1922, 578.

26 Founded as the Plague Research Laboratory in 1899 by Haffkine, it was renamed the Bombay Bacteriological Laboratory (BBL) in 1906. The BBL, still later named Haffkine Institute in 1925, became a provincial laboratory for general diagnosis and research activities, providing diagnostic services to Bombay hospitals.

27 In addition, 155 men and 132 women were inoculated twice. S.M. Kaka, *Report on the Effect of Preventive Inoculation with Prof. Haffkine's Plague Prophylactic*, Karachi: Municipal Commissioner's Office, 1899.

28 *RN, Kesari*, 1 August, 1899, 22 August, 1905.
29 B.K. Bhatvadekar, *M. Haffkine's Plague Prophylactic*, Bombay: Tattva Vivechaka Press, 1898, no page no.
30 *RN, Indian Spectator*, 4 November, 1905.
31 *RN, Maratha*, 8 September, 1907.
32 H.N. Kunzru (ed.), *Gopal Krishna Devadhar*, Poona: Servants of India Society, 1939, 134–9.
33 *RN, Bombay Samachar*, 26 August, 1908.
34 *RN, Indian Spectator*, 4 November, 1905, *Vrittasar*, 3 April, 1911.
35 *Report of Sanitary Commissioner, Bombay Presidency* (hereafter *RSC*), Bombay: Government Central Press, 1915, 15.
36 *The Bombay Sanitary Association and the Sanitary Institute* in GD, 938, 1917–1918.
37 *RSC, 1916*, 28.
38 GD, 826, 1920, Report of the Deputy Sanitary Commissioner on the *ashadhi* fair, 1919.
39 *BMJ*, 31 March, 1926, 569.
40 N.H. Choksy, 'The Serum Therapy of Plague', 120–5; 'The Symptomatic Treatment of Plague', 125–32; 'Relapsing Fever', 168–94, in W.E. Jennings (ed.), *Transactions of the Bombay Medical Congress, 1909* (hereafter *TBMC*), Bombay: The Times of India Press, 1909.
    For a discussion of Choksy's contribution, see Mridula Ramanna, 'N.H. Chosky: A Pioneer of Controlled Clinical Trials', *Journal of the Royal Society of Medicine*, 107, 3 (2014), 120–2.
41 Raghunath Row, 'Observations on the Development of Flagellated Organisms from the Parasite of Oriental Sore', *TBMC*, 204–8.
42 K.E. Dadachanji, 'Purity of Water and Measures Necessary for the Purity of Water', *TBMC*, 337–50. N.N. Katrak, 'The Standard of Water Purity for India', *TBMC*, 350–2.
43 Charles A. Bentley, *Report of an Investigation into the Causes of Malaria in Bombay and the Measures Necessary for Its Control*, Bombay: Government Central Press, 1911, 137.
44 Ibid., 138–9.
45 *BMJ*, 4 November, 1911, 1229.
46 *Report on Malaria Operations*, April 1912–March 1913, *ARMCB, 1912–13*, Bombay: The Times of India Press, 1913, 171.
47 Ibid., 178.
48 Ibid., 181.
49 *RN, Rast Goftar*, 7 July, 1912.
50 GD 156, 1912, 4 April, 1912.
51 GD 156, 1912, 'War on Phthisis: The Bombay Campaign'.
52 Rakhamabai, 'Purdah – The Need for Its Abolition', in Evelyn C. Gedge (ed.), *Women in Modern India*, Bombay: Taraporewala Sons & Co, 1929, 144–48.
53 GD, 1070, 1915, *Annual Report of King George V Anti-T.B. League for 1914*, Bombay, 1915, 35–6.
54 *BMJ*, 5 July, 1913, 44.
55 Roy Porter, *The Greatest Benefit to Mankind: A Medical History of Humanity*, London: W.W. Norton & Company, 1997, 441.
56 GD, 1070, 1915, *ATL Report, 1914*, 28.

57 John A. Turner, 'The Anti-Tuberculosis Campaign in Bombay, India', *The British Journal of Tuberculosis*, ix, 2 (April 1915), 51–5.
58 GD, 1070, 1915, *Report of the Medical Officer, ATL*, 25.
59 The City Improvement Trust was established in 1898, as a consequence of the plague epidemic to deal with the city's unhealthy environment, to clear slums, broaden roads and build *chawls* (tenements).
60 Sorab Engineer, 'Some Factors Necessary for the Prophylaxis of Tuberculosis in Bombay', *Report of the Bombay Medical Union, 1911–12*, Bombay: 1912, 89–99.
61 R.B. Billimoria, 'Specific Treatment of Pulmonary Tuberculosis', *Report of the BMU, 1915*, 31–9.
62 M.B. Soparkar, *Indian Journal of Medical Research*, April, 1917, 635.
63 B.S. Kanga, 'The Prevention and Cure of Tuberculosis', 125–31; F.N. Moos, 'The Present Position of Tuberculosis and Its Prevention', 131–44, in *Report and Proceedings of the All-India Social Service Conference*, Bombay: Servants of India Society, 1924.
64 Doctors in the 1880s, led by K.N. Bahadurji, had spearheaded a campaign against this monopoly. For details, see Mridula Ramanna, *Western Medicine*, 217–30.
65 *RN, Indu Prakash*, 26 August, 1911.
66 *Bombay Legislative Council Debates*, xxiv, 1928, 1264.
67 *HP*, November, 1896, 168.
68 *HP*, October, 1908, 191.
69 For detailed discussion of the Bombay experience, see Mridula Ramanna, 'Coping with the Influenza Pandemic, 1918–1919: The Bombay Experience', in Howard Philips and David Killingary (eds.), *The Spanish Influenza Pandemic of 1918–19, New Perspectives*, London: Routledge, 2003, 86–98.
70 Kantak, 'Vaccination Systems', *Indian Medical Congress*.
71 *BMJ*, 29 September, 1923, 577.

13 Tracking *kala-azar*

The East Indian experience and experiments

Achintya Kumar Dutta

Epidemic diseases in colonial India have attracted a host of foreign and Indian scholars. David Arnold, Ira Klein, I.J. Catanach, Paul Greenough, Mark Harrison, Sanjoy Bhattacharya, Rajnarayan Chandavarkar and V.R. Muraleedharan are the major authors among them. There has been much discussion over the epidemic diseases by these scholars. David Arnold has dealt with plague, cholera and smallpox; Ira Klein with malaria; Catanach and Chandavarkar with plague; Greenough and Bhattacharya with smallpox; Harrison with cholera and so forth. These studies have enriched medical historiography of colonial India. Surprisingly, *kala-azar* has not so far been taken up as a case study. This chapter is an attempt to situate the case of *kala-azar* (visceral leishmaniasis) epidemics in the medical historiography of British India.

I Colonial infrastructure and dissemination of the disease

In the postcolonial literature, India has been seen as the quagmire of lethal diseases and epidemics. Plague, malaria, cholera and smallpox have been consigned as Indian epidemics thriving on her enervating climate, untidiness, obscurantism and lack of social services among the people. But many of these constructs are empirically untenable. Most of the diseases stated above were of global occurrence. European countries had been attacked by plague in the sixth century during the reign of the Emperor Justinian of Byzantium. The 'Black Death' (bubonic plague) occurred throughout Europe in the fourteenth and fifteenth centuries and continued until the seventeenth century.[1] Smallpox occurred as epidemic in 581 in northern and western Europe and was still rampant in the seventeenth century.[2] Cholera and malaria were also endemic in parts of Europe and America. On the contrary, colonial rule is held responsible for the outbreak of epidemics in India. Plague became an epidemic due to official negligence. Other epidemics like malaria were very much connected with British railway expansion in India, immigration of labour and their concentration in unhygienic labour colonies of British plantations, mines and factories and inadequate network of hospitals and dispensaries. Many of these diseases, once widespread, have been pushed back to the warmer and poorer parts of the world by the success of hygiene and preventive measures in the more developed parts of the world.[3]

The tropical climate was considered to be the prime cause of European ill health. India was conceived as a land of dirt, disease and sudden death, where the Englishman was not likely to enjoy a healthy life. Philip Curtin has described India as a home of all dreadful diseases and epidemics where the ruling class migrated only to face death,[4] highlighting the binary contrast between the West and the East. This has also been reflected in the writing of colonial medical officers and imperial politicians, which underlines that the East was dark, while the West was 'enlightened', 'modern' and 'civilized'.

Presumably, the tropical climate seemed to have not abruptly changed its character in colonial India. It was the same tropical climate that existed in pre-colonial India too. But the outbreak of epidemics occurred repeatedly during colonial rule only, affecting the subcontinent as a whole. Some of these lethal diseases also continued to act as endemic for quite a long time in the areas traversed by the epidemic during the colonial administration. Though we get references of severe outbreak of pestilence in a few parts in pre-colonial India, they were occasional phenomena. For instance, in 1575, Gouda, once the magnificent city of India and the seat of wealth and luxury, was humbled to the dust owing to the outbreak of a pestilence, the cause of which was unknown, killing thousands of people.[5] In 1574, there was a virulent epidemic of smallpox in Assam in the course of which many people died.[6] But they occurred occasionally and remained confined to a particular region. Epidemics became frequent with the coming of colonialism.

Until the germ theory of disease was recognized towards the end of the nineteenth century, the health officials of India generally believed in the miasma theory of diseases,[7] that is, diseases were caused by some poisonous chemical brought by certain weather conditions, except in case of smallpox and contagious diseases. This hypothesis proved to be incorrect in the light of the germ theory of disease, which confirmed that the real causes of disease were specific living microorganisms. The germs were everywhere and consequently the disease. But disease became a part of wider condemnation of African and Asian backwardness.

However, recent writers are much more critical about colonialism itself, which is regarded as a major health hazard for indigenous people. Colonialism introduced Old World diseases among vulnerable populations, often with fatal consequences.[8] Some epidemic diseases are said to have been brought by the Europeans in their colonies, as revealed by the scholar that, for instance, plague was brought to India in the 1890s by the Europeans as smallpox and measles accompanied the Spanish conquests of Mexico and Peru in the early sixteenth century.[9] British citizens who travelled to India carried incipient germs in them and these flared up in the inter-communicating zone when they met the 'native' population. The Europeans brought venereal diseases, such as syphilis which was called *firangi roga* (disease of the Europeans). The white soldiers were potent disseminators of this disease about which Ballhatchet in his *Race, Sex and Class under the Raj* has so vividly written.

In fact, European commercial and political penetration in the nineteenth century, and the creation of colonial infrastructure – roads, railways, the system of labour migration and so forth – facilitated the spread of disease vectors – the mosquitoes, flees and lice by which epidemics were communicated – and dissemination of diseases.[10] The unhygienic coolie lines where the labourers were forced to stay by the British capitalists in the plantations, mines and factories facilitated diffusion of the epidemic diseases. The reason for cholera epidemics in India was attributed to the unsanitary conditions in the villages. But the common people and the raiyats should not be blamed for the lack of sanitary consciousness. The apathy and negligence of the government cannot be overlooked, because none of Bengal's villages possessed a single road to remove the filth. On the contrary, the spread of cholera was aided by newly introduced faster modes of communication like steamships and railways.[11] There is no gainsaying the fact that the nature of colonial economic exploitation and the consequent ecological changes brought about far-reaching and enduring effects on public health. Ira Klein has stated that expansion of irrigation canals and construction of railway embankments created favourable habitats for malaria-carrying mosquitoes in India.[12]

Kala-azar, or Black Fever, has also been attributed to climate, but the climatic influence on *kala-azar* occurrence in India is not convincing. For, this disease was not only confined to India and even occurred in the temperate zones. It was prevalent in China, the Mediterranean basin and in European countries like Italy, France, Spain, Portugal and

Greece. It became a global disease, but Indian 'backwardness' was blamed for it.

The global occurrence of *kala-azar* would seem to indicate that its vector, the sandfly, had a worldwide existence. As the sandflies, which have existed for 30 million years in the world, developed the habit of sucking blood for protein, they transmitted infection first to reptiles and then to mammals, and finally to humans.[13] Of the biting insects, sandflies were often more annoying in Assam, existing there long before the outbreak of the *kala-azar* epidemics.[14] So the possibility of the spread of the disease transmitted by sandflies cannot be ignored. They must have had a suitable atmosphere for further breeding after plantations sprung up during the Company's rule. Though very little is known about the disease, such as dropsical effusions, fever or ague with enlargement of the spleen could have been malaria or *kala-azar* that existed there even in the 1830s. But there was not the diffusion of fever in any alarming degree. Black fever broke out in epidemic form in Assam only after the extensive commercial enterprise of tea plantations in the forested territories of upper Assam was undertaken in the second half of the nineteenth century. This disease spread to the adjoining states, particularly Bengal and Bihar, after European commercial and political penetration in the nineteenth century, and the creation of colonial infrastructure – roads, railways, the system of labour migration – facilitated the spread of the disease vector by which epidemics were communicated and disseminated. The unhygienic coolie lines where the labourers were forced to stay by the British capitalists in the plantations, mines and factories facilitated diffusion of the epidemic diseases.

Kala-azar is believed to have appeared in the Garo Hills around the year 1869. Thence, it spread up the Assam Valley during the next three decades. In fact, the spread of *kala-azar* rapidly followed in the wake of the opening up of communication by rail and road in connection with British commercial and military penetration. The disease moved along the lines of communication in Bengal and Bihar. The fatal Burdwan fever epidemic, in which both *kala-azar* and malaria ravaged the country simultaneously, spread over Bengal districts following the main lines of communications. During the course of his investigation in 1910 in Assam, Leonard Rogers had predicted as a result of railway communication an extension of *kala-azar* sooner or later into the populous Golaghat area and the spread of the disease up the remainder of Assam Valley. His prediction proved to be true after a few years. The progressive opening up of tea plantations in large areas of Assam, the coming and going of the tea-garden coolies and accelerated movement of the people from infected areas to uninfected ones also facilitated its dissemination. It had been pointed out in a well-known medical journal in 1913 that the movement of the tea-garden workers caused the diffusion of the disease not only throughout Assam, but to other parts of India.[15] The unhygienic coolie lines in the tea plantations where the labourers were forced to stay by the British capitalists facilitated spread of this epidemic disease.

II Combatting kala-azar

There is controversy amongst scholars on the colonial health policy and impact of Western medicine on Indian society. Indian scholars are much more critical of it. Scholars like Radhika Ramasubban, Poonam Bala, Anil Kumar, Kabita Ray, V.R. Muraleedharan, Chittabrata Palit, Deepak Kumar and others are of the view that colonial medical policy privileged the needs of Europeans and the military.[16] The rulers primarily concentrated on how to provide sanitary and medical facilities to the military. Gradually it extended to urban areas and civil lines of European population and mines, plantations and factories. They argue that diseases like cholera, malaria, influenza and *kala-azar* threatened the security of British troops and civilians and high rate of mortality from these diseases prompted health measures across the subcontinent.

Ramasubban adds that the British developed a distinctly colonial mode of healthcare, characterized by residential segregation and neglect of the indigenous population.[17] David Arnold has also observed that Western medicine remained too closely identified with the requirements of the colonial state and so was remote from the needs of the people. It failed to make the transition from state medicine to public health. He also holds a critical opinion on the British India government for devolving much of the responsibility for sanitation and health to poorly funded and inexperienced local authorities.[18] Mark Harrison, however, raises questions over the claim that the limited scope of colonial medicine was chiefly a consequence of governmental neglect and inadequate funding from the state. He does not agree that deficiencies of medical and sanitary provisions in India can be attributed entirely to the colonial mode of healthcare. He points out that the state was much more active in the provision of public health by funding health measures, which was rather constrained by indigenous indifference or, even, hostility to medical and sanitary intervention.[19] Dismissing the view of Ramasubban, Roger Jeffery holds that the most substantial urban improvements (water supply and drainage) were designed to improve the living conditions of Indians and that the army and European civil population did not need so many hospitals and dispensaries.[20]

It is argued that the government's role to combat epidemic diseases in India was not commendable. Anti-malaria measures were found to be inadequate and unsatisfactory, and hence 100 million people suffered from it, of which 20 million died every year even in the 1930s. C.A. Bentley noted that only a very small proportion of malaria-affected people of Bengal received proper treatment. The vast majority of the sufferers from malaria received either no medical attention whatsoever or entirely depended on the treatment of village practitioners. Though quinine was supplied by the government agencies in the 1920s and 1930s, all the sufferers did not receive quinine in adequate doses. Even the government could not check the supply of spurious quinine in the market. The picture was very gloomy in southwest Bengal. Moreover, all the malaria-affected people of Bengal were not brought within the purview of treatment facilities in the late nineteenth century and in the early twentieth century. The non-government agencies, including the individual Bengalis, had undoubtedly tried to provide anti-malaria drugs to the affected people, but they had also certain limitations. Since the European population was concentrated in the town of Calcutta, attempts were made to insulate the British population in the town from the ravages of epidemic malaria.[21] V.R. Muraleedharan has referred to the lukewarm response of the government against malaria in Madras, illustrating that malaria was more severe in the countryside where little anti-malaria operations were taken up compared to urban areas.[22] Similarly, the weaknesses of anti-plague measures of the government have also been exemplified. There was segregation and forced hospitalization merely on suspicion of the native population during plague epidemics in the 1890s, and the measures to control plague are said to have been more militaristic than medical. It may, however, be pointed out, in this context, that there is ongoing controversy amongst scholars over the plague control policy of the British India Government in the late nineteenth century, and the argument goes in this way that the government reluctantly had been compelled by the contemporary situation to introduce draconian measures to control plague or there had been an increase in public expenditure by the government since 1896 on public health, sanitation and medical research.[23] In regard to the medical policy to control smallpox, Sanjoy Bhattacharya argues that though the colonial medicine in urban contexts catered to the European element and richer sections of Indian society, the situation in the countryside was markedly different. Official measures in rural areas were not targeted solely at its European inhabitants or select

Indians, and concerted efforts were made, most visibly during epidemics, to ensure vaccination of the rural people. This work was impeded by the deficiencies of technology.[24]

Interestingly, the debate on the efficacy of the medical policy to control epidemic disease seems to be unending. Let us see, in this context, what happened in the case of *kala-azar*. *Kala-azar* was a major health problem in British India, affecting the subcontinent for nearly a century. *Kala-azar* appeared to be an unknown disease to the people under colonial rule. The Garos of North-East India described it as *Sarkari Bemari* or British Government disease, owing possibly to its appearance being contemporaneous with that of British rule. It was a very severe and lethal disease with a high mortality rate of more than 95 per cent. *Kala-azar* ravaged a large part of eastern and northeastern India and the worst affected areas were Assam, Bengal and Bihar.

Kala-azar unleashed utter devastation on the population in terms of mortality and morbidity. During 1921–40, it took a toll of 234,931 lives in the Bengal Presidency.[25] The *kala-azar* situation was acute in Bihar in the first half of the twentieth century, killing a large number of people. Its incidence rapidly increased in the 1900s, affecting the districts of Patna, Gaya, Sahabad, Munghyr and Darbhanga. It caused havoc in Assam from 1880 to 1920. It was reported in a renowned medical journal that in three tea-growing districts – namely, Nowgong, Darrang and Kamrup – from 1891 to 1911 the deaths of no fewer than 152,000 persons were ascribed to this terrible disease.[26] These are only approximate estimates. The mortality from *kala-azar* was so serious in Assam that it was difficult to gain any exact idea of the absolute number of deaths it had caused. Depopulation and desertion caused by *kala-azar* adversely affected cultivation and land had lost its value. The decrease of cultivation also resulted in a corresponding loss of revenue.

Kala-azar became a matter of concern for the government from the early 1880s when it became a serious menace in certain parts of Assam. The rapid progress of the disease towards the areas close to tea gardens alarmed the government. British investment in tea plantations might be at stake if the garden workers and surrounding areas of the gardens were infected by this disease. It was also causing heavy depopulation in the tea-growing districts of Assam. Therefore, the government, in order to arrest its diffusion, immediately organized special measures of medical relief by starting dispensaries at several suitable centres and employing a number of medical subordinates to travel about and visit the people at their houses.

However, these measures were found to be ineffective, because there was no known remedy. Preventive measures like segregation and evacuation and disinfecting operations, such as fumigation of houses with burning sulpher, washing of beds with strong boiling carbolic lotion, could not reduce the infection and *kala-azar* continued to take its toll.[27] The health officials of Assam convened meetings to explain to the *panchayats* and *gaonburas* (village headmen) the nature of this disease and the method of preventing its spread. As a further method of control, in 1917 the Government of Assam enacted certain regulations under the provisions of the Imperial Epidemic Diseases Act of 1897 (Act III of 1897). But they could not check the disease.

British medical intervention against *kala-azar* succeeded after 1920 with the introduction of antimony treatment in the form of tartar emetic.[28] This treatment by tartar emetic was recommended as a method of prevention by Knowles, IMS, in 1920 and the result of its trial was encouraging.[29] With this the era of effective treatment for *kala-azar* cases may be said to have begun in India. A special hospital for the treatment of *kala-azar* was built at Nazira in the Sibsagar district in 1919 where treatment with tartar emetic started.[30] Soon afterwards, the number of special *kala-azar* hospitals and dispensaries rapidly increased. The Sanitary Department laid emphasis on providing treatment facilities in as many areas as possible, and 146 special *kala-azar* centres were running under this department in 1920.[31] *Kala-azar* cases were even treated at the hospital attached to the Pasteur Institute in Shillong. Besides these, there were government dispensaries, Local Board dispensaries and travelling dispensaries of the Medical Department for the treatment of this disease. By the mid-1920s more than 400 hospitals and dispensaries were working in Assam for the treatment of this disease.[32] Treatment with this drug also started in Bengal and Bihar. Numerous centres for the free treatment of this disease were opened in several districts in Bengal and trained doctors were appointed. All District Board dispensaries were made centres of treatment with requisite medicines and instruments.[33] A total of 92,000 cases of *kala-azar* were treated in the hospital and dispensaries of Bihar in 1939. Five *kala-azar* centres were opened in North Bihar, where the incidence of the disease was highest, in that year, and doctors were sent to Patna Medical College for receiving training in the technique of *kala-azar* serum tests.[34]

Thus, organization for treatment rapidly grew and active operations started. By that time some more efficacious drugs like urea stibamine and neostibosan to tackle it more effectively were also found and used by the doctors. Urea stibamine was a 'dramatic medical breakthrough' in tropical medicine and became the routine treatment in India with its many thousands of cases.[35] The Government of Assam started mass free treatment with this drug from 1927and it was found to be successful. The government also made the treatment compulsory under the revised *kala-azar* regulations in 1920 framed under the Epidemic Diseases Act.[36] Under the new regulations *kala-azar* patients were ordered to undergo a complete course of treatment. But keeping in mind the implications of the ruthless anti-plague measures in Bombay, the government of Assam abstained from taking any drastic action to force the patients to undergo treatment. Penal power under the regulations had been used very sparingly. Regulations would mainly be effective as a lever to induce the sufferers to take treatment without resort to prosecution.[37] All persons refusing or discontinuing treatment before a complete cure were reported to magistrates, who took steps to induce the patients to resume the treatment. This seems to have facilitated the survey operation for detecting the cases of interrupted treatment and bringing them again under regular treatment. Treatment with urea stibamine proved to be very effective and popular in Bengal and Bihar too. All these steps resulted in a decline of mortality due to *kala-azar*.

Thus, the fatal impact of the disease is said to have been brought under near-control as diagnostic, curative and preventive measures including technology were implemented.[38] The treatment spread and intensified through propaganda campaigns, legal measures and medical research. The Kala-azar Commission was appointed by the Government of India in April 1924 with S.R. Christophers as its director to study the disease in Assam. The *kala-azar* research wards of the Pasteur Institute and Medical Research Institute at Shillong were actively involved in their chosen field. Their recommendations led the government to initiate mass treatment with efficacious drugs. Researches on this disease continued under the auspices of the Indian Research Fund Association (IRFA) until the end of British rule at the Pasteur Institute, Shillong and at the School of Tropical Medicine and Hygiene, Calcutta. Experiments conducted in these institutions on the vector's behaviour, early diagnosis of *kala-azar* by easy pathological tests, new drugs like SAG and so forth until the mid-1940s had obviously added to the knowledge about this fatal disease. At the same time quite a large number of people were brought under successful treatment and their lives were saved.

This case study underlines that in Assam the government gave priority to the control of *kala-azar*. This was thanks to the health officials of Assam, who felt the nature of the holocaust caused by it and repeatedly appealed to the government to tackle it successfully. Assam was more notoriously affected by *kala-azar* than any other part of India. *Kala-azar* was more prevalent there than malaria at least until 1930. Moreover, the British government had a stake in the smooth running of Assam tea plantations, which was threatened by this fatal disease. Therefore, its protection seemed to have been the primary objective of the government, and hence anti-*kala-azar* measures received priority. In Bengal and Bihar, the government perhaps underestimated the intensity of the sufferings and invalidity caused by this disease and more attention was given to combat malaria than *kala-azar*.

III A critique of the policy of containment

But the other side of the story reveals that despite all the probable methods of controlling *kala-azar*, including the efficacy of modern insecticides such as DDT against the *kala-azar* vector, the sandfly, that were known, little had been done by the state to utilize this knowledge, and the disease was far from under control. In Bengal, the recorded incidence of *kala-azar* (which is probably a fraction of the actual incidence of the disease) had been more or less steady for twenty years during 1924–43. Though the disease was showing signs of regression in certain districts in western Bengal, the trend of incidence was towards an increase in a number of districts in East Bengal, particularly in Chittagong, Dacca and Faridpur districts in 1944.[39] It may be noted here that anti-*kala-azar* measures, both preventive and curative, were adopted to control *kala-azar* in Bengal as a whole, but the measures seemed to have not been effectively implemented in all the affected places. The preventive measures were not well organized and curative measures, such as treatment through temporary *kala-azar* dispensaries, are said to have been withdrawn in the places where the incidence of the disease was low. Consequently, *kala-azar* flared up in these places gradually. Moreover, the prevalence of insanitary and unhygienic conditions and the construction of roads and embankments causing an impediment to drainage added to the increase in incidences of the disease. In fact, there had been a widespread increase of incidences in different areas of Bengal from 1945, and it became so rampant in Bengal and its incidence was so high that it could still be regarded as a grave public health problem. Even in Calcutta where a well-marked focus of infection was discovered in about 1920–21, the disease was not only more prevalent in 1947 in that area but it had spread to other areas of the town as well.[40] In Assam there had been an increase in outbreaks of *kala-azar* in the 1940s. A number of *kala-azar* cases (91,552) were treated there in the years 1941–45, whereas it was 78,811 during 1936–40.[41] In Bihar there was an epidemic of *kala-azar* from 1939 to 1941. The situation in north Bihar was appalling in the 1930s and 1940s. In many villages in or near the Kosi belt in Darbhanga District, no children of 3 to 4 years of age could be found, and pregnant women did not survive for long.[42] The incidence of *kala-azar* was actually much higher than it was supposed to be. Surprisingly, with all the knowledge of the disease – its cause, diagnosis, treatment and prevention – *kala-azar* was widely prevalent in many parts of east and northeast India with an increasing trend towards the end of British rule. Mortality due to *kala-azar* continued to rise. The number of deaths due to it in Bengal rose from 16,766 in 1925 to 21,642 in 1938 (though it is only an approximate estimate).[43]

Though *kala-azar* treatment was found to be successful in the 1920s with the help of effective drugs saving a large number of patients, it is difficult to get an exact idea about what percentage of affected people were brought under treatment, because the actual number of sufferers and mortality due to it seems to have been unknown to the health officials. Unfortunately, any attempt to identify *kala-azar* mortality is hampered by the absence of statistical records before 1890 and also by the dubious reliability of the data thereafter. It is learnt that mortality from 'fevers' had been increasing in Assam from the early 1880s, and *kala-azar* seemed to have been the principal cause of this increase.[44] Deaths due to it had been registered under 'Fevers' all the years previous to 1890. Fevers (intermittent and others) were the most severe of the prevailing diseases and exceedingly common among the people and sepoys in the nineteenth century.[45] *Kala-azar* might have occupied the largest share in the mortality supposedly caused by 'Fevers', because both sandflies and fever with unusual enlargement of the spleen were very common in colonial Assam. In malaria cases, the spleen does not get so extraordinarily enlarged as in *kala-azar* cases. Moreover, health officials' reports reveal that malaria was not so rampant in Assam as *kala-azar* was before 1930.

Statistics regarding mortality due to epidemic diseases especially in rural areas were unreliable because the method of recording the cause of death was highly dubious. There was dearth of medical men, except in towns and *Thana* (police station) headquarters, and the diagnosis of the cause of death was made by the *gaonburas* (village headmen) in Assam or village *chaukidars* in Bengal and Bihar or by the patients' relations. Statistics were maintained on the basis of their verbal reports. There was no arrangement to keep local records for checking them on the spot. Little improvement was effected on this method of collecting vital statistics even in the twentieth century.[46] Moreover, for want of better diagnoses, especially in the village dispensaries, many *kala-azar* deaths were attributed to other causes like anaemia, beri-beri or anchylostomiasis, which were somewhat common amongst *kala-azar* cases. In fact, prior to the discovery of the *kala-azar* parasite in 1903, medical men confused it with other diseases. For instance, Dr. Giles concluded that *kala-azar* was the same disease that was known as 'beri-beri of Ceylon', and a case of *kala-azar* in Upper Assam would be called anaemia of coolies, or beri-beri.[47]

The official reports cannot provide the actual number of *kala-azar* cases. Captain James, IMS, who was appointed by the Government of India to investigate *kala-azar* in Assam in 1904, was of the opinion that it was much more prevalent than was generally thought to be the case. In a village within 2 miles of Guahati dispensary James found that over 20 per cent of the people were suffering from it, but only eight cases of diseases had been recorded in the books of the Guahati dispensary as having been treated during 1903.[48] Many cases, which were formerly diagnosed as 'fever', were later found to be *kala-azar*.[49] The disease was actually more prevalent than the reports indicated. In 1923, the *Indian Medical Gazette* revealed that the conditions in Bengal seemed to indicate such widespread and heavy incidence of the disease that *kala-azar* rather than malaria appeared to be the chief public health problem of rural Bengal.[50]

It might have been thought before 1920 that *kala-azar* was a problem of little importance in Bengal. But as the Calcutta School of Tropical Medicine (CSTM) started working from 1920, there had been a steady and constantly increasing influx of *kala-azar* cases from all over Bengal, some even from Orissa. It was observed from peripheral blood examination, the aldehyde test and spleen puncture at the laboratory of the CSTM, that not less than 60 per cent of all cases of fever with enlarged spleen which attended the general out-patient clinic were cases, not of malaria, but of *kala-azar*. Perhaps the most striking evidence of the widespread incidence of *kala-azar* in Bengal was the splendid work of the Bengal Anti-kala-azar League under Dr. N. Bhattacharji, a work which was widely acclaimed. The survey report of the League reveals that no less than 80 per cent of patients with fever and enlargement of the spleen attending the treatment centre of the League in the 24-Parganas (1923) proved to be cases of *kala-azar*. On the basis of this survey report and data collected from other sources in the same year, L.E. Napier estimated that the total number of cases of *kala-azar* in Bengal was at least 1.5 million. It may, however, be doubted in this context that a sample survey based on the findings in one or two areas can give the exact picture of the incidence of the disease in the whole province, as the incidence of the *kala-azar* was not uniform in all the districts of Bengal, and the figures published by the Public Health Department seem to have been quite reliable for the estimation of the relative prevalence of the disease. But in calculating the incidence of the disease in Bengal, the figures would fall short of the actual number of cases because a large number of patients from the districts would come to Calcutta for treatment. As per the hospital and dispensary records, the incidence of *kala-azar* in Bengal during 1931–40 was also alarming, amounting to more than 1.1 million.[51] More importantly, very few rural dispensaries had the efficiency to detect whether the cases with fever and enlarged spleen were of *kala-azar*, and therefore in most cases these were misdiagnosed as malaria, and thus actual estimation of the number of *kala-azar* cases was constrained. In fact, the incidence of *kala-azar* was so high in Bengal that it was no less a grave problem than malaria to the medical and public health authorities.

It would not be an exaggeration to say that quite a large number of these sufferers did not receive the benefits of successful treatment. The government had actually failed to provide *kala-azar* treatment facilities to the affected villagers. Thousands of them were left untreated. The government might possibly have faced certain constraints, geographical, technological or social, to bring all the sufferers, particularly in the remote villages, under treatment. But deficiencies in the medical policy of the government cannot be overlooked. The measures adopted by the government to tackle this disease in India are said to have been too limited. After 1920, the responsibility of the situation was left to the local authorities – District Boards, Union Boards and so forth. The District Boards in the affected districts of Bengal were actively engaged in treating *kala-azar* cases. But lack of funds continued to be the chief problem with them. Financial grants for controlling *kala-azar* to these bodies were far from adequate.[52] In fact the District Boards were not in a position to cope with the situation. Compared to the number of affected people, the number of *kala-azar* centres was very small in Bengal. A large number of special *kala-azar* centres and dispensaries within a convenient distance of each other were required. But that remained a dream to the people. What is more, most of the *kala-azar* dispensaries were not in good shape, lacking qualified doctors, medicine and necessary equipment. Even Sir Arthur Dash, the secretary to the government of Bengal, noted in 1927 the wretched condition of a *kala-azar* dispensary in Bengal, which was equipped with unskilled medical practitioners.[53] A large number of *kala-azar* patients would come to Calcutta for treatment, resulting in overcrowding of the city hospitals. Many patients were even turned away.[54] *Kala-azar* patients flocked to the School of Tropical Medicine and Hygiene, Calcutta, in such a huge number that available staff was unable to deal expeditiously with all the cases.[55] Moreover, since the facilities for pathological investigation for diagnosis were inadequate or almost non-existent in the village dispensaries, *kala-azar* cases were generally treated as malaria. It resulted in prolonged suffering of the patients and a fatal end of their lives. Local demands for free supply of *kala-azar* specifics could not be met and consequently many of the *kala-azar* centres had to be closed down.[56]

The application of a large-scale survey and curative treatment as a prophylactic measure against *kala-azar* could be a successful venture. But that was not the case, as it could involve huge money which the government did not spend. Even Rogers had noted that with sufficient funds and medical staff, a very great deal could be done to eradicate this terrible disease.[57] But this was lacking. The problem of medical relief for the rural areas in Bihar had not been sufficiently tackled. Though the people had come to understand the efficiency of treatment by tarter emetic for *kala-azar*, it was not possible for the majority of the poor rural patients suffering from this ailment to get the benefit of this treatment for want of dispensaries in the vicinity.[58] Treatment of *kala-azar* needed a careful technique as regards preparation and an experienced doctor. Both were lacking in the village dispensaries of the affected districts of Bihar. These were available in big hospitals[59] in the towns where effective treatment was carried on. Health organization was poor indeed. The Public Health Report of Bihar reveals that without effective health organization and staff, effective control of the epidemic was hardly possible. Timely adequate measures were urgent for combating epidemics, but these were found to be absent.[60]

There was no dearth of people's cooperation in combating *kala-azar*. People of Assam, Bengal and Bihar were not opposed to *kala-azar* treatment and Western medicine. They attended the hospitals for successful medication. In different instances, *kala-azar* patients in Assam arrived at the hospital unexpectedly for treatment on their own initiative, at their own expenses after selling up their property to provide themselves with funds.[61] People cooperated with the health officials in maintaining regulations under the Epidemic Diseases Act for checking the progress of *kala-azar*. The villagers reported *kala-azar*, requested for medical assistance and attended anti-*kala-azar* campaigns conducted by the Health Department. Patients from distant villages of Bengal walked many miles and stood in the queue for urea stibamine injections in the urban hospitals. But the health policy of the government had a very limited coverage. People's voluntary work was not lacking in the domain of public health in Bengal and other provinces, especially in anti-*kala-azar* and anti-malaria activities. Certain voluntary associations like the Central Co-operative Anti-Malarial Society and the Bengal Health Association opened numerous centres where gratuitous treatment was given to *kala-azar* patients. But the government assisted them with very small grants.[62]

The grants sanctioned by the government for *kala-azar* treatment were not adequate. Bihar received a meagre amount to tackle it in the 1920s and 1930s, when the disease was widely prevalent. It was 10,150 rupees in 1926, 5,000 rupees in 1927, 7,500 rupees in 1932 and 10,000 rupees in 1933. A lot more money was required for the treatment of *kala-azar* cases in Bihar, but the medical budget was low indeed.[63] It was widely prevalent for a long time in North Bihar. But as it was believed to be a slightly infected area, adequate attention was not given to this disease here.[64] The Medical Department, perhaps more than any other, had felt the effect of the financial stringency. There was fund retrenchment and their activities restricted. The condition of most of the hospitals in the rural areas was deplorable because of financial restrictions.[65] In 1943, the expenditure per head on medical relief and public health for India was between 3 and 4 *annas* per annum. Of this, only one-third was spent on preventive medicine. It was very small compared to the UK where 54 rupees/per head per year were spent on medical relief alone.[66]

The apathetic attitude of the government of India to medical research has been criticized by the researchers like Ross, Haffkine and also by the Bhore Committee (1943). Medical research in India did not receive priority, and it was secondary to political and economic imperialism.[67] The post-war Health Survey Committee was of the opinion that the influence of the central government in the matters of epidemics, medical educational standards and research in the provinces seemed weak.[68] Recent studies have been critical of it and argue that the research structure that eventually evolved was the result of a piece-meal and adhoc response to sudden epidemic emergencies, and there existed no enduring foundation for the growth of medical science in the country.[69] But the argument does not claim acceptance by some contemporary Western scholars. Mark Harrison is of the view that much of the government's plan for a more extensive network of laboratories remained on paper, but it is unfair to claim that research laboratories provided no enduring foundation for the growth of medical science in India.[70]

In this context, it may be pointed out that laboratory research in the colonies received a new dimension by the end of the nineteenth century as a result of the emergence of Pasteurian bacteriological science and germ theory when a shift from clinical medicine to laboratory medicine was found. The British in India set up several bacteriological laboratories, such as the Imperial Bacteriological Laboratory in Poona (1890), Plague Research Laboratory in Bombay (1896), the Pasteur Institute of India in Kasauli (1900), Central Research Institute at Kasauli (1905) and others for promoting bacteriological and prophylactic research, providing opportunities to scientists to make experiments and observation.[71] These colonial medical research institutes had undoubtedly contributed to the extension of medical knowledge in British India, and it is hard to deny their contributions even in post-independence India. But the development of medical science and the public health system in British India was not an organic one.

The government seems to have been reluctant to provide requisite funds for *kala-azar* research in India. Grants recommended for *kala-azar* research at the Calcutta School of Tropical Medicine, Medical School in Darbhanga (Bihar) and Pasteur Institute Shillong were not sufficient.[72] Medical research in the India Research Fund Association (IRFA) also faced financial constraints. Even the financial assistance from the government was too small to run a teaching academic centre like Carmichael Medical College, Calcutta. The matter was raised even in the Bengal Legislative Council in 1930 by Rev. B.A. Nag, moving a resolution for increasing the annual recurring grant to this college, when he referred to the joint inspection report by Col. R.A. Needham and Sir Norman Walker on behalf of the British General Medical Council which stated that ever since its establishment, this college had never received adequate financial support to enable it to fulfill its obligations as an academic institution.[73]

Actually, the apathy of the government to medical research because of financial involvement was not singularly seen in this disease. The same attitude was observed in the case of some other diseases as well. The suggestion of Col. W.G. King, Sanitary Commissioner of Madras, for undertaking investigation as to the differentiating various types of fever and their etiology in 1904, which could be of much scientific interest, was not considered. Though his suggestion was brought in the context of anti-malaria surveys and research, the Madras government ignored King's suggestion for large-scale measures apparently because of its financial implications.[74]

It would not be an exaggeration to say that the British India Government never demonstrated any liberal gesture in incurring financial liabilities for promoting medical research or public health in India compared to enormous sums spent for other departments like defence and police. Even the government was reluctant to see the IMS scientists engaging in medical research. In fact, research on preventive and curative measures did not receive greater attention of the government. The government undertook only some palliative measures when necessity arose.

No effective means of prevention, based on true epidemiology of the disease, had been devised. The measures for vector control had not been found even after 1942 when the mystery of transmission of *kala-azar* infection was finally explored, and the Director of Public Health, Assam, advocated further preventive measures mainly for controlling the vectors. The fact that the sandflies were sensitive to DDT, pyrethrum, was also known. But the government seldom used this knowledge to control them. There was neither any short-term nor any long-term projects for vector control, either by spraying insecticides or by providing better sanitation even after the war. Consequently, its occurrence and recrudescence could not be prevented.

Improved sanitation, as was suggested by Leonard Rogers, could be a remedy for *kala-azar*. Improvement in sanitation in rural areas and liberal use of lime wash in the habitats of sandflies might possibly have been effective in making conditions unsuitable for the *kala-azar* vector. But improvement in this field was very meagre.[75] Neither the Sanitary Boards nor the District Boards could make much headway in this regard. On the contrary, Indians were blamed for their apathy and resistance to sanitary programmes and other health measures. The conservative and superstitious beliefs of indigenous people might possibly have stood in the way of sanitary reforms to some extent. But this cannot be a defensive argument for inadequate sanitary measures. The government did not think of tackling these constraints and was reluctant to make any financial commitments for sanitary improvement.

Conclusion

The foregoing analysis leads to this observation that the policy of the government to control *kala-azar* had certain deficiencies. What was required was a more concerted effort targeted at prevention and eradication of this disease. It is true that anti-*kala-azar* measures adopted by the government had a bearing upon the incidences of the disease. But the question does arise as to the adequacy of these measures and the efficacy of epidemic control policy as well. Arguably, Western medicine had the efficacy to successfully fight against it. Research on *kala-azar* sponsored by the colonial administration added to the knowledge of disease control. In 1924, a special Kala-azar Commission was appointed by the Government of India to make further experiments on this disease. Investigation on the *kala-azar* transmission problem, which was resolved in 1942, was undoubtedly a great achievement of medical research in India. Experiments and researches conducted on this disease under the auspices of IRFA at the Pasteur Institute, Shillong and the School of Tropical Medicine and Hygiene, Calcutta, on the vector's behaviour and new drugs like SAG have obviously provided knowledge and tools for its conquest. But the disease could not be eradicated. It is argued that governmental measures to control it were too limited. There was lack of proper measures for its prevention and eradication, and a disease control programme was launched on a very small budget.

But amazingly, India could not be free from *kala-azar* even after 1947 when colonial complexities were no longer prevalent. It is still prevalent in India, posing serious threat to her people. Health policy changed following India's independence in 1947 and control of epidemic diseases received priority. *Kala-azar* occurrence and mortality due to it in India declined rapidly in the 1960s as a result of the collateral benefit of extensive DDT spraying under the National Malaria Eradication Programme (1958).[76] Effective treatment of detected cases also added to it. But it resurged in the mid-1970s and assumed epidemic proportions in North Bihar in 1976–77, with an extension to West Bengal, affecting thousands of people. The disease was, however, never extinct, and all through 1960 to 1975 transmission at a low level was going on in the areas where sporadic cases were reported, particularly in Bihar.[77] In fact, adequate and organized control methods had never been undertaken in those areas. DDT spraying ceased as and when *kala-azar* transmission reduced and death due to it reached almost nil. Thereafter, *kala-azar* transmission continued, resulting in more than 250,000 cases and several thousand deaths until 1990. The National Planning Commission approved a centrally sponsored scheme for *kala-azar* control from the year 1990–91 with liberal financial and material assistance. Specific funds were made available for its control during 1990–91 and subsequently the budget was enhanced. Besides, the WHO and UNICEF have also provided medical, technical and financial assistance for its control and elimination. But it is yet to be eradicated.

Kala-azar does not receive priority in the health policy of the government. The governments (central and the states) allocate meagre funds for its prevention and eradication. It might be argued that since *kala-azar* affects only a small part of the subcontinent and a small number of people, it gets little importance in the health agenda. But the disease management and eradication programme of India as a whole is not laudable. Malaria is much more prevalent than *kala-azar*, posing a serious threat to the people. Tuberculosis is nearly 100 per cent curable, yet thousands of people continue to die every year in India. The persistent neglect of health matters in public policy is evident by the abysmally low level of expenditure on health. Disease eradication programmes have therefore been affected by the overall shortage of funds. Central grants for disease control programmes fell from 41 per cent in 1984–85 to 29 per cent in 1988–89, and to 18.5 per cent in 1992–93.[78] The government gives low priority to prevention of disease and protection of health. The health service in general has therefore been deteriorated.

Notes

1 Frederick F. Cartwright, *A Social History of Medicine*, New York: Longman, 1977, 61–2.
2 Ibid., 75.
3 Chittabrata Palit, 'Epidemics and Empire: A Critique of Public Health Policy in Colonial India', in Chittabrata Palit and Achintya Dutta (eds.), *History of Medicine in India: The Medical Encounter*, New Delhi: Kalpaz Publications, 2005, 35–47.
4 Philip D. Curtin, *Death by Migration: Europe's Encounter with the Tropical World in the 19th Century*, Cambridge: Cambridge University Press, 1989, chaps. 1–3.
5 Charles J.S. Montagu, *A Concise History of Bengal from the Earliest Period*, edition 1840, 31, in Records of Past Epidemics in India, no date and place of publication [National Archives of India (hereafter NAI)], 2; Acharya Prafulla Chandra Ray and Prabodh Chandra Bandopadhyay, 'Kala-Azar O Tar Pratikarer Itihas' (in Bengali) [History of Kala-azar and Its Remedy], Bharatvarsha, Bhadra 1348, B.Y (1941), 305–7.
6 E.A. Gait, History of Assam, edition 1906, 100 in Records of Past Epidemics in India, 2.
7 Ralph Shlomowitz and Lance Brennan, 'Mortality and Migrant Labour in Assam, 1865–1921', *Indian Economic and Social History Review* (hereafter IESHR), 27, 1, (1990), 85–110.
8 Madhav Gadgil and Ramchandra Guha, *This Fissured Land*, New Delhi: Oxford University Press, 1993, 117.
9 David Arnold (ed.), *Imperial Medicine and Indigenous Societies*, New York: Manchester University Press, 1988, Introduction, 3–5.
10 Arnold, *Imperial Medicine*, 5.
11 Anil Kumar, *Medicine and the Raj: British Medical Policy in India 1835–1911*, New Delhi: Sage Publications Pvt. Ltd., 1998, 171.
12 Ira Klein, 'Malaria and Mortality in Bengal 1840–1921', *IESHR*, 9, 2 (1972), 132–60.

13 P.E.C. Manson-Bahr, 'Old World Leishmaniasis', in F.E.G. Cox (ed.), *The Wellcome Trust Illustrated History of Tropical Diseases*, London: Wellcome Trust, 1996, 206–17.

14 John M. Cosh, *Topography of Assam*, Calcutta: Bengal Military Orphan Press, 1837, 52.

15 'Kala-Azar in Assam', *The Lancet*, (July 5, 1913), 33.

16 Radhika Ramasubban, 'Imperial Health in British India, 1857–1900', in Roy Macleod and Milton Lewis (eds.), *Disease, Medicine and Empire; Perspectives of Western Medicine and the Experience of European Expansion*, London: Routledge, 1988, 38–60; Poonam Bala, *Imperialism and Medicine in Bengal: A Socio-Historical Perspective*, New Delhi: Sage Publications Pvt. Ltd., 1991, chaps. 1–3; Kumar, *Medicine and the Raj*; Kabita Ray, *History of Public Health: Colonial Bengal 1921–1947*, Calcutta: K P Bagchi & Co., 1998, chaps. 1–3; V.R. Muraleedharan, 'Malady in Madras: The Colonial Government's Response to Malaria in the Early 20th Century', in Deepak Kumar (ed.), *Science and Empire, Essays in Indian Context (1700–1947)*, New Delhi: Anamika Prakashan, 1991, 101–14; Palit, *Epidemics and Empire*; Deepak Kumar, *Science and the Raj 1857–1905*, New Delhi: Oxford University Press, 1997, 165.

17 Ramasubban, 'Imperial Health', 38–42.

18 David Arnold, *Colonizing the Body: State Medicine and Epidemic Disease in Nineteenth Century India* (Indian edition), New Delhi: Oxford University Press, 1993, 3; also see, Mark Harrison, *Public Health in British India Anglo-Indian Preventive Medicine 1859–1914*, New Delhi: Foundation Books, 1994, 233.

19 Harrison, *Public Health*, chaps. 6–8 and conclusion; also see, Biswamoy Pati and Mark Harrison (eds.), *Health, Medicine and Empire: Perspective on Colonial India*, New Delhi: Orient Longman Limited, 2001, Introduction, 4.

20 Roger Jeffery, *The Politics of Health in India*, Berkeley: University of California Press, 1988, 101.

21 For details, see C.A. Bentley, *Malaria and Agriculture in Bengal*, Calcutta: Bengal Secretariat Book Depot, 1925, chaps. VI & VII; Ray, *History of Public Health*, 103–29; Arabinda Samanta, *Malarial Fever in Colonial Bengal 1820–1939: Social History of an Epidemic*, Kolkata: Firma K L M Pvt. Ltd., 2002, 120.

22 Muraleedharan, 'Malady in Madras', 103.

23 For details, see Kumar, *Medicine and the Raj*, 190–203; Harrison, *Public Health*, 152–57.

24 Sanjoy Bhattacharya, 'Re-Devising Jennerian Vaccines?: European Technologies, Indian Innovation and the Control of Smallpox in South Asia, 1850–1950', in B. Pati and M. Harrison (eds.), *Health, Medicine and Empire*, (details of publication stated in note no 19) 217–69.

25 The number of *kala-azar* deaths has been calculated from the Bengal Public Health Report for the Years 1921–40 (hereafter BPHR).

26 *The Lancet*, 5 July 1913, 33.

27 Upendranath Brahmachari, *Gleanings from My Research Kala-azar, Its Chemotherapy*, Vol. I, Calcutta: University of Calcutta, 1940, 186.

28 Leonard Rogers introduced tartar emetic first in India in 1915 for the treatment of *kala-azar* cases. This drug gained some reputation in 1918 in

Calcutta. Then it was used for *kala-azar* treatment in Assam. See D Murrison, 'Treatment Campaign against Kala-azar, Assam', Health Bulletin No. 9, Calcutta, 1927, 1.

29　Upendranath Brahmachari, *A Treatise on Kala-Azar*, London: John Bale Sons & Danielson Ltd, 1928, 158.

30　*Annual Sanitary Report of the Province of Assam for the Year 1920*, Shillong: Assam Government Press, 1921, 13 (hereafter ASR, Assam).

31　*ASR, Assam for the Year 1920*, 14.

32　Murrison, *Treatment Campaign*, 5; *Annual Public Health Report of the Province of Assam for the Year 1926*, Shillong: Assam Government Press, 1927, 16 (hereafter APHR, Assam).

33　Resolutions Reviewing the Reports on the Working of District & Local Boards in Bengal during the Year 1925–26, Calcutta, 1927, 3.

34　*Annual Public Health Report of the Province of Bihar for the Year 1938*, Patna: Superintendent Government Printing, 1939, 18 (hereafter APHR, Bihar).

35　MSS/EUR: H.E. Shortt, 'In the Days of the Raj and After, Doctor, Soldier, Scientist, Sikari', 73, British Library [hereafter, BL]; Triennial Report on the Working of the Dispensaries in Assam for the Years 1926, 1927 & 1928, Shillong Assam Government Press, 1928, 5.

36　*APHR, Assam for the Year 1927*, 16.

37　*ASR, Assam for the Year 1920*, 16.

38　Government of Assam, Medical Department (Medical), June 1931, Proc. No. 52, BL; Reports of the Kala-azar Commission, India, Report No. II (1926–1930), Calcutta: Indian Research Fund Association, 1932, 47.

39　P.C. Sengupta, 'History of Kala-azar in India', *The Indian Medical Gazette* (May 1947), 281–6.

40　Sengupta, 'History of Kala-Azar', 285.

41　For details, see Achintya Kumar Dutta, 'Kala-Azar in Assam: British Medical Intervention and People's Response', in Amiya Kumar Bagchi and Krishna Soman (eds.), *Maladies, Preventives and Curatives Debates in Public Health in India*, New Delhi: Tulika Books, 2005, 15–31.

42　The Searchlight, September 2, 1944, 1–3; for details see, Achintya Kumar Dutta, 'Black Fever in Bihar: Experiences and Responses', *Economic and Political Weekly*, XLIII, 12 & 13 (2008), 47–53.

43　BPHR for the Year 1926, Calcutta: Bengal Secretariat Book Depot, 1927, 52; *BPHR for the Year 1939*, 74.

44　*ASR, Assam for the Year 1890*, 16.

45　Cosh, *Topography of Assam*, 26.

46　Government of India (GOI), Home Department (Sanitary), January 1910, Proc. No. 157, NAI; APHR, *Bihar and Orissa for the Year 1929*, Patna: Superintendent Government Printing, 1930, 9.

47　ASR, *Assam for the Year 1891*, 19–20; GOI, Home Department (Sanitary), January 1910, Proc. No. 183, NAI.

48　*ASR, Assam for the Year 1904*, 7; *Annual Report of the Sanitary Commissioner with Government of India for 1903*, Calcutta: Superintendent Government Printing, India, 1904, 96.

49　*APHR, Assam for the Year 1924*, 14.

50　The Indian Medical Gazette (hereafter IMG), July 1923, editorial, 318.

51 IMG (1923), 517–18; P.C. Sengupta, 'Kala-Azar in Bengal: Its Incidence and Trends', *IMG* (November 1944), 547–49.

52 Resolutions Reviewing the Reports on the Working of District & Local Boards in Bengal during the Year 1923–24, Calcutta, 1925, 6.

53 MSS/EUR, The Memoirs of Sir Arthur Dash, pt. 2, 43, BL.

54 Ray, *History of Public Health*, 73.

55 *Annual Report of the Calcutta School of Tropical Medicine Institute of Hygiene and the Carmichael Hospital for Tropical Diseases for the Year 1924*, Calcutta, 1925, 9.

56 Ray, *History of Public Health*, 72–3.

57 Leonard Rogers, *Recent Advances in Tropical Medicine*, London: J & A Churchil, 1928, 33–4.

58 Government of Bihar and Orissa, Local Self Government (Medical), October 1921, Proc.No. 7, Resolutions, BL.

59 *Annual Returns of the Hospitals and Dispensaries in Bihar and Orissa for 1920*, Patna: Bihar Government Press, 1921, 3 (hereafter Annual Returns of Hospitals, Bihar and Orissa)

60 *APHR, Bihar for the Year 1937*, Patna: Superintendent Government Printing, 1938, 15.

61 Report of the Pasteur Institute, Shillong, Third Annual Report for the Year ending December 1919, 7.

62 BPHR for the Year 1923, 65; Ray, *History of Public Health*, 71–2.

63 *Triennial Report on the Working of the Hospitals and Dispensaries in Bihar and Orissa for the Years 1932, 1933 and 1934*, Patna: Bihar Government Press, 1935, 11, 14; *Annual Returns of Hospitals, Bihar and Orissa for 1926, 1927, 1932*, 3, 3, and 2, respectively.

64 Reports of the Kala-azar Commission, India, Report No. 1 (1924–1925), Calcutta: Thacker Spink & Co, 1926, 277; APHR, Bihar for the Year 1938, 18.

65 *Annual Report of the Working of Hospitals and Dispensaries under the Govt. of Bengal for the Year1933*, 11.

66 Papers on Health Survey Committee, India by Dr. Janet Vaughan, 1944, Pt. I, 7 (hereafter Health Survey Committee Papers).

67 Kumar, *Medicine and the Raj*, 207.

68 Health Survey Committee Papers, 11.

69 Radhika Ramasubban, Public Health and Medical Research in India: Their Origins Under the Impact of British Colonial Policy, SAREC report, Stockholm, 1982, 32.

70 Harrison, *Public Health*, 157.

71 Pratik Chakrabarti, *Medicine and Empire 1600–1960*, London and New York: Palgrave Macmillan, 2014, 111–12.

72 Report of the Scientific Advisory Board of the Indian Research Fund Association for the Year 1938, 1939, 1940, 1943, New Delhi, 1939, 1940, 1941, 1944, relevant pages.

73 *Annual Report of the Working of Carmichael Medical College, Belgachia, Calcutta for 1930–31*, Calcutta: Bengal Government Press, 1931, 6–7.

74 Muraleedharan, 'Malady in Madras', 101–14.

75 Andrew Balfour and H.H Scott, *Health Problems of the Empire Past, Present and Future*, London: W Collins, 1924, 128; *APHR, Assam for the Year1944*, 14.

76 W. Peters and L.S.N. Prasad, 'Kala-Azar in India – Its Importance as an Issue in Public Health', Proceedings of the Indo-UK Workshop on Leishmaniasis, Patna, 1982, New Delhi: Indian Council of Medical Research, 1983, 5–9.

77 The Leishmaniasis Report of a WHO Expert Committee Technical Report Series, 701, WHO: Geneva, 1984, 56–7; C.P. Thakur et al., 'Kala-Azar Hits Again', *Journal of Tropical Medicine and Hygiene*, 84 (1981), 271–76.

78 Rama Varu, 'Health Sector Reforms and Structural Adjustment: A State-Level Analysis', in Imrana Qadeer et al. (eds.), *Public Health and the Poverty of Reforms: The South Asian Predicament*, New Delhi: Sage Publications, 2001, 211–34.

Index

Page numbers in *italics* indicate to figures and those in **bold** indicate tables